JUL X X 2015

Public Health Ethics

Key Concepts and Issues in Policy and Practice

D0711583

Public Health Ethics

Key Concepts and Issues in Policy and Practice

Edited by
Angus Dawson

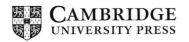
CAMBRIDGE
UNIVERSITY PRESS

CAMBRIDGE UNIVERSITY PRESS
Cambridge, New York, Melbourne, Madrid, Cape Town,
Singapore, São Paulo, Delhi, Tokyo, Mexico City

Cambridge University Press
The Edinburgh Building, Cambridge CB2 8RU, UK

Published in the United States of America by
Cambridge University Press, New York

www.cambridge.org
Information on this title: www.cambridge.org/9780521689366

First published 2011

Printed in the United Kingdom at the University Press, Cambridge

A catalogue record for this publication is available from the British Library

Library of Congress Cataloging-in-Publication Data

Public Health Ethics : Key Concepts and Issues in Policy and Practice /
edited by Angus Dawson.
    p. cm
  Includes bibliographical references and index.
  ISBN 978-0-521-68936-6 (pbk.)
1. Public health–Moral and ethical aspects.   I. Dawson, Angus.
  RA427.25.P8285 2011
  362.1–dc22

                                                            2010050335

ISBN 978-0-521-68936-6 Paperback

Contents

Contributors

Richard Ashcroft
Queen Mary, University of London,
London, UK

Bengt Brülde
University of Gothenburg, Gothenburg,
Sweden

Norman Daniels
Harvard University, Boston, MA, USA

Angus Dawson
Keele University, Staffordshire, UK

Stephen John
Cambridge University, Cambridge, UK

Anthony Kessel
London School of Hygiene and Tropical
Medicine, London, UK

John McMillan
Flinders University, Adelaide, Australia

Ainsley J. Newson
University of Bristol, Bristol, UK

Carolyn Stephens
London School of Hygiene and Tropical
Medicine, London, UK

Marcel Verweij
Utrecht University, Utrecht,
the Netherlands

Stephen Wilkinson
Keele University, Staffordshire, UK

James Wilson
University College London, London, UK

Preface

This book serves to introduce a number of central concepts and key issues in public health ethics. Each chapter is written by an expert in the field and they seek to both introduce and discuss critically at least some of the relevant literature related to their topic or theme. However, this book is not merely a textbook, as each chapter also seeks to advance (or in some cases re-frame) academic debate and practical reflection upon these topics in public health. This book will be of interest to everyone working in public health and related fields, policy makers, as well as students in philosophy, ethics, public health ethics, medicine, public health and critical social science.

Acknowledgements

First, I would like to extend my warmest thanks to the many colleagues and friends that contributed their chapters to this collection of papers. Public health ethics is a relatively young discipline but the explosion of high-quality activity in this area in recent years has been extraordinary. I am very grateful that many of the best minds working on these topics were able to contribute some of their work to this volume.

Second, I would like to thank everyone at Cambridge University Press who made this collection possible. Their patience, support and expertise have all been exemplary. Particular thanks are due to Nick Dunton.

Third, I would like to thank Melissa Williams, Ross Upshur and all at the Centre for Ethics and the Joint Centre for Bioethics, for providing the opportunity to spend time at the University of Toronto and complete work on the manuscript.

Fourth, I would like to thank Trevor King and Bev Sykes for their help in preparing the manuscript for publication.

Finally, I would like to thank the editor of the Hastings Center Report and Wiley for their generosity in granting permission to re-publish material that had previously appeared. Chapter 8 is a revised and extended version of: Dawson, A. (2007) Vaccination ethics. In *Principles of Health Care Ethics*, 2nd edn, ed. R. Ashcroft, D. Dawson, H. Draper and J. McMillan. Chichester: Wiley and Chapter 11 is a very slightly modified version of: Daniels, N. (2006) Equity and population health: toward a broader bioethics agenda, *Hastings Center Report*, **36**(4): 22–35.

Angus Dawson

Resetting the parameters

Public health as the foundation for public health ethics

Angus Dawson

Introduction

In this chapter I introduce a number of different approaches to public health ethics. However, I do this in a deliberately provocative way. I argue that we need a revolutionary, rather than evolutionary, approach to the development of public health ethics: in other words, we ought to reset the parameters that frame this area of applied ethics. I attempt to argue for this conclusion in the three sections of this chapter. First, I outline and defend what I consider to be a necessary condition to be met by any adequate theory of public health ethics. Second, I suggest what I call the traditional liberal approach, currently dominant in much medical ethics, fails to meet this condition because of the primacy it accords the idea of non-interference. I also suggest that various proposed alternatives, although offering some welcome broadening to this traditional liberal position, ultimately remain restricted by their implicit or explicit acceptance of the parameters set by the liberal approach. Third, I briefly outline a range of areas where I argue that future work ought to be directed as a means of developing a sufficiently rich account of public health ethics: a substantive account that meets my condition. I suggest that such an account must accept a view of human interests as intrinsically social. My primary focus in this chapter is a general argument in favour of the re-orientation of the field of public health ethics. I do not defend any particular theoretical perspective, beyond a general defence of what I term 'substantive' accounts of public health ethics.

I begin this discussion with the observation that if you approach public health from the perspective of much contemporary medical ethics, many public health policies and activities are likely to be viewed as ethically dubious. This is for a number of reasons but will include the following: public health's primary focus on populations rather than individuals; public health's assumptions about necessary features of the human good; and a broader focus on other values beside non-interference. Consider just a few examples of core public health activities: cancer screening programmes are designed to reduce the number of cases in a given population, through the early discovery of asymptomatic cases. This focus might mean that informed consent and individual decision making are less of a priority than in some other areas of health care. Most preventive vaccination programmes seek to reduce the risk of individuals being infected with harmful diseases, through the creation and maintenance of a population effect called herd immunity. Such programmes aim to maximize participation because if

Public Health Ethics, ed. Angus Dawson. Published by Cambridge University Press. © Cambridge University Press 2011.

insufficient individuals contribute, then this important protection cannot be achieved. A healthy environment with adequate sanitation, clean water and good air quality requires the coordinated activity of the whole community, through the day-to-day action of relevant civil or public agencies. This may impose significant cost on some industries and individuals. Health promotion can seek to change people's preferences in relation to issues such as smoking, exercise and food choices, with the aim of reducing the chronic disease burden in a population through the promotion of healthier lifestyles. Many public health research activities are focused on populations, where epidemiological work to determine risk factors for disease may require the analysis of personal health information without the consent of individuals. Preparing for and responding to public health emergencies may require infrastructure for disease surveillance and legal structures to compel behaviour and seize property (in at least some circumstances). Health inequities are the result of many different socio-economic determinants and can often be addressed only through structural and societal level policy initiatives (that may in turn restrict or negate individual choice).

If the currently dominant views in contemporary medical ethics are applied to these public health activities there is a danger that such routine public health actions will be seen to be wrongly prioritizing population over individual interests. One possible response is to accept this critique and argue that much public health activity is actually unethical because it fails to prioritize individuals and their choices, as well as the moral principles that have evolved within the field of medical ethics to protect these considerations such as informed consent and patient confidentiality. However, an alternative approach is to argue that public health is a vitally important activity and that its ends are legitimate and can only be attained through such population-level interventions. On this view, the 'problem', assuming it is one, lies with the perspective derived from traditional medical ethics, not with public health practice itself. On this latter view, it is certainly possible for public health actions to be unethical, but the mere fact that they do not easily fit within a medical ethics framework does not *make* them unethical; and we certainly have no a-priori reason to hold public health to be intrinsically unethical. In this chapter, I argue that we face an important dilemma. Either we explicitly accept the consequences of our liberal framework (and damn much routine public health practice) or we choose to re-set our parameters and rethink our ethical theories, thereby ensuring that public health activities and their justification move closer to the core of ethics. In this chapter I argue that it is time for us to move towards the latter view.

A necessary condition for any adequate account of public health ethics

In any clash between a chosen moral theory and public health practice and policy we have no reason to assume that it is the practice or policy that is problematic rather than the theory. In this section I will argue that we ought to accept a necessary condition for something being an adequate theoretical perspective in relation to public health, and that this condition ought to be applied as a filter in choosing an appropriate ethical theory for public health. I will call this condition the *nature of public health* condition. I have suggested that meeting this condition is a necessary feature of an adequate theory. What this means is not that we can rule out those moral views that fail to meet it, but that the consequences of embracing any view that does not meet the condition is likely to be too great (in the sense that it will entail excluding a substantial amount of public health policy and practice, which we otherwise find appealing and arguably is necessary to establish the conditions for living a good life). What is the nature of public health condition? The main idea behind it is the thought that any adequate account of public health ethics must begin with a clear articulation and defence of a concept of public health. I suggest this is the case because the aims, nature and methods of public health appear to be different from those of much clinical medicine. If this is true, then we have good reason to be cautious in simply applying our methods and results from clinical medicine (the main focus of most discussions in contemporary medical ethics) in the sphere of public health. However, this focus on the definition of public health is more difficult than might at first appear because the concept is itself a contentious one. What do we mean when we talk of 'public health'? What are the legitimate aims of public health (Munthe, 2008)? There is, of course, a huge literature discussing the concept of 'health' and a smaller but growing literature discussing the concept of 'public health' (Brülde, Chapter 2).

In previous joint work with Marcel Verweij we explored many of the most influential definitions of public health that have been offered. Our own rough account of public health focuses on this area of activity as being characterized by 'collective interventions that aim to promote and protect the health of the public' (Verweij and Dawson, 2007: 21). This is further articulated in terms of two different but equally important senses of 'public' being contained in the notion of public health. These two senses of 'public' in public health can be structured around, first, the idea of the health of *the public* as a social entity or a target for an intervention (that is, a population, community or group) and, second, public as a description of the *mode of intervention*, which requires some form of collective action. As a result, on this approach, we end up with a particular view of the elements of public health, but also with an agenda for some of the issues to discuss within public health ethics. There are many issues that require clarification, but I will consider only three important central issues here. First, public health is focused on populations (not just individuals). Second, much public health work is preventive rather than curative. Third, most public health improvements cannot be brought about by individuals on their own: the attainment of public health ends requires collective efforts.

First, public health activity is concerned not just with the health of individuals but, rather, primarily focuses on the health of the population or community. What does this mean? When we think of a population it is tempting to consider it as merely a collection or aggregation of particular individuals. There is an important sense in which this is true. If we have a population and we keep taking away individuals, we will ultimately have nothing left: the 'population' does not exist as an entity independently of the individuals that collectively constitute that population. However, while this is important, it cannot be the whole story. First, this model fails to take into account such things as the way that unequal socio-economic determinants influence health. You are not just an individual, but an individual with a particular position in a society; and that position has a significant impact upon your health status. Second, we can think of different populations or societies as having better or worse health than others and we can think of a particular population's health improving or worsening over time (perhaps because they have lower or higher inequities or a lower or higher overall disease burden). Both of these examples might be used to express a concern about the public's health in these populations, and may provide a basis for aiming to improve a population's health through population-level interventions. Third, population health cannot merely be viewed as an additive correlate of the health of the constituent individuals. For example, it looks as though, paradoxically, in targeting population health we can improve the health of the individuals in that population, but if we target the individuals as individuals then we may not improve that population's health. This is one of the many things we can learn from the work of Geoffrey Rose (1992) and his focus on the complexities of the relationship between population health and individual health. One of his examples focuses on the influence of drinking 'cultures' on individual behaviour in relation to alcohol consumption and associated adverse medical consequences. The relationship between the population and individual is a complex one. While no one would deny that there may be 'individual' factors such as an individual's genetic makeup that contribute to the risk of being a 'heavy drinker', it is important to see that the behaviour of individuals in relation to alcohol consumption is very strongly influenced by population factors such as social attitudes to alcohol and the resultant legal and political climate. The more that is drunk by the average citizen in a population, the more 'heavy drinkers' there will be. Indeed, even more specific correlations can be drawn between alcohol and disease at the population level in some situations, such as the drop in cases of cirrhosis in France during times of reduced access to wine during the two world wars (Rose, 1992: 85). What this suggests is that lifestyle choices are not simply within the control of individuals. If this is true, then we should take care in attributing causation (and therefore responsibility for lifestyle behaviour) to individuals alone.[1]

Second, public health activity focuses on seeking to prevent, reduce or ameliorate harm, not just treat patients after a negative event has occurred. This is an intuitively powerful idea. Such interventions require an inference to be drawn from known population risks and applied to the lives of individuals. This, in turn, will require interventions focused on asymptomatic individuals, and this can generate anxiety and other harms (Newson, Chapter 7). Such harms, then, need to be weighed against the benefits of prevention. The scope for prevention is vast, and it is important for public health to intervene only where it is appropriate. However, deciding when this is the case is difficult. For example, what limits ought we to place on the idea of harm? What kind of harms are relevant (Dawson, 2007; Verweij, Chapter 6)? Public health operates with a broader notion of harm than that commonly employed in contemporary medical ethics. For example, public health is concerned not just with the immediate factors that impact upon people's lives but also with the prevention and reduction of harm as well as the wider determinants of health and many of the factors that shape the kind of society within which we wish to live. Such influences upon our health are often best described in terms of probabilities and risks, and so public health is often motivated by a concern for uncertainty and precaution (John, Chapter 4). The more complex or broader the notion of harm as the focus of public health, the more likely it is that the benefits and burdens calculations will become increasingly difficult (and contentious). If it is true that much public health can only be performed through collective activity, then the bringing about of such ends will entail coordinated action (and, if the end is judged to be sufficiently important, perhaps, in some cases, coercion too).

---

[1] See, also, Paul (2009) for an excellent discussion of how Rose's work may help us rethink HIV prevention.

Third, public health requires collective action, as many desired public health ends are impossible to achieve for individuals by themselves. In reality, collective activity usually means state action on behalf of society as a whole. This fact can often result in the charge of paternalism, with the state taking an active decision-making role in relation to the best way that people should live their lives. Of course, we might question if such activities are really paternalistic, if this is the only way to secure these ends for the good of the whole population (Nys, 2008). But, even if the charge of paternalism is fair, we can still ask the question whether such paternalistic action is always wrong. We have no reason to just assume that all cases of paternalism are wrong by definition (in the absence of an argument to establish this rather odd conclusion).

How will these considerations work out in practice? Consider a brief example related to the key contemporary policy concern of rapidly rising rates of obesity in many parts of the developed world. First, with this approach it is important to see that this is a population problem (as well as being a concern for individuals). It is a population problem in a straightforward epidemiological sense, as we can measure obesity at the population level by analysing the differences between countries and within countries and relate these differences to other population features such as socio-economic factors. I do not mean to suggest that obesity is simply a matter of poverty: it is not. But it looks as though there is an association between obesity and socio-economic status, in that more affluent individuals are less likely to be obese (probably for very complex reasons: better access to information, better quality and variety of food, greater opportunities to exercise in stimulating ways, etc.). Second, prevention is central to obesity because we have enough empirical evidence to suggest that while prevention of obesity is difficult, treatment is virtually impossible (except for surgery, which carries risks significant enough for this to be an option only for those at very high risk from their obesity). Third, and relating back to the fact that obesity is a population problem, collective interventions will be vital if we are serious about tackling the issue of obesity. Such interventions will have to be at the societal level and are likely to include profound changes to a number of factors including the nature of work and schooling, the built environment, transport policy, the regulation of the food industry and the possible restriction to food advertising (especially in relation to children). We might argue that such interventions do not count as paternalism (as the focus is on the collective) or that they do (but they are still justifiable). In either case, it might be argued that such collective interventions may be permissible.

In conclusion to this section, it is vitally important to be clear about what we mean by public health before we begin to explore public health ethics. Any theoretical perspective orientated towards public health must, I argue, be responsive to the aims and nature of public health: too often discussions on public health ethics fail this test. Attempting to construct a public health ethics without a substantive notion of public health will inevitably result in error. Setting the correct parameters is the first step in trying to attain the correct perspective upon this vital area of health care practice.

The inadequacy of liberal medical ethics as a means of thinking about public health ethics

One important aim of this chapter is to argue that much of the work that has been done on public health ethics so far, even that explicitly aware of the need for something more than a liberal approach, has remained locked within the parameters set by the traditional medical ethics framework. I argue here that we need to re-frame the way that we think about public health ethics and move away from the assumption that public health ethics ought to be structured in terms of debates about non-interference and the subsequent central pre-occupation with apparent conflicts between individual and population. This approach, which I will label as 'liberal', encourages the idea that a particular value or set of values, primarily attached to individuals and their decision making (such as liberty and autonomy) has priority in our moral deliberations. Approaching things in this way places the onus on those seeking to argue that such values should not always hold sway in public health to justify situations where it is appropriate to restrict or interfere with an individual's liberty. In this chapter I argue that this way of conceptualizing things is part of the problem and is so dominant that it tends to be assumed without argument. I will begin by discussing what I term 'narrow' or 'pure' liberal views and then move on to what I call 'moderated' liberal views.

Narrow liberal views

The exact meaning of the term 'liberal' can, of course, be disputed. However, I will take it here to imply a set of commitments, long dominant in contemporary medical ethics, that draw upon a particular and narrow reading of the harm principle taken to be derived from John Stuart Mill's *On Liberty*. Within this view, the only ground for coercive interference in the decision making of individuals is when their actions may have negative consequences for others. Any action to reduce or prevent harm to an individual, once they are aware and informed of the relevant danger, is held to be a case of paternalism and thereby morally wrong. Within this view, liberalism is seen as centrally concerned with non-interference.[2] However, there are a number of problems with this view. First, it is not clear that this is really Mill's considered view. He explicitly includes action to preserve public goods within the list of acceptable reasons to restrict liberty. In this sense, Mill is not a 'Millian' liberal in the way that many imply (Dawson and Verweij, 2008). Second, as mentioned before, when we talk of the concept of 'harm' in relation to public health practice and policy we are interested in much more than harm to others as traditionally conceived. Public health actions are designed not merely to prevent harm, but also to reduce or ameliorate it. The relevant notion of harm implicit in routine public health activities is much broader, more contextual, more interested in the social reality of actual lived lives, and more about the conditions that are required to live a healthy life. As a result the traditional distinction drawn in much medical ethics between beneficence and non-maleficence is less obviously relevant (Dawson, 2007), and if this is true, this makes it more difficult to defend the very coherence of the idea of 'non-interference'. At the very least advocates of the 'Millian' view need to defend such a narrow conception of harm, and it is not clear that this is possible. Even if it is, we might still argue that discussion of public health requires a broader conception (that is one that permits harm prevention and harm reduction) to make sense

---

[2] When I write of 'liberalism' in this chapter I just mean the dominant 'Millian' strand that dominates much contemporary medical ethics. There are, of course, ways of formulating richer versions of liberalism, such as that due to Raz (1986). If anyone is offended by my characterization of liberalism they can read my text as referring to a very particular type of liberalism (perhaps, one to be thought of as liberalism*). I will also leave to one side the possibility of other options in choosing one's political philosophy, such as varieties of republicanism (Jennings, 2007a).

of the very idea of public health.[3] So, for both these reasons, an appeal to the 'harm principle' will not result in as clear a policy directive as may be assumed: public health ethics (and, in my view, medical ethics in general) cannot be built upon such shaky foundations.

However, let us assume, for the sake of argument, that this is not the case and the idea of non-interference (allegedly derived from the harm principle) is robust. The first thing to note is that quite a lot is built upon the idea of non-interference. For example, priority will be given to individual freedom or autonomous decision making because it is for individuals to decide what they should do. Liberals tend, also, to support the importance of maintaining a clear distinction between the private and the public. The private represents an area where the state or its representatives have no legitimate reason to trespass. With this approach, it is easy to see how public health ethics can get conceptualized as being about protecting the sphere of the individual from the interference of state power. An example of this might be a view of the limits of ethical health promotion as being related to the provision of information as a means for individuals to make their own decisions about what to do. People's existing preferences are to be respected because they are *their* preferences, and as a result the state ought to be neutral and not promote particular views of the 'good life'.[4]

Liberals need not see liberty as the only value that matters or the value that always takes precedence (perhaps it is that which distinguishes them from libertarians). However, there is a problem here for the advocate of non-interference that I will briefly explore. The problem arises from a failure to recognize that non-interference or neutrality towards all other values is itself a value. There are two coherent options here. First, assume that non-interference itself can be given a different status to other values. The advocate of non-interference looks as though they ought to embrace this option, but then we need an argument to establish why we ought to see non-interference as a higher or second-order value (and this account must also explain how such a higher value can cohere with other values). Second, and alternatively, while non-interference and its cognates, such as autonomy and liberty, are seen as important values, we have no good reason to assign them any special status. In this view, we have a range of important values of equal status that can be weighed against each other. Each of these values may take priority over the others in some contexts. Sometimes liberty is the winning value, but at other times it is not. With this view it makes no sense to frame the discussion of these issues in terms of only liberty. A non-privileging account of values in public health ethics will allow liberty to be legitimately defeated on at least some occasions, perhaps because there will in turn be more liberty further down the way or because other values are just more important on that particular occasion. If this second approach is true, as I think it must be, then non-interference as a privileged value is not a coherent option.

---

[3] Public health is, of course, often concerned with what we can think of as the 'background conditions' for living healthy lives. It is quite a stretch (perhaps even incoherent) to think of many of these activities as *coercive*, and so it might be argued, once again, that non-interference is too narrow a principle to capture all that is relevant to public health. Thanks to Adrian Viens for discussion on this point.

[4] Dan Wikler's work (1978) is a good example of a 'Millian' approach to the ethics of health promotion. Holland (2007) provides another well-worked out position defending a liberal approach to public health ethics more broadly. See Jennings (2007b) for a critical perspective upon liberal approaches to public health ethics.

In addition, a common inference from the liberal non-interference approach to framing debates in public health ethics is an assumption about responsibility. It is usually assumed that individuals have the freedom to make choices (whether or not they in fact do), and therefore responsibility for the consequences of those choices is attached to the individual choice-makers. The danger is that we are offered a rather simplistic view of both choice and responsibility (one that tends to ignore the way that many 'choices' are partly or even largely the product of factors beyond the individual's direct control [such as socio-economic, historic, geographic or cultural factors]). The liberal faces a dilemma in such a case. Either the individual is not free because they do not make choices in the relevant sense (but this may mean that no one is free) or we begin to take seriously the social construction of choice (in which case, it turns out that the degree to which we can be free is restricted in some sense. Perhaps there are only a sub-set of choices that are free, or each choice is only free to some extent). Of course, it has long been recognized that the relationship between causal and moral responsibility need not be a straightforward one. However, if it looks as though the causes of behaviour are not merely the result of an individual's 'choice', then it is clearly not appropriate to attribute responsibility for the consequences of such lifestyle 'choices' to individuals in any meaningful sense. What this raises is the possibility that many liberals are working with a deeply implausible view of human psychology and a potentially morally problematic view of responsibility attribution.

So leaving these more theoretical concerns about non-interference to one side, I now turn to some possible reasons for why the liberal framing has been so powerful. I think the liberal tradition in contemporary medical ethics has been supported by at least three features: the history of medical ethics as a discipline; its relation with the law; and a set of assumptions about pluralism. These features are partial explanations as to why the parameters are set in their current position. However, I suggest that none of these three reasons provide any convincing justification for why we must remain locked within such a framework.

First, as many people have now noted, the history of medical ethics from its early years was focused very much on dyadic clinical relationships between doctor and patient and a very narrow set of issues either related to such a relationship (for example, consent and confidentiality) or a view of ethical theory and principles focused on individual patient rights and autonomous decision making. The consensus that health care was too paternalistic resulted in the *de facto* establishment of respect for individual autonomy as the dominating principle in medical ethics. Other areas of bioethics, related to animals and the broader environment, tended to be downplayed. The other factor that has driven much ethical discussion is the apparent glamour of new technologies and cutting-edge medicine. Much contemporary medical ethics can be seen as dwelling in one of two camps: those with a tendency to see technology as providing solutions and those suspicious of it. More recently, many writers in medical ethics have started to shift their focus, and there is now growing interest in issues relating to infectious disease (particularly due to SARS, pandemic influenza, tuberculosis, etc.), the impact of social disparities upon health at the national and international level and the renewed interest in global justice, particularly in relation to arguments surrounding the impact of intellectual property issues upon access to medicines. As I have already mentioned, many others have said that medical ethics must be revised to accommodate these issues. However, I want to go further and suggest that many of those that have argued that medical ethics needs to 'expand', often apply traditional frameworks to issues in public health, and thereby fail to capture what is special or different about public health ethics.

The second feature that has tended to support the liberal approach is a set of assumptions about the relationship between law and ethics. There is a common tendency to confuse the two, and this may relate to the apparent obsession that many working in medical ethics seem to have with the issue of regulation of health care practice (often with the assumption that anything is and ought to be permitted unless it is explicitly squashed by law, resulting in the focus, too easily, becoming one of ensuring that regulation is minimal). The relation between law and ethics is a complex one, but the main point is that the two are distinct, although they may be related. The problem with confusing the law and ethics in relation to public health is that the law too often works with narrow accounts of both causation and responsibility, with a focus on individual action. This can be seen, for example, in relation to both tort and crime (Coker and Martin, 2006; Martin, 2009), although the law may also be used in other ways to promote public health (Gostin and Stone, 2007).

Third, there is an assumption in much contemporary medical ethics that as we cannot agree in our moral judgments we, therefore, ought to be committed to pluralism in ethics in general. It is then concluded that we must focus on process values rather than pursuing substantive answers to ethical questions. The relation of these ideas to liberalism is the thought that we can remain neutral in terms of values and allow individuals to make their own decisions and pursue their own view of what is morally appropriate. However, all of these commitments can be contested. First, the fact that different perspectives exist upon an ethical issue does not on its own have any implications for our normative views. There needs to be further substantive argument to establish such a claim. Second, we need to take care when talking about pluralism. This is not *value* pluralism (there is more than one morally relevant value) but *judgment* pluralism (there is more than one 'answer' to a moral issue). The former does not imply the latter, and it is the latter that the supporters of such relativistic pluralism need to establish. It should also be noted that you can be both a value pluralist (there is more than one value) and a moral realist (there are objective answers to moral questions) at the same time. Third, one thing that drives the liberal 'neutrality' view here is a commitment to tolerance. However, it often seems to be missed that judgment pluralism cannot easily be combined with a coherent defence of a value such as tolerance. Indeed, a commitment to tolerance is most easily defended from a realist tradition (that is we ought to be tolerant, even if other people think differently). Fourth, a commitment to procedure over content is not remaining neutral about values, but just choosing to adopt a particular account of ethics: one committed to procedural values as though this were not just a commitment to a particularly thin set of substantive values.[5]

Whether or not the liberal approach is an appropriate one for public health, and therefore for public health ethics, it is certainly the case that if we adopt this kind of liberal framing of public health ethics, many aspects of routine public health practice will be ruled out as unethical and this approach will not be able to capture the more substantive notion of public health outlined earlier. In other words, narrow liberal views will fail to meet my suggested condition for an adequate theory of public health ethics.

---

[5] Of course, all of these issues are much more complex than I suggest here. My intention is just to illustrate how the easy moral relativism of our times fits with the alleged 'neutrality' of liberalism.

Moderated liberal positions

Are moderated liberal views any more successful? I call such views 'moderated' liberal positions as they clearly suggest dissatisfaction with a simple liberal position (for example, one built solely upon an appeal to non-interference or the harm principle) in regard to an adequate public health ethics. However, I suggest that these views are still too cautious or modest. They remain locked within liberal parameters: with, despite their apparent pluralism, an implicit commitment to giving priority to the 'liberal' values of freedom and autonomy. The first three views that I discuss here, Upshur (2002), Childress *et al.* (2002) and Gostin (2005) are 'principled' approaches. They are essentially attempts to highlight a useful and pragmatic set of issues, with a clear focus on practical implementation for those working in public health practice and policy. This is a laudable aim. However, I suggest that there are specific problems with each view and there are general problems for any principled approach. Lastly, in this section, I outline and discuss the recent proposal for a 'stewardship model' described by the Nuffield Council of Bioethics (2007). I classify the latter view as a modified liberal view because, like these three principled approaches, it seems deeply committed to working within liberal parameters.

I will begin by just stating the three 'principled' views. First, Upshur (2002) offers us a set of four 'principles for the justification of public health interventions' as follows:

1. harm principle;
2. least restrictive or coercive means;
3. reciprocity principle;
4. transparency principle.

Second, Childress *et al.* (2002) in a paper involving ten authors, many of them well-known names in public health ethics, are much more ambitious, in that they are interested in sketching out an account of public health ethics, in the course of which they outline a set of moral considerations 'generally taken to instantiate the goal of public health' as follows:

1. producing benefits;
2. avoiding, preventing, removing harms;
3. maximizing utility.

They then offer five 'justificatory conditions' for interventions to promote such public health goals:

1. effectiveness;
2. proportionality;
3. necessity;
4. least infringement;
5. public justification.

Third, Gostin (2005) outlines a set of what he terms public health values as follows:

1. transparency;
2. protection of vulnerable populations;
3. fair treatment and social justice;
4. the least restrictive alternative.

In my comments I will concentrate on general remarks about this kind of approach, rather than focusing on each account in any detail. The first thing to notice is that while there is some overlap between the features picked out, there are also some significant differences. This is partly due, no doubt, to the different aims of each of these three perspectives but also the different way they are presented. Upshur explicitly calls them 'principles', Childress *et al.* call them 'considerations' and Gostin calls them 'values'. So this leads to the first set of questions related to the status of these different elements. Are they in fact 'principles' at all? They are clearly supposed to be normative in some way – but how? All three accounts combine both procedural (transparency, proportionality, public justification, etc.) and substantive (harm principle, least restrictive, social justice, etc.) elements. Do these different elements have equal status or value? Are they *prima facie* principles or values or more 'substantive' than this? These questions then lead on to the second set of issues related to how they are to be used. Are they to be literally applied to cases or are they just things to be kept in mind? Are they to be used as justifications for actions as suggested by Upshur and Childress *et al.*? How are they to be combined? What happens when they conflict? If a potential action that would bring about greater social justice is more restrictive is this permissible or not (Gostin)? If a satisfactory implementation of our obligation of reciprocity seems to require a more restrictive option is this permissible (Upshur)? If a possible option is likely to be more effective but will be a greater infringement is this justifiable or not (Childress *et al.*)? Is the order of the principles significant? Upshur places transparency last, whereas Gostin has it first. There are many different possible options when it comes to ordering and ranking principles and we are owed some account of the justification of the weighting to be given to the relevant principles and an explanation about how deliberation ought to occur (Dawson and Garrard, 2006).

Of course, it will be argued that this discussion is unfair as these approaches are not supposed to be well worked out theories of public health ethics. This is true. Perhaps they are best thought of as frameworks for thinking about issues.[6] But, even so, the problem is that such approaches are taken very seriously. They are taken up by busy people and influence the way that people operate and think about these issues. In the end, of course, they perhaps say most about the dominant values in society, and in this sense, I would argue, they illustrate my point about the dominance of liberal assumptions. So, for example, all three views mention the idea of least restrictive or coercive means/alternative/infringement. This clearly points at the high value to be assigned to individual freedom (in the sense of both autonomy and liberty). There is no corresponding mention of the common good, public good or community benefit. There is no statement that captures the two senses of 'public' in public health as outlined

---

[6] Although they do have more normative content than some other proposed frameworks, such as that proposed by Kass (2001). Kass seems to think that her approach, and perhaps frameworks in general, can be normatively neutral. However, her framework incorporates many values and assumptions (mostly ones clearly deriving from a liberal approach). The distinction between a theory and a framework is not a clear one, but we might, roughly, think of a theory as providing normative justification and a framework as being more focused on aiding deliberation. The framework must, of course, be supported ultimately by normative commitments, even if they can be put to one side at the moment of deliberation. The best framework will capture all of the relevant issues: ones that are partial will not produce the appropriate answers. For more on frameworks, see Dawson (2009).

above: public as a social entity (to which every individual belongs) and as requiring collective action. These three accounts seem to broadly accept the minimalism and individualism of liberal approaches, except for Upshur's invocation of reciprocity and Gostin's mention of social justice (and, perhaps, his idea of protecting vulnerable populations). So while each of these three views has details specific to it, and to be fair, they should be considered in more detail, they all share a particular approach. Although they are an improvement upon the narrow liberal view, they inherit and share too much of the general liberal approach, and for that reason they fail my condition for an adequate public health ethics.

The last view I will consider in this section is explicitly a modified liberal view. It is called the stewardship model and is proposed by the Nuffield Council of Bioethics (2007). They argue that an approach built upon a narrow reading of the harm principle is inadequate, as they draw attention to the importance of being able to justify support for government action in relation to health care provision to ensure a framework for adequate equality of health care access. They suggest that a fuller liberal approach can be supported by what they term the stewardship model. They do not really explain what this view is in any detail and provide little support for it in a theoretical sense. They focus instead on sketching out what such a model would support in practice. It is explicitly said to be a 'revised' liberal approach. It is certainly wedded to strong liberal assumptions (visible in their 'intervention ladder' and their discussion of suggested policy options) and it clearly fails my condition. There is some discussion about what they mean by the concept of 'public health', but it does not seem to be carried over into the development of the stewardship model. Does it move beyond the 'Millian' paradigm that it is critical of? I think not (Dawson and Verweij, 2008).

I have argued that, despite their differences, both narrow and moderated liberal views fail to meet my condition of adequacy because they share a common set of assumptions that frame the way that ethical decision making is viewed. Progress can only be made in public health ethics by seeking to overcome the hold that this framing has on our deliberations. Fortunately, there are many different options that are still open to us, and I will explore some of these in the next section.

Resetting the parameters: in defence of a substantive public health ethics

A revolutionary or what we might call a 'substantive' account of public health ethics will begin elsewhere: not with the individual and the assumption of liberty as our prime value, but with a *set* of values that try to capture the *public* nature of public health. This approach will begin with some defence of the different normative factors that might be used to take seriously what we share in common as human beings and social creatures. Taking this as the basis of public health ethics will lead to a re-orientation of much of the field of discussion and to the re-setting of the parameters as envisaged by the core metaphor of this chapter. This change in perspective will, in turn, set a clear agenda for the work of public health ethics.

If we are serious about defending public health activities from the traditional criticisms drawn from the direction of medical ethics, then we need to think about how we can justify a more population- or community-orientated approach to ethics. However, this does not just mean an easy flip into some form of communitarianism. Although communitarianism is one option, there are many other ways of attempting to capture the 'publicness' of public health through the exploration of a series of theoretical questions. How does public health relate to such concepts as social justice, solidarity and reciprocity? Can we seek support from moral theories such as contractarianism, welfare forms of consequentialism, or accounts of human flourishing and capabilities? Can we capture the idea of public goods and common goods in our approach? In other words, reflection upon the nature of public health practice, and the ethical issues that arise there, is also likely to result in a welcome development of our moral theories. However, before we proceed any further, it is worth sounding two notes of caution.

First, of course, (at least some of) these views may be combined with liberal values or even be integrated into a more sophisticated version of liberalism.[7] The account of liberalism that I have criticized is a fairly simple, if influential, one. The claim about using the 'substantive' approaches discussed here for a re-setting of the parameters for public health ethics is based on the idea that such approaches (to varying degrees) make no assumption that we ought to begin with individuals or individual decision making, nor that liberty or individual autonomy ought to be treated as having a special status in a set of values. Of course, this does not mean that liberty or autonomy are not important values. The argument is about the special or privileged status that these values are often given in discussions. I argued above that approaches to public health ethics that focus on such values alone will fail to meet my condition for adequacy, but this does not mean that these values are without merit and ought not to play a role in a developing public health ethics.

Second, it is worth stressing, again, that in the course of this chapter, I offer no defence of any particular substantive approach to public health ethics. What I do want to do is briefly show how there is plenty of potential for exploring how we can use these theories and ideas to begin to ground an account of public health ethics that meets the criterion for public health ethics I outlined above. It should also be noted that these approaches are not mutually exclusive and that they may well, eventually, cohere into a well-rounded theory of public health ethics.

Substantive notions of the good

First, I begin with a broad family of theories that support the idea of an approach to ethics based around a substantive notion of the good. Perhaps the most discussed such theory in relation to public health is consequentialism. Consequentialism is really a family of theories with a common focus on the goodness of outcomes of actions. This family will include the classical utilitarianism of Bentham, with its focus on maximizing pleasure and minimizing pain, but is not limited to it, as it will include preference-satisfaction and objective list forms of consequentialism (Parfit, 1984: Appendix I; Griffin, 1986). This is not the place to discuss the relative merits of these approaches, but we should note that both the last two options can be used to capture a complex and pluralistic account of welfare that may satisfy many of the requirements we are looking for in the field of public health ethics. Furthermore, some non-consequentialist theoretical positions may be seen to be related to such accounts because of their commitment

---

[7] For one discussion of what such a broader liberalism might mean for public health ethics, appealing to the work of Raz (1986), see Coggon (2008).

to a substantive notion of the good such as human flourishing or a particular notion of the good life or the capabilities that are necessary to live a good life.[8]

It remains to be seen how these views might be used in the context of public health ethics, but they surely offer a rich source of enquiry because they are all seeking to promote a substantive notion of the good by providing the conditions not just for health, but for a good life. Public health as an activity is concerned with exactly such a notion by seeking to prevent, minimize or remove harms, including those that can best or only be tackled through collective action. This means that such accounts can meet my suggested condition for an adequate theory for public health ethics.

Collective values: interests, goods and harms

Second, many of the values that are the focus of public health activity are collective in nature. It is important to see that such collective values are of different types, including collective interests, goods and harms. I suggest that at least some of these can only be pursued and attained through joint or common activity, but this is a complex notion. In this section, I draw on the work of Postema (1987) to offer a taxonomy of the different ways that we might use the idea of what we have in common.[9] This is a necessary simplification, as a first step to exploring in more detail what normative implications such distinctions might have.[10]

I begin by defining three related terms: goods, harms and interests. The goods I am interested in here are those things that are *good for* humans (or allow human flourishing or the good life).[11] They will include some of the same things that are often appealed to during the formulation of arguments over the objective list forms of consequentialism (for example, autonomy, pleasure, health, etc.). Whatever these goods are (and this will be a matter of vigorous debate), all human beings have an interest or a stake in attaining a sufficient level of each good to ensure the basis of a flourishing life. Any setback to such interests will count as a harm (Feinberg, 1984).[12] It should be noted that some interests in certain goods will remain even if they are not desired by the individual. In other words, desiring something may create an interest, but not all interests require that they be desired for them to exist as interests for that person.

I suggest that when we think of collective values we can distinguish at least three senses of interest and three correlated notions of goods. Public health (as an activity) will be interested in all three pairings, even if (as I suggest below) only one is genuinely a *common* good, because all relate to the idea of protecting and promoting the health of the public through directed activities that will require collective action as a means of attaining the satisfaction of the

---

[8] There are many options to explore here, but they will include: Sen (1999), Nussbaum (2000) and Kraut (2007).

[9] I have found Postema's (1987) paper inspiring, and in this brief discussion I borrow much of his terminology. However, I find at least some of his discussion rather confusing, so I deliberately simplify and adapt his ideas. I do not explore how exactly my views contrast with his.

[10] Note that my interest here is a far broader one than that of public goods in the economists' sense. They are perhaps just one particular form of the collective entities I am exploring here. I think it is to be regretted that sometimes people use the terms 'public goods' and 'common goods' interchangeably. Hardin (1968), for example, is really interested in the provision of public goods when he discusses 'the commons'.

[11] I leave other kinds of possible goods (and bearers of goods) to one side.

[12] Although I agree with Postema (1987) that we need to allow for the notion of collective harms that is only weakly present (at best) in Feinberg's work.

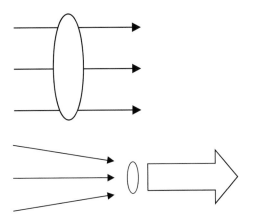

Figure 1.1 Congruent interests. The ellipse represents the structures that need to be in place for our individual interests (represented by the thin arrows) to be attained.

Figure 1.2 Convergent interests. The ellipse represents the shared end that needs to be in place for our individual interests (represented by the thin arrows) to be attained through the public good (represented by the thick arrow).

relevant interest. I build upon Postema's work to offer a hierarchy of these collective values and attempt to make clear the degree of commonness required to create and maintain them. I will discuss three sets of collective interests: congruent, convergent and common interests.

The first two of these senses of interest are well described by Postema (1987) in his contrast between congruent and convergent interests. Congruent interests are the same kind of interests that we have as individuals in the same kind of thing. Such interests essentially run in parallel with each other and require some minimal collective response as a means of meeting them (see Figure 1.1). An example might be the enforcement of safe food preparation techniques in restaurants and food processing plants. Such congruent interests are not merely a group of separate private interests, as they require public structures, processes or regulations to be in place for these individual ends to be attained. However, they are only very weakly public. It is convenient or more efficient to meet such parallel interests through the action of public health departments.

Convergent interests, by contrast, are interests that converge on the same end and are more strongly public (see Figure 1.2). Indeed, they will include the kind of things that economists mean when they talk of public goods. What the relevant criteria are for something to count as a public good is disputed. However, they often include non-excludability (people cannot be excluded from the enjoyment of the public good once it is created); indivisibility (the relevant public good cannot be 'broken up' into individual goods, without destroying the good itself). They often, also, depend upon the cooperation of a large number of people to create and maintain them (Dawson, 2007). Convergent interests may be expressed in terms of our individual interests, but as it turns out the only way to bring about their fulfilment is through the production and maintenance of such public goods. As a result, the attaining of such goods will often require some potential means of enforcement to avoid the problems of free-riding. A good example of a public good, and therefore of a convergent interest, is the creation and maintenance of herd protection through sufficient vaccination within a community as a means of protecting individuals from harm (Dawson, 2007). Such convergent interests require a 'coming together' in a more substantive way than congruent interests: they require the attainment of a collective end as well as public provision. Contrast vaccination for tetanus (a disease that cannot be transmitted person-to-person and therefore herd protection is impossible) and measles (a highly transmissible disease where we can attain herd protection). Public health will be interested in both, even though the former is fulfilling a congruent interest

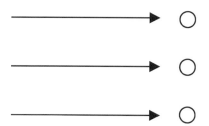

Figure 1.3 Private interests. The circles represent the chosen ends for each individual private interest (represented by the thin arrows).

and the latter a convergent interest. The former requires the infrastructure to be in place to satisfy the interest, but the latter can only be satisfied if 90% of the population participate through individual vaccination.

Just before I move on, it might also help to say a brief word about private interests (that is, those that are in no way public) (see Figure 1.3). It looks as though, in the end, the only private interests we can make sense of will be quite trivial wants (for example, the fact that you want strawberry and I want vanilla ice cream). This is because it is hard to think of the satisfaction of any more substantive interests, without them collapsing into one of the forms of collective interests (particularly congruent interests). For example, if I decide to aim to become a professional ice hockey player or a scientist, the satisfaction of either interest will require substantive public provision of infrastructure (for example, ice rinks, laboratories and schools). In these cases although I might claim to be pursuing my own private interests, I can actually only do so through taking advantage of various collective goods. What this suggests is that the satisfaction of many of our interests, and certainly most of our health-related interests, actually requires *essentially* collective provision. If this is true, then it pulls public health closer to clinical medicine, and so, public health ethics closer to clinical ethics: but it is public health ethics, not clinical ethics, that ought to be dominant and frame the debate (because of public health's core concern with the satisfaction of the various relevant collective interests).[13]

However, I now turn back to the third type of non-private interests: common interests. They are an example of the strongest form of collective values, and it is they that are related to what I think of as genuine common goods (see Figure 1.4). Collective interests relate to the common goods that that *we* necessarily and irreducibly share as a group or community.[14] It will be remembered that I defined goods as those things that are *good for* humans. Common goods will include the shared norms and behaviour that create and maintain rich and substantive social values, such as solidarity and trust. Such goods are good for all humans. Neither the relevant goods nor the corresponding interests are the result of individual consent and so do not need to be consciously adopted by each individual; indeed, many people might not even be aware of the operation of such common interests (and the value of the corresponding common goods) in their lives despite the fact that they benefit from them. Some of these aspects are the result of the type of society within which we live, but we do not have reason to hold them to be mysterious. Examples might include the way that one society may be more or less accepting of diversity than another; or the fact that a society has lower HIV rates as a result of particular attitudes to the disease; or, to return to my earlier example, that changes in relation to societal attitudes, food production and consumption, work patterns and lifestyle changes result in greater rates of overweight and obesity. Many of

---

[13] I think the best expression of something close to my views here is that to be found in Cribb (2005).
[14] Once again, much of the way this is phrased is borrowed from Postema (1987).

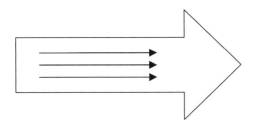

Figure 1.4 Common interests. Our individual interests represented by the thin arrows are part of, and jointly constitute, the common interests we have.

these factors can be captured by the kind of population effects that were explored in the work of Rose (1992) as outlined above. Our attitudes and behaviour as a society can result in positive or negative results for individuals. The causal mechanisms for this are complex and seeking change (if needed) will be difficult. But we need to see that such common goods (and the corresponding harms) are largely emergent properties of the relevant social group, rather than the product of consensual creation or assent. This is an important justification for collective action as an individual does not have total control of all the factors that influence their life. Public health interventions can reinforce, shape and change some of these factors and this fact provides a potential normative justification for such interventions when they seek to prevent or reduce harm or bring about or reinforce common goods. An awareness of the importance of such goods, that are neither a mere aggregation of individual goods nor public goods in the traditional sense, is one reason why the notion of community is a concept that is often invoked in such discussions. Those with parameters set by liberal medical ethics are often dismissive of such a notion, but the concept of community captures the vital collective and emergent aspects of such important social and common goods.[15]

Conceptions of social justice

Third, social justice is at the core of much public health activity, both nationally and internationally (Anand *et al.*, 2004; Faden and Powers, 2006). This concern is an option for the development of substantive public health ethics because of the way that inequalities (and therefore their impact on health) can be thought of as a population effect. Such a harm is not brought about by individual action (although, of course, this may contribute) but partly (perhaps even largely) by one's place within a society (Marmot and Wilkinson, 2005). Again, this is an excellent illustration of the reason why population-level analysis is vital to public health, and therefore, why it ought to be central to public health ethics (see Daniels, Chapter 11, and Wilson, Chapter 12). It can also be argued, as it is by O'Neill (2002), that a concern for justice in public health will have clear implications for the kinds of interventions that may be justified. She argues that the obsessive focus on individual autonomy in medical ethics may result in a negative impact upon the public's health, and that compulsion, even coercion, is necessary at times to achieve the desired aims of public health policy. In other words, a concern for justice may well result in actions that a 'Millian' liberal may find uncomfortable because in those situations liberty is not the core value. Sometimes a concern about equality may result in the sacrifice of individual liberty. A judgment about whether this is appropriate will have to be made in an individual situation, but the point is

---

[15] For further discussion see, for example, Cribb (2005), Jennings (2007b) and Baylis *et al.* (2008). One area for potential fruitful development in the future is to consider how social ontology and public health ethics may be mutually supporting.

that there is no a-priori reason to give priority to liberty. Of course, there is a huge literature on notions of justice, but I raise it here because of its importance in public health work and the fact that accounts of public health ethics committed to the idea of social justice will be able to meet my suggested condition.

Conclusion

Public health ethics is enjoying a surge of interest. The work of this discipline is not only to help to explore the ethical issues that emerge in public health practice, policy and research, but also to consider how medical ethics and ethical theory may need to be rethought and revised as a result of taking public health and public health ethics seriously. There is no a-priori reason for thinking that public health ethics ought to develop as a separate discourse, distinct from that of medical ethics or bioethics more generally, and on the whole I think we have good reasons to retain or seek theoretical unification. While there is a lot of interesting work going on at the moment in the field of public health ethics, there is much still to be done. It is almost certainly too early to outline a satisfactory account of what public health ethics ought to be. Despite this we can say something about the areas that we need to explore in the future. The core values will be some of those I have identified above as belonging to the list of factors that might be used as the basis for building a substantive public health ethics: the concepts of group, community, population, public goods, common goods, solidarity, reciprocity, welfare, well-being and justice. This predominantly social focus need not mean that we can ignore individual concerns, or that individuals are sacrificed for the sake of populations. The way forward is surely a sufficiently rich and pluralistic account of public health ethics that does not feel the need to embrace such dichotomous thinking. Individuals are neither just individuals, nor merely constituent parts of groups, societies, communities and populations. What we need is a public health ethics, and in turn a bioethics, that is both sensitive to and grounded in the reality of relevant social relationships.

Acknowledgements

I am very grateful to the following for their critical comments on a previous version of this chapter: Cecile Bensimon, John Coggon, Alan Cribb, Ross Upshur and Adrian Viens.

References

Anand, S., Peter, F. and Sen, A. (eds). (2004) *Public Health, Ethics & Equity.* Oxford: Oxford University Press.

Baylis, F., Kenny, N. P. and Sherwin, S. (2008) A relational account of public health ethics. *Public Health Ethics*, **1**, 3: 196–209.

Childress, J. F., Faden, R. R., Gaare, R. D., *et al.* (2002) Public health ethics: mapping the terrain. *The Journal of Law, Medicine & Ethics*, **30**, 2: 170–8.

Coggon, J. (2008) Harmful rights-doing? The perceived problem of liberal paradigms and public health. *Journal of Medical Ethics*, 34: 798–801.

Coker, R. and Martin, R., eds (2006) *Public Health*, **120**, Supplement 1: The Importance of Law for Public Health Policy and Practice.

Cribb, A. (2005) *Health and the Good Society.* Oxford: Oxford University Press.

Dawson, A. (2007) Herd protection as a public good: vaccination and our obligations to others. In *Ethics, Prevention and Public Health*, ed. A. Dawson and M. Verweij. Oxford: Oxford University Press.

Dawson, A. (2009) Theory and practice in public health ethics: a complex relationship. In *Public Health Ethics & Practice*, ed. S. Peckham and A. Hann. London: Polity Press.

Dawson, A. and Garrard, E. (2006) In defence of moral imperialism: four equal and universal prima facie duties. *Journal of Medical Ethics*, 32, 4: 200–4.

Dawson, A. and Verweij, M. (2008) The steward of the Millian state. *Public Health Ethics*, 1, 3: 193–5.

Feinberg, J. (1984) *Harm to Others*. Oxford: Oxford University Press.

Gostin, L. O. (2005) Public health preparedness and ethical values in pandemic influenza. In *The Threat of Pandemic Influenza: Are We Ready?* Institute of Medicine, ed. Washington: National Academies Press.

Gostin, L. O. and Stone, L. (2007) The health of the people: the highest law. In *Ethics, Prevention and Public Health*, ed. A. Dawson and M. Verweij. Oxford: Oxford University Press.

Griffin, J. (1986) *Well-Being: Its Meaning, Measurement and Moral Importance*. Oxford: Clarendon Press.

Hardin, G. (1968) The Tragedy of the Commons. *Science*, 162, 3859: 1243–8.

Holland, S. (2007) *Public Health Ethics*. London: Polity Press.

Jennings, B. (2007a) Public health and civic republicanism: toward an alternative framework for public health ethics. In *Ethics, Prevention and Public Health*, ed. A. Dawson and M. Verweij. Oxford: Oxford University Press.

Jennings, B. (2007b) Community. In *Principles of Health Care Ethics*, ed. R. Ashcroft, A. Dawson, H. Draper and J. McMillan, 2nd edn. Chichester: Wiley.

Kass, N. E. (2001) An ethics framework for public health. *American Journal of Public Health*, 91, 11: 1776–82.

Kraut, R. (2007) *What is Good and Why: The Ethics of Well-being*. Harvard, MA: Harvard University Press.

Marmot, M. and Wilkinson, R., eds (2005) *Social Determinants of Health*, 2nd edn. Oxford: Oxford University Press.

Martin, R. (2009) The role of the law in public health. In *The Philosophy of Public Health*, ed. A. Dawson. Aldershot: Ashgate.

Mill, J. S. (1859) *On Liberty*. (Many editions).

Munthe, C. (2008) The goals of public health: an integrated, multidimensional model. *Public Health Ethics*, 1: 39–52.

Nuffield Council on Bioethics. (2007) *Public Health: Ethical Issues*. London: NCB.

Nussbaum, M. C. (2000) *Women and Human Development*. Cambridge: Cambridge University Press.

Nys, T. (2008) Paternalism in public health care. *Public Health Ethics*, 1: 64–72.

O'Neill, O. (2002) Public health or clinical ethics: thinking beyond borders. *Ethics & International Affairs*, 16, 2: 35–45.

Parfit, D. (1984) *Reasons and Persons*. Oxford: Oxford University Press.

Paul, C. (2009) The common good argument and HIV prevention. In *The Philosophy of Public Health*, ed. A. Dawson. Aldershot: Ashgate.

Postema, G. J. (1987) Collective evils, harms, and the law. *Ethics*, 97: 414–40.

Powers, M. and Faden, R. (2006) *Social Justice: the Moral Foundations of Public Health and Health Policy*. Oxford: Oxford University Press.

Raz, J. (1986) *The Morality of Freedom*. Oxford: Oxford University Press.

Rose, G. (1992) *The Strategy of Preventive Medicine*. Oxford: Oxford University Press.

Sen, A. (1999) *Development as Freedom*. New York: Knopf.

Upshur, R. E. G. (2002) Principles for the justification of public health interventions. *Canadian Journal of Public Health*, 93, 2: 101–3.

Verweij, M. and Dawson, A. (2007) The meaning of 'public' in 'public health'. In *Ethics, Prevention and Public Health*, ed. A. Dawson and M. Verweij. Oxford: Oxford University Press.

Wikler, D. I. (1978) Persuasion and coercion for health: ethical issues in government efforts to change lifestyle. *Millbank Memorial Fund Quarterly*, 56, 5: 303–38.

Chapter

2

Health, disease and the goal of public health

Bengt Brülde

Introduction

What is the ultimate goal of public health activities, such as health promotion, health education or health protection? Or rather, what *should* these activities aim at, what 'values' should public health workers try to realize or maximize?[1] To suggest that the goal of public health is to promote or improve population health is not very informative, at least not before we establish what is meant by 'population health' in this context, or rather, what the phrase *should* mean in this context. Moreover, there might be some appropriate goals that are not really possible to subsume under this heading, at least not without stretching the ordinary meaning of the phrase a little too far. That is, the central question of this chapter cannot be regarded as conceptual.

To come up with a reasonable view on what the ultimate goals of public health are, we need to look at what more specific suggestions have been made. Among the different goals that have been suggested, there are at least three that are worth considering more closely, namely (1) to improve the average level of health (or the like) in the relevant population, (2) to reduce health inequalities between groups or individuals and (3) to create certain types of opportunities for health, most often equal opportunities. It is possible that we should add (4) to improve the health level of the worst-off groups.[2,3]

---

[1] To assess the quality and effectiveness of different public health strategies (practices, interventions or efforts) is, to a large extent, a matter of determining to what extent these ultimate goals have been attained. It is worth noting that most operative public health goals, for example, to reduce the consumption of alcohol or the percentage of smokers, are not ultimate or final in this sense, but 'merely' instrumental.

In my view, the question of what the ultimate goals should be is one of the three most central issues in public health ethics. The other two are (i) the question of what interventions are morally acceptable, for example, in what ways it is morally permissible or legitimate to influence people's choices or to manipulate the social determinants of health; and (ii) the question of how the resources available should be allocated or distributed, for example, whether the allocation of resources should be based on considerations of need or on considerations of cost effectiveness. Both these questions are intimately related to the question of the ultimate goals.

[2] Like (2), this is a distributive concern, but it is not identical to (2). It might be combined with (2), however, for example, if the goal is to reduce health inequalities *through* improving the health of the worst-off groups. In the following, I will discuss (4) in connection with (2), that is, I will, for the time being, not treat it as a goal in its own right.

Public Health Ethics, ed. Angus Dawson. Published by Cambridge University Press. © Cambridge University Press 2011.

Assuming that (1)–(3) constitute a pretty comprehensive view of the goals of public health, let us now take a closer look at how exactly they should be understood.

To improve the average level of health

To improve the average level of health in a population is to improve population health in the most narrow sense of the term, or alternatively, to make an improvement in what Verweij and Dawson (2007) refer to as the aggregative dimension of population health.[4] This goal reflects the plausible idea that public health activities should aim to benefit the individuals in the relevant population, and the more these people are benefited the better. However, it is less clear in what way the individuals should be benefited, that is, in what dimension or dimensions. For example, to suggest that public health should promote or maintain individual *health* is far from sufficient. To prevent disease and injury (to reduce morbidity) is a second way in which public health should benefit people and to prolong people's lives (to reduce mortality) is a third possibility. There are more views than these of what the relevant individual outcomes should be, for example, empowerment (people's ability to control the determinants of health or to make healthy choices),[5] responsibility, autonomy, dignity, integrity (Buchanan, 2000), well-being (quality of life) or health-related quality of life. In short, it is an open question how exactly public health should benefit the individuals in the relevant population, that is, what individual 'health outcome' it should aim to improve or maximize. I return to this question below.

To reduce health inequalities

To reduce health inequalities is to make an improvement in what Verweij and Dawson (2007) refer to as the distributive dimension of population health. This suggestion also gives rise to a large number of questions. First, we need to ask what inequalities should be reduced, that is, what the relevant individual 'health outcome' is. In my view, we can safely assume that it is the same outcome as above, that is, the outcome that public health should also try to improve or maximize. (The concern with social inequality as a means to equality in health does not belong here, but in (3).) Second, we need to ask what distributive

---

[3] Many of the standard epidemiological measures are strongly related to (1), properly construed (see below). For example, most traditional morbidity and mortality measures tell us to what extent (1) has been attained. However, there are also a number of traditional measures that are, at best, *indicators* of population health. It might be worth considering whether public health should try to improve these measures as well, for example, whether it should also try to reduce the utilization of health services, the number of sick days per capita and year, or the amount of early retirements due to illness.

[4] Few theorists regard this as the only goal of public health, but Rose (1992) seems to be an exception. It is worth noting that if this were the case (that is, if there were no distributive goals), then health care and public health resources should simply be allocated so as to maximize the health benefits they produce, and it would be sufficient to use cost effectiveness analysis alone to set priorities (Brock 2004). It is also worth noting that if maximization of aggregate health were the only goal, then we should be indifferent between small benefits to a large number of persons and large benefits to a small number of persons (regardless of people's initial health states).

[5] In this context, it is worth noting that empowerment has a rather complex role in this context: the term does not just denote a goal (a state to be achieved), but also a certain kind of process, viz. a process characterized by a high level of client influence and participation (Tengland, 2007).

considerations are most plausible. There are other possible distributive considerations besides the aim to reduce health inequalities, for example, (4) to give priority to those with the worst health or shortest life expectancy, to reduce health inequities (those inequalities that are unjust) or to ensure that no one falls below a certain critical level. It is not quite clear how these other considerations are related to the goal of reducing inequality, and what we should do if different distributive considerations pull in different directions. Maybe we should abandon egalitarianism altogether, and replace it with some version of (4), such as the priority view. In any case, we need to ask what inequality is, and how it should be measured in this context. Without doing so it is hard to formulate a plausible distributive goal for public health activities.

To create (equal) opportunities for health

This goal corresponds, at least in part, to Verweij and Dawson's (2007) third dimension of population health. If this dimension is formulated as a goal, we get the suggestion that public health should 'improve those conditions that are relevant for the health of everyone' (2007: 26), for example, that it should try to contain and control those environmental (and perhaps social) risk factors that might affect the health of everyone, that it should aim to exclude these factors from the population. (An example of this is to achieve herd immunity against certain diseases by vaccination.) The idea that public health activities should aim to create equal opportunities for health seems to include more than this, however, viz. that these activities should also attack other central risk factors or determinants, risk factors that might affect the health of many but not everyone. For example, it might be argued that public health should try to improve the social conditions of the worst-off groups, or to reduce socio-economic inequalities. (This is a central goal of what Seedhouse (1997) refers to as 'social health promotion'.) The idea that health promotion should aim to empower groups or communities (not just individuals) might belong here as well.[6]

Regardless of what exactly is included under this heading, it is clear that success in this area does not automatically manifest itself in improved aggregative or distributive figures: a decrease in average health or an increased inequality in health is not *necessarily* a sign of failure.[7] Now, it is rather obvious what this might mean on the individual level,

---

[6] This goal is sometimes qualified in different ways. For example, Munthe (2008) thinks that this goal has weight only when the average level of health is acceptable. Another possibility is that the goal to create equal opportunities for health is not really ultimate, for example, that it should only be pursued when this is expected to result in better population health.

[7] According to Verweij and Dawson (2007), this suggests that the health of a population can improve even if no one becomes healthier and even if the inequality in health is not reduced. I prefer a somewhat different language, however. In my terminology, public health work may have other goals besides improving population health, for example, to protect population health, and can thus be 'successful' even if there is no improvement in population health. In my view, the health of a population is solely a function of average level and distributive features. (Which implies that population health can be improved by selectively aborting everyone with a below average life expectancy.) Or alternatively put, the health of a population is a function of the actual health states (life expectancy, etc.) of its members: if we know how healthy the relevant individuals are (including how individual health is distributed in the population), we can (in principle) determine the health of the population. It can also be argued that the question of how population health should be measured is really an evaluative question, that the question of how different health distributions should be ranked with regard to population health cannot be distinguished from the

for example, the fact someone has a good opportunity to stop smoking does not imply that they will in fact stop smoking. However, what counts as an opportunity in this context, how do we determine how 'big' a certain opportunity is, and how big a gap can there be between people's opportunities for health and their actual health states? (Does being informed about the dangers of smoking count as an opportunity for health?) I will not pursue these questions any further. Neither will I discuss to what extent the third goal is reasonable, but it is worth noting that considerations of autonomy suggest that we cannot ignore this goal.

Towards a conception of the goals of public health

It is important to note that the above three goals can conflict in several different ways. For example, aggregative considerations can conflict with distributive considerations: that the health of the best-off group is improved is desirable from an aggregative perspective but might be undesirable from a distributive perspective. A theory of the goals of public health cannot be complete unless it tells us how we should deal with these conflicts. One way to do this is to create a goal structure (Brülde, 2001) and another (perhaps more promising) way is to create a summary measure; to combine the different concerns into a single measure.

In summary, several questions need to be answered if we want to arrive at a well-founded and reasonably complete view of the goals of public health. In the following, I will restrict myself to two of these questions: (1) In what respect or respects should public health try to benefit the relevant individuals? What individual 'health outcomes' are most relevant in this context, that is, what exactly should public health try to maximize and distribute fairly or equally in the relevant population? In connection with this I discuss central concepts such as 'health', 'disease', 'quality of life', 'health-related quality of life' and 'quality-adjusted life years'. I will also offer a few reflections on how valuable different health gains and life extensions are from a public health perspective, and whether it is possible to combine the relevant variables (for example, health and life expectancy) into a single measure. (2) What is the most plausible distributive goal for public health activities? For example, is it to reduce all health inequalities, or only those inequalities that are unjust or unfair? Is the priority view more plausible than strict egalitarianism? Is there a critical level, such that it should be regarded as especially important that people do not fall below this level? There will also be a short discussion on how aggregative concerns might be weighed against distributive concerns. I will devote more space to the first question than to the second. The two questions will, to a certain extent, be treated separately, but not fully: we can hardly arrive at a reasonable individual summary measure unless some distributive considerations are incorporated into this measure.

The relevant individual outcomes

In what dimensions should public health activities try to benefit the members of the relevant population? There are several different possibilities here, for example, to promote health, to prevent disease and injury, to prolong lives, to promote well-being or health-related quality of life, and to promote (individual) empowerment, responsibility or autonomy. In my view, goals such as individual autonomy and empowerment are either

---

question of how they should be ranked with regard to *value*. This suggests that there is little or no point in trying to define 'population health', that it is far more important to focus on what the legitimate goals of public health activities should be.

constitutive parts of well-being and/or mental health, or they belong to the third goal (to create opportunities for health) and thus they need not be treated separately in this context. (It can also be argued that these outcomes are only desirable from a public health perspective if they are conducive to better health or a longer life; Tengland, 2006.) The other possibilities are worth looking into, however. Let us start with the perhaps most frequently used measure of the health status of a population, namely life expectancy at birth.

To prolong lives

How long we live obviously matters, not just from our own perspective but also from a public health perspective. But how much does it matter, and in what way? A key issue here is whether we should always attribute the same value to an additional life year (whether we should regard each life year as equally important) or whether we should give different moral weights to life years at different ages. In my view, we can safely assume that each life year is equally valuable to the person who is living the life (with one possible exception, see 5 below), but it is not clear whether public health professionals ought to evaluate each life year equally (or whether each life year gives an equally large contribution to the health of a population). Should each life year be given the same weight, regardless of when during the life cycle it occurs? There are at least five simple answers to this question (see also Figure 2.1):[8]

1. Each life year added is equally valuable (given an acceptable level of health, etc).
2. The older the person is, the less is the value of an additional year, that is, the marginal value of a life is diminishing with increasing age.
3. After a certain age, an additional year is worth nothing from a public health perspective. 'Years of potential life lost' is a measure that reflects this view, since it only counts the years lost before a certain (arbitrarily determined) age, for example, 75 years.
4. After, for example, the age of 75, each additional year still has value, but it is worth less (from a public health perspective) than it was before this age.
5. Each of these four views can be modified as follows: a life year has less value in the beginning, when we are infants, for example, because we're lacking in crucial capacities.

There are also more complex views on this matter, for example, the age-weighting used in the so-called GBD (Global Disease Burden) formulation of the DALY measure (Murray, 1996; Anand and Hanson, 1997; Murray and Acharya, 1997).[9] In this measure, age is weighted 'according to a (somewhat) bell-shaped curve whereby a year of life during young adulthood counts for more than one, peaking at 1,5 during one's early twenties, and a year of life counts for almost zero when one is close to birth or death' (Selgelid, 2008).[10]

---

[8] It is worth noting that these answers are, to a large extent, distributive considerations. Or more specifically, that they are combinations of aggregative and distributive considerations. They can therefore be regarded as partial answers to question (2) above.

[9] This particular DALY measure was only used in the first GBD study (in 1990), there was no age-weighting in the DALY measure that was used in the 2001 study.

[10] It is important that the question of age-weighting be carefully distinguished from another 'temporal' question, namely whether it is appropriate to *discount future life years* when making decisions in the present, that is, to regard future life years as less and less important as the years in question fall further into the future. Time discounting is often used in health economics, and future life years were discounted by 3 per cent in both the 1990 and the 2001 GBD studies. This can hardly be

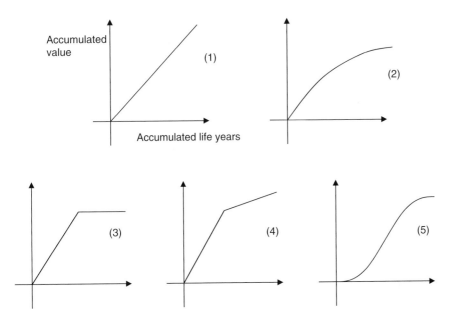

Figure 2.1 Graphical representations of positions (1)–(5). Note that the measure on the x-axis is longevity (accumulated life years) and that the measure on the y-axis is accumulated value.

This kind of age-weighting can only be justified instrumentally. A healthy life year at the age of 30 is regarded as more valuable than a healthy life year at the age of 70 because 30-year-olds are typically more productive and because others typically depend on them economically. As Murray and Acharya (1997: 719) put it, the health of some groups 'is instrumental in making society flourish: therefore collectively we may be more concerned with improving health status for individuals in these age groups'.[11]

To justify a certain age-weighting in this manner is ethically problematic (Brock, 2004). Moreover, it leads to double-counting (Anand and Hanson, 1997). When assigning value to different life years, we should not evaluate these years instrumentally, but intrinsically. Does this mean that all age-weighting is unjustified, that is, that we should accept (1) above? I think not. In my view, a combination of (2) and (5) seems most plausible, and for the

---

justified. The usual arguments for discounting money do not apply to discounting healthy life years, and it seems absurd to discount public health measures that reap their health benefits years into the future, like vaccination programmes. Future benefits are appropriately discounted when they are more uncertain than proximate benefits, but (even) this consideration does not require the use of a discount rate (Anand and Hanson, 1997; Brock, 2004; Selgelid, 2008). There is also a third 'temporal' question that needs to be addressed when assessing disease burden or cost effectiveness, namely what 'ideal' life expectancies should be used (Brock 2004; Selgelid 2008). For example, should we use the same uniform measure (for example, life expectancy in Japan) when calculating disease burden as in resource allocation contexts, for example, when calculating the benefits of life saving interventions (that is, the number of life years gained)?

[11] It has also been pointed out that life years lived as a young or middle-aged adult are valued more by people in general: one QALY for a 30-year-old is regarded as equal in value to three QALYs at age 50 or to nine QALYs at age 70. We should be grateful that these people are not running the health care system!

following reasons. The reason why we should accept (5) is that life of an infant has less quality. Now, it might be argued that we may deal with this 'on the qualitative side', but since *full quality* for an infant is not as high as full quality for an adult, it is more manageable to incorporate this on the 'temporal side': in this way, we can regard full quality at the age of 1 as equal in value to full quality at the age of 30, which makes it much easier to construct plausible summary measures (see below). To see why we should accept (2), let us first note why (4) (and perhaps (3)) is more plausible than (1). A good reason for this is the 'fair innings argument' (Williams, 1997). Given that our resources are limited, equality of opportunity requires that society gives lesser weight to a year of life extension beyond the normal life span. The reason why we should prefer (2) to (3) and (4) is simply that it involves no arbitrary cut-off point.

To differentially weight life years in this way might be irrelevant in a public health context, however, we can probably stick to life expectancy at birth here. In any case, to prolong life is certainly a plausible individual goal of public health.

Summary measures that combine 'quality' and 'quantity'

Now, it is quite clear that life expectancy is not the only relevant individual outcome in this context. How long we live is not all that matters: it also matters how healthy our lives are. And we cannot assume that most or all life years are healthy, especially not in rich societies, where we are good at prolonging unhealthy lives, and where increases in life expectancy are not always accompanied by increases in health. This suggests that we need a complex measure that does not just take the duration of life into account, but also some measure of its quality (broadly understood).

The most straightforward summary measure is to simply count the number of years with 'full health' or 'full quality'. Here, equal weight is given to health and life expectancy, that is, one year in full health is given the same value as two years lived in 50 per cent of full health (whatever this means). There are several summary measures of this type, for example, QALY's (quality-adjusted life years), HALE's (healthy life expectancy), DFLE (disability-free life expectancy) and DALE (disability-adjusted life expectancy). What is measured here are the years of life expected to be lived in full health, in full quality or without disability. It is also possible to measure the number of healthy life years lost through illness, disability or death, for example, as in the case of DALY's (the number of years lost because of death and disability in relation to some arbitrary standard age, for example, 82.5 for women and 80 for men). The basic idea is the same in all these cases: Public health should not just maximize people's life expectancy, but also try to make sure that the life years lived are healthy life years of good quality. To illustrate this idea, we can represent each life graphically, where the number of life years (or weighted life years) are represented on the x-axis, and where the person's health state (or quality of life) is represented on the y-axis (Figure 2.2).

What should be maximized is (roughly) the area below the curve. This idea gives rise to two important questions, however. First, what exactly should be represented on the y-axis, that is, what are the relevant qualitative individual outcomes? And second, once this has been decided, how should the scale be calibrated, for example, what level of health should count as full health, or as 50 per cent of full health? In this contribution, I focus on the first question, but first a few remarks on what might be meant by 'full health' in this context.[12]

---

[12] Thanks to Niklas Juth, who made me aware of the importance of this question.

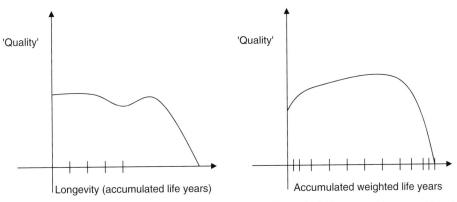

Figure 2.2 An example of what a graphical representation of a life can look like in a health context. Note that the measure on the x-axis is the number of weighted life years in the graph to the right, and that these weights can be represented by making the more valuable life years 'broader' (and thus more weight when the area below the curve is calculated).

What is full health? And is there a notion of full health that makes the HALE view (the view that public health should try to maximize the number of years with 'full health') plausible? One possibility is to conceive of 'full health' as 'maximal health', but this possibility is hardly plausible. Such a view would imply that few people are in full health, and that public health should try to benefit people who are very healthy (but below the maximum). Such a view would also make it quite difficult to make trade-offs between health and longevity. Another possibility is to conceive of 'full health' as 'acceptable health', where acceptable health may vary over time and across nations. Since many people's health is better than acceptable, this view implies that if these people's health is improved, there is no corresponding improvement in HALE, that is, that such improvements have no value from a public health perspective (assuming that HALE is the relevant individual outcome).[13]

However, to present the problem as a choice between different notions of full health is quite misleading. The question is really how we should value different improvements in health from a public health perspective, a question that is analogous to the question how we should value different life years depending on when during the life cycle they occur. (Moreover, we want to calibrate the health scale (functioning scale, or the like) in a way that makes it possible to compare life years lost to premature death with life years lived in a reduced health state, for example, in a way that makes it possible to translate a number of years lived with a certain disability into an equivalent time loss. Only then does it make sense to say that we ought to maximize the area below the curve.) There are at least four possibilities here, possibilities that correspond to (1)–(4) above:

1. Each improvement in health of a certain magnitude is equally valuable (from a public health perspective), regardless of where on the scale it occurs. (This is the view we are likely to adopt if we combine the HALE view with the idea that full health equals maximal health.)

---

[13] This is not to deny that it can have instrumental value to improve people's health above this level, however, since this might prolong their lives, or postpone the time when they sink below acceptable health. The observation is Per-Anders Tengland's.

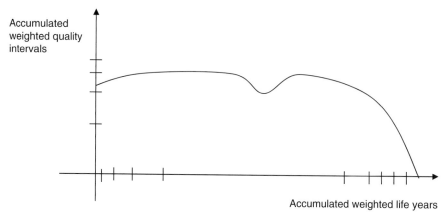

Figure 2.3 An example of how a life can be represented graphically if we are looking for a measure of weighted QALY or HALE. Note that the measures on both axes are weighted, which can be represented by making the more valuable life years and the more valuable 'quality intervals' broader: they are thus given more weight when the area below the curve is calculated.

2. The better a person's health is, the less is the value of a certain improvement, that is, the marginal value of health is diminishing.
3. Once a certain level of health has been attained, a further improvement is worth nothing from a public health perspective. Public health should do nothing for those people who have reached this level (and who can be expected to stay on this level). (This is the view we get if the idea that full health equals acceptable health is incorporated into the HALE view.)
4. Improvements beyond acceptable health still have value, but they are worth less (from a public health perspective) than improvements below this level.

Now, the HALE view cannot be made sufficiently precise unless we take a stand on this issue. In my view, (2) is most plausible. If this idea is accepted, we get the following modification of the HALE view: We represent each life graphically, in the form of a curve (Figure 2.3). The number of weighted life years are still represented on the x-axis, but we no longer measure people's health states on the y-axis. The y-axis is no longer a straightforward heath scale, but a 'health value scale' that consists of 'weighted health units'. It is the area below *this* curve that we should try to maximize, that is, weighted HALEs (QALYs, or the like). But again, this maximizing idea only makes sense if the health value scale is calibrated in a way that makes it possible to make trade-offs between health and longevity, for example, to determine how many life years lived with a certain disability that is equivalent in value to one life year lived in 'full health'. The calibration question will be discussed later.

Let us now return to the first question, that is, what exactly should be represented on the y-axis. The perhaps most natural answer to this question (an answer that has been taken for granted in the above) is *health*. There are several views of what health is, however, one of which is the absence of disorders or maladies (that is, diseases, injuries and defects). To suggest that public health should promote health in this sense is to suggest that it should aim at preventing disease and injury. (As we will see, this goal is central regardless of what notion of health is chosen, but if 'health' is defined in terms of functioning or well-being, this is because disease is regarded as a common *cause* of ill health.) Let us therefore start with the goal to prevent disease or injury.

To prevent disease and injury

This is obviously a plausible goal of public health. But to find out what it means more exactly, and how it relates to the other goals (for example, whether it is an instance of the goal to promote health or a means to promoting health), we need to know how the term 'disorder' (or 'malady') can and should be defined.

What is a disorder? Or alternatively put, what conditions should be categorized as disorders, mental or somatic? How should we draw the line between pathological and non-pathological conditions?[14] There are many reasons why it might be of practical importance how we define the concept (Brülde, 2003; Brülde and Tengland, 2003). In this context, the most important practical purpose is that a definition of 'disorder' can help us specify the proper goals of medicine, and maybe also of public health activities. It seems reasonable to assume that one of the central goals of public health is to prevent diseases and other disorders, which suggests that a well-founded definition of 'disorder' can help us specify the goals of public health, and that it can perhaps help us (at an institutional level) to demarcate the special responsibilities of public health professionals from those of other professionals.

Disorders as internally caused undesirable conditions

It is generally assumed that disorders are physical or mental states or processes (for example, underlying anatomical or physiological pathologies or abnormalities) that typically manifest themselves in different kinds of undesirable symptoms. On this view, a condition is a disorder if and only if (1) it is undesirable or bad (either in itself or because of its consequences) – let us call this the *value component* of the concept – and (2) the proximate cause of the symptoms is some type of internal state or process (for example, a lesion or a part dysfunction), that is, something inside the individual's body or mind – let us call this the *factual or explanatory component.*[15]

This mixed or hybrid view has been challenged in three different ways. First, there is the view that the concept of disorder (particularly mental disorder) is a purely evaluative concept, that is, that there is really no need for a factual component (Wakefield, 1992). Second, it has been argued that the concept is a purely factual or scientific concept, that the presence of the right kind of internal cause is not just necessary for disorder, but also sufficient (Boorse, 1975). For example, on the so-called traditional medical model (or 'machine-fault model') of disorder, disorders are 'machine-faults', for example, underlying structural or functional abnormalities. The presence of a machine-fault is not just necessary for disorder, but also sufficient, and it is often assumed that the presence of such an

---

[14] The main reason why the question is best phrased in terms of *disorder* rather than in terms of *illness* or *disease* is that the most practically relevant category is a broader category that also includes injury, retardation, and so on. The practically important thing is obviously how we distinguish disorder from non-disorder, and not how we draw the line between for example, disease and injury, or between illness and disease.

[15] This rudimentary conceptual theory of disorder offers us truth conditions for disorder statements, that is, it tells us under what conditions a disorder is present. This leaves it open what kind of thing a disorder *is*, however, for example, whether it is (1) the condition that is *caused by* an underlying dysfunction (or the like), that is, some kind of syndrome, (2) the internal cause that produces the symptomatic manifestations or (3) the whole complex, that is, the underlying pathology *plus* the symptoms.

abnormality can be established in an objective and scientific way. Third, it has been suggested that the value component and the factual component should be supplemented by a third component, for example, the idea that a disorder is, by definition, a condition that health professionals treat, or a condition that (we think) should be treated by health professionals or by medical means (Reznek, 1987).

All these suggestions fail, but for slightly different reasons (Brülde, 2003). That is, it seems reasonable to accept the general idea that disorders are undesirable conditions immediately caused by internal states and processes. This assumption gives rise to two questions: (1) How should the evaluative content of the concept of disorder (its value component) be characterized? (2) What kind of internal proximate cause is essentially involved, that is, how should the factual component of the concept be characterized?

The value component: harm and other bad things

With the possible exception of a few machine-fault theorists and a number of physicians, it is generally agreed that we have to rely on value judgments to distinguish disorders from other conditions. It is not quite clear how, however. To clarify this, we need to know more than to what extent attributions of disorder are dependent on values. In particular, we have to know what kind of evaluations we have to rely on to identify the class of disorder. If disorders are by definition bad, in what way are they bad?[16]

The most obvious answer is that we have to rely on considerations of harm. Disorders typically involve some kind of harm to the individual who has the disorder, for example, distress or disability. As Wilkinson (2000: 289) puts it, 'we have a *prima facie* reason for believing that a condition is a disorder if it is a state of persons which causes them to be harmed (for example, through death or pain)'. This suggests that the connection between disorder and harm is conceptual rather than contingent, that is, that we rely rather heavily on considerations of harm when we want to determine whether a certain condition should be regarded as a disorder. The specific harms that are most often involved in disorder are of three different kinds, viz. (1) displeasure (for example, pain), (2) disability and (3) significantly increased risk of suffering the harms mentioned in (1) or (2), or of suffering premature death.

Many theorists (for example, Wakefield, 1992) claim that harm to the individual is a necessary condition for disorder. Some theorists (including Wakefield) also claim that we don't have to rely on any other kinds of evaluative considerations to delineate the class of disorder, that is, that harm for the individual is also sufficient for disorder given that the condition has the right kind of proximate cause. However, it seems that we sometimes need to rely on other evaluative considerations, particularly in the case of mental disorder. In my view, there are at least two additional evaluative considerations that are of relevance when we want to determine whether a certain type of condition should be regarded as a mental disorder, namely (1) judgments about what is bad or harmful for others, and (2) judgments

---

[16] In my view, there are at least two more questions that any reasonably complete theory of the 'evaluative content' of the concept of disorder need to answer, namely (1) whether attributions of disorder contain any implicit reference to some specific evaluative standard and (2) whether the concept of mental disorder is value laden in the definitional or in the epistemic sense. In Brülde (2007a) I argue (1) that there should be no references to any specific evaluative standards at all, and (2) that even though disorders are necessarily undesirable, 'disorder' may well be a descriptive phrase.

about abnormal functioning on the holistic level, for example, the idea that the person's behaviour deviates from some standard of good or normal functioning (where this standard is not fully derived from or based on considerations of harm, for example, as in attributions of severe irrationality). In this view, the presence of harm for the individual is neither necessary nor sufficient for disorder (given that the factual component is in place). The main reason for this is there seem to be mental disorders that are either not associated with such harm, or not considered disorders primarily in virtue of being associated with such harm, for example, paedophilia and antisocial personality disorder (Brülde, 2007a). If these conditions are correctly classified as mental disorders, then this is not by virtue of being harmful for the individual who has the condition, but rather because these conditions are abnormal and/or harmful to others.

The factual component: 'machine faults' and other internal causes

On the hybrid view, the undesirable symptoms are by definition caused by the right kind of internal factor. But what kind of proximate internal cause is 'essentially' involved in disorder? There are at least five possible answers to this question.

The first two views are both based on the assumption that the relevant internal cause can be fully characterized in objective, scientific or essentialist terms: (1) In the lesion view, all disorders are essentially lesions, that is, structural or anatomical abnormalities. A person can only have a disorder if some structural part of the organism (like a cell, a tissue, or an organ) is 'damaged'. (2) In the dysfunction view, disorders are essentially part dysfunctions, for example, physiological or biochemical abnormalities or disturbances that may or may not be caused by lesions. These two ideas are both versions of the so-called traditional medical model of disorder. Disorders are regarded as 'machine-faults', that is, underlying abnormalities (structural or functional) that tend to cause problems on the holistic level. This view has two central features, namely: (1) The reductionist idea that the symptoms are caused by some kind of 'underlying' or 'lower-level' pathology. The machine as a whole does not function because there is a fault somewhere in the apparatus. (2) The view that these machine-faults are abnormalities, that is, deviations from normal structure or function, where normality is understood in terms of species design.

Since the dysfunction view is more plausible than the lesion view (see for example, Brülde, 2003), let us restrict our attention to this view. There are at least two different views on the nature of dysfunction: the first idea is that dysfunctions are statistical abnormalities that give rise to biological disadvantage (where the notion of biological disadvantage is understood in evolutionary terms, viz. in terms of reduced survival or lowered reproductive fitness [Boorse, 1975; Kendell, 1975]). If this notion of dysfunction is incorporated into the concept of disorder, we get the idea that a disorder is (roughly) a condition that tends to reduce longevity or fertility. The second view of dysfunction (Wakefield's view) is also inspired by evolutionary theory. Here, a dysfunction is regarded as a failure of some internal mechanism to perform its natural function, where a natural function of a mechanism is an effect of this mechanism that explains why it was naturally selected (Wakefield, 1992, 2000). Both dysfunction views have been heavily criticized, for example, Wakefield's evolutionary view has been criticized by Lilienfeld and Marino (1995), Murphy and Woolfolk (2000a, 2000b), Nordenfelt (2003) and many others. Most of the objections to Wakefield's theory purport to show that dysfunction (as defined by

Wakefield) is not *necessary* for disorder, that is, that someone may well suffer from a disorder even when there is no 'evolutionary malfunction'. In my view, all traditional medical (essentialist) dysfunction analyses of disorder are highly problematic and should be rejected (Brülde, 2003).

A major problem with the traditional medical dysfunction view is that it is most probably too narrow. If dysfunction (defined in evolutionary terms) is necessary for disorder, this seems to exclude too many consensual disorders from the category of disorder. Conversely, it seems quite clear that if someone has a disorder, this means that something has gone wrong with the person. So how should we specify the central notion of 'going wrong', now that we can no longer appeal to dysfunctions? There are at least three non-essentialist answers to this question: (1) A dysfunction view that appeals to failed Cummins-functions, where a so-called Cummins-function of a structure or mechanism is its causal contribution to the overall operation of the system that contains it (Cummins, 1975). (2) The idea that *any* internal cause will do, or more specifically, that any *type* of internal cause will do. On this type of view, diseases and other disorders are, by definition, internal conditions that tend to compromise people's health, where 'health' is, as a rule, defined in terms of functional ability. (3) In Culver and Gert's (1982) view, disorders are (roughly) internally caused harmful conditions, and the phrase 'internally caused' is specified in terms of the absence of a distinct sustaining cause. In this view, a person can only have a disorder (malady) if the distress or disability he is suffering does *not* have a sustaining cause which is clearly distinct from the person.

The appeal to failed Cummins-functions tends to collapse into (2), the idea that any internal cause will do (Brülde, 2003). In this type of view (adopted by for example, Nordenfelt, Pörn, Reznek, Whitbeck and Sedgweck), a disorder is, by definition, an internal condition that tends to compromise people's functional ability. This view gives rise to several difficulties, for example, how to distinguish the internal from external, or more specifically, how to determine whether a certain incapacitating condition is caused by internal factors or whether it is 'merely' a reaction to environmental factors. How can internally caused conditions be distinguished from externally caused conditions in a way that helps us to delineate the concept of disorder? Culver and Gert (1982: 72) offer an interesting answer to this question when they specify the phrase 'internally caused' in terms of the absence of a distinct sustaining cause: 'We could say that to be a malady, the evil-producing condition must be part of the person. However, for reasons of conceptual rigor, a more formal negative statement is preferable: the person has a malady if and only if the evil he is suffering does *not* have a sustaining cause which is clearly distinct from the person'. The notion of a distinct sustaining cause is defined as follows: X is a distinct sustaining cause of a condition C if and only if (1) X is a cause of C, (2) X is not part of the person with C, that is, it is distinct from this person and (3) if X were removed, C would cease to exist almost immediately, that is, X is necessary for sustaining C (Wilkinson, 2000: 301). That is, the idea is that if a condition has a distinct sustaining cause, then it is externally caused (in the relevant sense) and cannot be a malady (disorder). This is not to deny that a malady may have been caused *originally* by factors distinct from the person. The important thing is that to be a malady, a condition is *not now* 'in a state of continuing dependence on those [external] factors; rather, it is present even in their absence' (Culver and Gert, 1982: 72).

This may well be the most adequate view of how the factual component of 'disorder' should be characterized. However, Culver and Gert do not draw the line between the pathological and the non-pathological where most people intuitively want to draw it. For example, their theory might be considered too inclusive, because it seems to imply that 'normal grief', unhappy love, ignorance or fanatical beliefs should be classified as mental disorders. It is hard to see on what grounds they can argue that fanatical beliefs or unhappy love are disorders. It is of course possible to refer to what is considered normal in the culture in which the condition appears, but this would really turn it into another theory, which includes a new evaluative element. Another possibility is to argue that ignorance or fanatical beliefs are only harmful in certain environments, and that they should therefore be conceived of as suboptimal behaviours (or the like) rather than as disorders. However, this strategy cannot explain why conditions like unhappy love or 'normal grief' should not be regarded as pathological. It is of course possible to accept the implications, and to regard grief as a mental injury and fanatical beliefs or infatuation as 'viruses of the mind', and that they should therefore be classified as mental disorders.

To conclude, Wakefield's idea that disorders are, by definition, caused by dysfunctions (defined in evolutionary terms) is a well-founded theory, but it tends to exclude some consensual disorders from the category of disorder. The most promising alternative to this analysis is the idea that a disorder is a harmful condition that does *not* have a distinct sustaining cause. However, this tends to include some more or less consensual non-disorders in the category of disorder. In my view, this strongly suggests that the different desiderata for a good definition are pulling in different directions. For example, it seems that if we rely on our linguistic intuitions, then we probably have to give up the idea that 'disorder' can be defined in terms of necessary conditions that are jointly sufficient. In fact, it seems likely that if we want to capture the concept of disorder as it is actually used in everyday speech, we should probably settle for some kind of family resemblance analysis or prototype analysis.

Disorder and public health

It can hardly be doubted that the prevention of different disorders is an appropriate goal of public health. The reason for this is partly that it is, by definition, bad to suffer from a disorder. To repeat, the harms that are typically associated with disorder are of three different kinds, viz. suffering, disability, and significantly increased risk of future suffering or disability, or of premature death. This strongly suggests that the severity of a disorder should be measured along these lines. The goal to prevent premature death has already been considered, however, which suggests that it is only the other two harms that can be added to the summary measure we are trying to construct. That is, it seems that the qualitative part of the relevant individual goal consists of trying to reduce (internally caused) suffering and disability. This idea is remarkably similar to the idea that public health should aim at *promoting health* (on the lower end of the health scale).

To promote health (physical and mental)

To understand what it means to promote people's health, we need to know how the concept of health can and should be defined in this context. We should not forget that a reasonable definition should take both somatic and mental health into consideration. It is easy to forget mental health, perhaps especially in public health contexts.

The concept of health can either be understood in terms of normal biological and physiological function, in terms of physical and mental functioning of the person as a whole, in terms of well-being, or pluralistically.

Biomedical definitions

It is sometimes claimed (for example by Boorse, 1977) that good health is the same as absence of disease or disorder. This definition is normally supplemented by a biomedical conception of disorder, that is, the machine-fault model. On this view, a person is in good health if there are no structural or anatomical abnormalities, and if there are no part dysfunctions. The objection that this leaves no room for variations in positive health is easily met. Even if there are no machine-faults, for example, even if all the parts of the apparatus are functioning 'normally', the apparatus can be in better or worse shape. This suggests that we can simply stipulate that a person (an organism) is in full health if its parts are in good order, and if the different physiological systems are working well. This is a 'reductionist' view, since the health of the whole is regarded as wholly dependent on the functioning (or 'health') of its parts.

If this view is adopted, how can a person's health be measured? Let us start with the negative case: If someone suffers from a disorder, it is often the severity of the symptoms that determine how severe the disorder is, that is, how much the person is suffering and to what extent they are disabled. (We should not forget the risk element, however, for example, a disorder can be severe in virtue of giving rise to a high risk of premature death). In the positive case, we can of course measure the ability to absorb oxygen or the like, but it seems easier to measure for example, athletic performance, that is, how the person is functioning as a whole. In short, the biomedical definition cannot help us to measure health; for this purpose, we have to rely on other criteria. Consider also the fact that many diagnoses are symptomatic in character, especially in psychiatry, which suggests that health is often the same as absence of symptoms. And since most symptoms are either sufferings or disabilities, this line of reasoning also suggests that we measure health in terms of functioning and/ or well-being. On the next two definitions, the clinical status of organs, tissues and cells is not conceptually related to health, but a determinant of health.

Functional definitions

On the functional view, to be in good health is (roughly) to function well as a whole person. However, this should not be taken to imply that every improvement in functioning is also an improvement in health. After all, there are abilities (such as the ability to read or to swim) that have nothing to do with health. A functional definition must therefore contain some idea of what abilities are health-related, for example, what it is that a healthy person can (by definition) do better than an unhealthy person. It must also contain some reference to the circumstances involved. That a person cannot walk is often considered a disability, but that he cannot walk in a hurricane is not. So, the question is under what kind of circumstances a person should be able to function well to be regarded as healthy.

Regarding the relevant circumstances, there have been four different suggestions: It has been suggested that a person cannot be regarded as fully healthy unless they are functioning well (1) in their actual environment, (2) under normal circumstances, (3) under reasonable or acceptable circumstances or (4) in many different types of circumstances (for example, the better they are functioning in adverse circumstances, the healthier they are). There is good reason to believe that the last two suggestions are most plausible (Brülde and Tengland, 2003; Chapter 9).

In response to the question of what abilities are health related, there are at least eight different suggestions. A person's level of health is at least partly dependent on to what extent they have the ability to (1) satisfy their basic needs, (2) realize their goals, (3) realize their vital goals, (4) acquire the ability to realize their vital goals, (5) live normally, that is, do the things people normally do, or (6) live a life that is normal for themselves. In my own view, a person's health is conceptually dependent on (7) what basic abilities they have, on the one hand, and (8) their ability to perform, that is (roughly) the ability to make use of the abilities one has, on the other (Brülde, 2000a, 2000b; Brülde and Tengland, 2003).[17]

Well-being definition

'Health' is rarely defined exclusively in terms of well-being, WHO's (1948) classical definition is an exception. Well-being is often regarded as one of several components of the concept, however. In this view, a person's level of health is, in part, conceptually dependent on their level of well-being. Or alternatively put, some improvements in subjective well-being are also, by definition, improvements in health. This should not be taken to imply that every improvement in well-being is also an improvement in health. If a person becomes happier as a result of winning the lottery or meeting a new partner, this has nothing to do with health. Just as in the functional realm, we need to know what feelings are health related. In my view, a pleasant or unpleasant mental state is health related if it is, to a considerable extent, internally caused, and associated with the ability to perform. This is a tricky issue, however, since a person's hedonic level is typically caused by both internal and external factors. Anyone can be happy under optimal circumstances, which suggests that circumstances should be normal (whatever that means). We should also remember that some people put themselves in positions that would make everyone suffer. In this case, however, the problem is really functional.

Pluralistic definitions

A definition is pluralistic (or multi-factorial) if two or more of the above considerations are combined into a single definition. In my own tentative view (Brülde, 2000a, 2000b), a person's position in the health-illness dimension is a function of their respective positions in five different dimensions, viz. (1) their clinical status, or organ function, (2) their 'ability to perform', to use the abilities they have, (3) to what extent they have certain relevant basic abilities, (4) what their health-related mood state is like and (5) how pleasant-unpleasant their health-related bodily experiences and emotions are. The first of these dimensions is 'biomedical', the following two are functional, and the last two concern the person's well-being.

Another way to accommodate all three definitions is to introduce a distinction between fundamental health and manifest health. A person's manifest health can vary from day to day, it gets worse when we catch colds, and it can be temporarily improved by different forms of doping or recreational drugs. To have good manifest health is roughly to be in good shape. A person's fundamental health is of a more dispositional or resource-like kind, and it remains intact when she is struck by the flu. Fundamental health is to a considerable extent a matter of how resistant and resilient one is, and it determines how

---

[17] Nordenfelt (1995: 148) defines 'health' in terms of functional ability only. In his view, '*A* is healthy if, and only if, *A* has the second-order ability, given standard circumstances, to realize all his vital goals [that is, the set of goals that are necessary and together sufficient for his minimal happiness]'.

disposed one is to fall ill or to die prematurely. Now, it seems that manifest health is mainly a matter of (health-related) functioning and well-being, whereas fundamental health is more of a biomedical matter. In this way, all three definitions can be accommodated.[18]

Health and public health

To promote health is clearly an appropriate individual goal of public health, at least up to a certain limit (see above), and as long as the individuals involved give their consent.[19] But is it an ultimate goal? It seems that subjective well-being is a better candidate than functioning in this regard, since it is good as an end whereas functioning is most likely merely good as a means. This suggests that functioning should only be promoted to the extent that it can be expected to have positive effects on well-being. Subjective well-being is more closely related to quality of life than to health, however, and this suggests that the ultimate individual goal of public health is to promote good and long lives rather than to promote long and healthy lives. But is it really a plausible goal of public health activities to promote people's quality of life? Is it a good idea to engage in what Seedhouse (1997) refers to as 'good life health promotion'?

A preference-based health index?

Before we take a closer look at this possibility, let us first look at the preference-based health index approach. (This approach can be regarded as something between the health approach and the quality of life approach.) By letting individuals themselves rank possible health states with regard to 'value', we can (for example, by calculating the average) create a preference-based 'health value index' in which a utility number is assigned to each possible health state. Here, it is possible to make use of the Rosser classification (Rosser and Kind, 1978), a two-dimensional system where health states are ranked with regard to disability (8 levels ranging from 1 = normal functioning to 8 = unconsciousness) and suffering (4 levels ranging from A = no suffering to D = severe suffering). We can assign the utility number 1 to health state 1A, and then make use of the individual preference rankings to calculate a utility number for the other 28 possible health states (8 B–D are not possible). This utility number may well be negative, for example, in the case of 7D, bedridden with severe suffering (Levin et al., 1991).

The individual rankings can be generated in several different ways, for example, by using Standard Gamble (SG), Time Trade-Off (TTO), Rating Scale or Magnitude Estimation (Karlsson, 1991). Let us call the health state we want to evaluate H. In SG, the individual is supposed to choose between H (with certainty) and a lottery (or gamble) with full health and death as 'prices'. The utility of H (for the individual) is calculated by

---

[18] It should be noted that all pluralistic approaches make it rather tricky to measure health. For example, how should one's position in the functioning dimension be combined with one's position in the subjective well-being dimension to yield a single measure? Maybe we should let each individual attach a weight to each dimension, assume that the dimensions are independent, let each individual place a value on the different levels in each dimension, and then use the average value to calculate the health level?

[19] The question of to what extent it is acceptable to promote health by paternalistic means falls outside the scope of this chapter.

finding at what odds the individual is indifferent between H and the lottery. In TTO, the choice is between being in H during a certain time and being fully healthy during a shorter time, for example, between 5 years in full health and x years in H. By finding the x-value where the individual is indifferent between the alternatives, we can assign a utility value to H. This method provides us with a way to balance health gains against life years gained, since this is exactly the kind of balancing the individuals are asked to make. This may well be the best solution to the calibration problem formulated above.

Utility values of different health states (or severity weights for different disabilities) can also be generated by the Person Trade-Off (PTO) method. Here, people are asked how many outcomes of one kind they consider equivalent in social value (for example, measured in terms of claims on resources) to x outcomes of another kind, where the outcomes are for different groups or individuals with different conditions (Brock, 2004). That is, people are asked to adopt the perspective of a policy maker. There are several versions of PTO. Let us assume that we want to determine the preference weight for a health state H, for example, a state of severe disability. One way to do this is to make trade-offs between life extensions for people in H and equal life extensions for healthy people, for example, by asking how many one year life extensions for people in H are equivalent in value to 1000 one year life extensions for healthy people (Murray and Acharya, 1997). Suppose we regard 8000 life extensions for people in H as equivalent in value to 1000 life extensions for the healthy. In this case, the value of H is 0.125. Another way to determine the value of H is to make trade-offs between raising those in H to perfect health for one year and extending life for healthy individuals for one year, for example, by asking how many improvements for people in H that are equivalent in value to 1000 one-year life extensions for healthy people (Murray and Acharya, 1997). Suppose we regard 5000 one-year long improvements for people in H (to full health) as equivalent in value to 1000 one-year life extensions for the healthy. In this case, the value of H is 0.2. It is worth noting that the PTO approach is designed to permit people to incorporate concerns for equity or distributive justice into their judgements about the social value of alternative health programmes (Brock, 2004: 221). The values generated by this approach are (most probably) strongly affected by distributive concerns, and they are thus unsuitable for assigning utility values to individual health states. It is better to use some other method to determine the relevant utility values, and then use the PTO method as a purely distributive device (Brock, 2004; and below).

There are several general objections to the preference-based health approach. First, we can ask how informed people's preferences are in this area. The value of a certain health state is mainly instrumental (it is good as a means rather than as an end), and it can be quite difficult to determine the consequences of different health states. One might try to avoid this problem by disregarding the preferences of non-disabled ordinary citizens, and instead appeal to the preferences of people who are well acquainted with the relevant health state, for example, the disabled. A problem with this approach is that the disabled tend to adapt rather well to their condition, which may result in evaluations that are 'too positive'. Another option is to rely on the preferences of independent health experts, but this suggestion is also problematic (Brock, 2004). It seems quite hard to determine whose preferences should be used to determine the values of different health states, and since different evaluative standpoints tend to give rise to different evaluations, this is rather problematic.

Second, we may ask what kind of value is assigned to the different health states. With the exception of the PTO approach, it seems quite clear that it is value for the individual rather than value from a public health perspective (the kind of value public health is supposed to promote or maximize). This suggests that the 'health-related utility values' that are generated by for example, SG or TTO have a diminishing marginal value in a public health perspective (see above). A third objection is that the restriction to health states is somewhat arbitrary. If we decide to appeal to people's preferences when we construct the relevant quality measure (the y-axis), why should we restrict ourselves to how people evaluate their *health states*? Why not start from how people evaluate their *lives* as wholes? This suggestion is very closely related to the idea that the most relevant 'qualitative' individual measure is quality of life.

To promote quality of life

The question of the good life (well-being, eudaimonia or quality of life) is one of the classical questions in philosophy. This question has been formulated in somewhat different ways, for example, 'What makes a life good for the person who lives it?' or 'What does ultimately make a life worth living?'. In order to make this question more precise, philosophers have formally defined the notion of well-being (quality of life) in terms of what has *final value for a person*. There are three important aspects of this formal definition. First, to claim that a certain life is good, or that it is of high quality, is to evaluate it in a positive way. That is, the question of the good life is a purely evaluative question, for example, it is not empirical. Second, the type of value that is of relevance in this context is *value-for* (or 'prudential value'). When we say that someone has a good life, we do not mean that their life is morally or aesthetically good, but that it is good for them. That is, the question of well-being is a question about what kind of life is good *for the person who lives it*. And third, the relevant prudential values are final values rather than instrumental values. On this view, the question of well-being is really a question of what is good for us *as ends* rather than as means. To have a good life is simply to have a lot of positive final value (and little or no negative final value) in one's life (Brülde, 2007b).

The different theories of the good life that philosophers have formulated and defended over the years can be classified in somewhat different ways. Most of the modern discussion of well-being is based on Parfit's (1984) distinction between three kinds of conceptions of the good life (or 'theories of self-interest'), viz. hedonistic theories, desire-fulfilment theories, and objective list theories.[20]

According to *the hedonistic theory*, the good life is identical with the pleasant or happy life. Well-being is the same as 'subjective well-being', to feel good. In this view, the prudential value of a life is a function of how much pleasure and displeasure (for example, suffering) this life contains. The more pleasure it contains, the better, and the more displeasure it contains, the worse.

There are other mental-state theories besides hedonism, however, such as *the happiness theory*. On the pure version of this theory, a person's quality of life is dependent on one thing only, viz. how happy that person is. Whether this theory is not just a mental state

---

[20] Parfit's (1984) classification is not the only possible classification, however. An alternative classification (closely related to Parfit's) has been proposed by Kagan (1992), who suggests that theories of the good life can be classified as subjective versus objective, on the one hand, and as internalist versus externalist, on the other.

theory, but also a hedonistic theory, depends on what conception of happiness is incorporated into the theory, for example, whether happiness is regarded as an attitudinal state (life satisfaction), an affective state (feeling good), or as a complex mental state consisting both of an affective and a cognitive component.

According to *the desire-fulfilment theory* (desire theory, or preferentialism), a person has a good life if and only if they have the kind of life that they themselves want to have. The only thing that has positive final value for a person is that their *intrinsic* desires are fulfilled (that they get what they want for its own sake), and the only thing that has negative final value for a person is that their (intrinsic) aversions are fulfilled, that is, that they get what they do not want. This is not a mental state theory, since whether a desire is actually satisfied depends in part on the state of the world.

Finally, according to *objectivist pluralism* (the objective list theory, or the substantive good theory), there are several objective values (besides pleasure or happiness) that make a life good for a person, independently of what they themselves think of the matter, and to have a good life is to have these values present to a high degree. Classical examples of such alleged objective values are knowledge, contact with reality, friendship, love, freedom, autonomy, to function well (for example, virtuously), personal development, meaningful work and rational activity. Health or empowerment are other possibilities, but these values are most often regarded as instrumental.

There are also mixed theories. The *modified happiness theories* are good examples of such theories, for example, the idea that a life cannot be really good for the person who lives it unless the cognitive part of their happiness (the positive value judgement) is informed and autonomous (this is Sumner's [1996] view), or the idea that a state of happiness is more valuable for the happy person if the relevant value judgement is based on true beliefs about her own life (this is a central part of my own view; Brülde, 2007c). On these mixed views (which are all based on the hybrid view of the nature of happiness), the presence of a happy mental state is necessary but not sufficient for maximal well-being, that is, these theories require that the happiness in question satisfies certain further criteria.

Well-being and public health

Now, is the promotion of well-being (on any of these views) a plausible goal of public health? It might be argued that it is. After all, that we live long and good lives is the only ultimate goal, and institutional arrangements should be created with this in mind. So, why not attribute this goal to public health activities? Here, it might be objected that a certain division of labour is necessary, for example, that society is best divided into separate spheres, and that each sphere (for example, the health care system) should focus on its own goals (Brock, 2004). It might also be objected that some kind of bottom-up method is most appropriate in this context, that is, that we should start from existing institutional arrangements and their existing goals, and then reflect on these arrangements in order to come up with suggestions for reform. For these reasons, I reject the idea that the promotion of well-being is a plausible goal of public health. The suggestion that public health should promote quality of life can only be plausible if this idea is qualified in several ways. For example, it would be rather unreasonable to suggest that public health should try to improve the quality of life in any respect (by relieving midlife crises) or by any means (by offering luxury holidays). It seems that public health can and should primarily promote quality of life *through* promoting health or *through* preventing disease or injury. But we may add that public health should (ideally) only try to promote health when this is expected to have positive effects on quality of life and/or life expectancy, since this is what matters ultimately.[21]

To conclude, it seems that health is the most plausible 'qualitative' measure we can find, especially if it is taken to include a well-being component. To promote health is not just a more plausible goal than preventing disease (since it includes the positive part of the health scale), it is also a more plausible goal than promoting quality of life. This suggests that something like HALE (healthy life expectancy) is the best individual summary measure we can find. To repeat, we can represent the relevant aspects of a life graphically, as follows. On the x-axis, weighted life years are represented, but the number of life years will serve as a good approximation. A person's position on the y-axis depends on her weighted (health-related) functioning and well-being. It is hard to combine a measure of each into a single measure, however. It is also hard to determine how much weight should be attributed to this combined (and weighted) health measure compared with the (weighted) longevity measure. In practice, it may well be necessary to make use of people's preferences on both counts, that is, first to create a single y-axis (as it were), and then to calibrate the resulting health scale in a way that makes it possible to weigh, health gains against life extensions. Only when this has been accomplished does it make proper sense to say that the individual goal of public health is to maximize the area below the curve. All other possible goals of public health, for example, to promote empowerment, are merely *instrumental* in relation to this complex ultimate goal.

What distribution?

I have suggested that it is HALEs that count. The higher the HALE average in a population, the better (from a public health perspective). The weighted HALE measure I have suggested already contains some distributive considerations (a certain version of the idea that we should give priority to the worst-off), but we may still ask how the HALE-levels of different individuals (or groups) should be distributed. Besides the idea that we should give priority to the worst-off ('the priority view' that has been incorporated into my weighted HALE measure), there are at least three possible suggestions in this area (given a certain average

---

[21] This suggests that *health-related quality of life* (HRQOL) might be the most appropriate individual goal of public health. This is a rather tricky notion, however, for example, does it refer to the part of a person's quality of life that depends on her health state, or to the part of a person's health that has a positive effect on her quality of life? In either case, it seems unnecessary to complicate matters by introducing such a notion, since we can say whatever we want to say in terms of health and/or well-being. Moreover, as the category HRQOL is normally understood, it is far too heterogeneous to be of any use. The instruments that purport to measure HRQOL normally contain both functioning and well-being variables, and sometimes also certain features of external circumstances, for example, vocational status. In fact, the phrase sometimes seems to denote everything that medicine should aim at, at least everything of a psycho-social nature. As O'Donoghue *et al.* (1998) point out, '[health-related] quality-of-life models typically consist of a mixture of physical symptoms (for example, pain or fatigue), assessments of emotional state (for example, happiness, anxiety and depression scales) and aspects of occupational and social functioning. Treating these disparate consequences of disease within a single framework causes difficulties.' They also add that the very complexity of the notion of HRQOL 'suggests that it may be helpful, when trying to understand the impact of therapeutic interventions, to focus on different "levels" separately' (1998).

level): to reduce health inequalities; to reduce health inequities; and to minimize the number (or percentage) of people below a certain critical level.

Now, there are at least two ways we can go to find out what distributive considerations are most plausible. The first way is to study the distributive aspect in and by itself, that is, to keep the average level (and population size) constant and then try to rank different (non-weighted?) HALE-distributions – where the HALE-levels of the different individuals are represented on the y-axis and where the population is represented on the x-axis, for example, from worse to better – with regard to value or population health. To focus exclusively on the distributive aspects of different HALE-distributions only takes us so far, since we also want to know how the most plausible distributive principles should be weighed against our aggregative concerns.

A more preferable approach is to study the distributive aspect in combination with average level, population size, etc. In this view, the central question is how we should rank different HALE-distributions with regard to value. (The reason why I phrase the question in terms of value rather than population health is to make it explicit that the question is to a large extent evaluative, which should come as no surprise given that its relevance is purely normative anyway.) Or alternatively put, how should we measure population health, for example, what changes should be regarded as improvements in population health?

Some distributive principles (for example, the priority view or the idea of a critical level) are straightforward (but partial) answers to this second question, whereas others (for example, to reduce inequality or inequity) are purely distributive. Let us start with the idea that the central distributive goal of public health is to reduce health inequalities.

To reduce inequality

It can hardly be doubted that health and other values are very unequally distributed in this world. What is inequality, and how can it be measured? And is the reduction of inequality a plausible goal of public health? If so, is it the only distributive goal? And how should it be weighed against the goal to increase the average?

On the standard egalitarian view, it is bad in itself that some *individuals* are worse off than others (through no fault of their own). This also holds when the worst-off are pretty well off in absolute terms. Should we also be concerned with equality between groups? I think not. In practice, we often need to concern ourselves with group inequalities, but this is mainly because some health inequalities between individuals are caused by social injustices, and because it is a more manageable political goal to try to reduce the latter. But we should also be concerned with inequality within groups.

So, how should we determine just how bad a certain unequal distribution is, that is, how should we rank different distributions in this regard? Temkin (1993) has found six relevant egalitarian considerations, three 'views of complaints' and three 'principles of equality', where each view of complaints can be combined with each principle of equality to yield a specific ranking of distributions with regard to how good or bad they are with regard to equality.

The three possible views of how individual complaints should be measured, of how serious a complaint is, are: (1) the relative to the average view of complaints (AVE); (2) the relative to the best-off person view of complaints (BOP); and (3) the relative to all those better off view of complaints (ATBO). The first view assumes that only those worse off than the average has a complaint, whereas the last two views assume that everyone worse off than the best-off person has a complaint.

There are also three principles of equality that tell us how distributions should be ranked with regard to value (given a certain view of complaints): (1) According to the maximin principle (MP), the larger the (average) complaint of the worst-off group is, the worse the distribution (or 'world') is with regard to equality. If the complaint of the worst-off is equally large in two worlds, the world where the worst-off group is smaller is better. If there is still a tie between two worlds, the procedure should be repeated for the next worse-off group, and so on. (2) On the additive principle (AP), the larger the sum total of complaints is, the worse is the inequality. (3) On the weighted additive principle (WAP), we should attribute larger weights to larger complaints before we add all the (weighted) complaints.

Temkin also points out that different traditional measures of inequality appeal to different views of complaints, on the one hand, and different principles of equality, on the other. For example, there are a number of measures that appeal to AVE and WAP, for example, the variance and the standard deviation, the coefficient of variation, the standard deviation of the logarithms and Atkinson's measure. To get the variance, we calculate the difference between each value and the mean, we then square these differences (so that larger deviations from the mean get more weight) and then add these squared differences up. In this measure, deviations above the mean and deviations below the mean are given the same weight. In the standard deviation of the logarithms, deviations from the mean are weighed before they are squared and added, so that deviations below the mean are given more weight than deviations above the mean. This measure has several plausible features, for example, it seems reasonable to attribute more weight to larger deviations from the mean (that is, to accept WAP) and to attribute more weight to deviations below the mean than deviations above the mean. The problem with the standard deviation of the log is that this is done in a rather arbitrary way.[22]

This is not the place to argue for any particular version of egalitarianism, or any particular view of how inequality should be measured. However, I strongly suggest that a plausible measure be based on moral considerations, for example, on some of the six egalitarian considerations listed above. That is, we first need to take a view on what the morally relevant aspects of inequality are. We can then find a way to measure each aspect. If there are more aspects than one, we also need to determine the relative importance of each aspect, give each (partial) measure a weight, and then combine them all into one single measure.

A few words need to be said on the relative importance of equality, however. How much does equality matter compared to for example, the average level? It is clear that equality is not all that counts: if it were, we could improve the value of a distribution by making things considerably worse for the best-off, for example, by injuring them. This is not plausible, however, and we therefore have to admit that the average level matters too, and that trade-offs are possible. But how should the level of equality be weighed against the average level, for example, is it ever possible to improve the health of a population by making the healthiest people a little less healthy? One way to find principled answers to such questions

---

[22] In a similar way, it can be shown that the range appeals to BOP and MP, the relative mean deviation appeals to AVE and AP, and the Gini coefficient appeals to ATBO and AP (Temkin, 1993). There are many possible equality measures besides these, however, where it is not as clear which egalitarian considerations are appealed to. Examples of such measures are the semiquartile range, the interquartile range, and comparisons between the top third (1/5, 1/10, etc.) with the bottom third (etc.) with regard to how much they have of the total share.

is to simply combine an aggregative measure and an egalitarian measure into one single summary measure. For example, Veenhoven and Kalmijn (2005) have suggested a measure of happiness in nations that combines utilitarian and egalitarian concerns (IAH = inequality adjusted happiness). Here, equal weight is given to the average level of happiness and the standard deviation (as a measure of disparity in happiness).

Egalitarianism versus the priority view

It is also possible to question egalitarianism altogether, that is, by arguing that people's relative standings are not morally relevant at all, that the important thing is that people live as long and healthy lives as possible, not how long or healthy these lives are relative to others. On this type of view, our legitimate egalitarian concerns are best captured by the idea that we should give priority to the worse-off. There are several possible versions of this idea. On the maximin version, we should give absolute priority to the worst-off, that is, the value of a distribution is almost wholly dependent on how well off the worst-off group is. The better off this group is, the better is the distribution, and the only way to improve population health is to improve the health of the most unhealthy group. This view is not plausible, since it suggests that we spend all resources on those who suffer most even when this is of little benefit.

A much more plausible version of 'the priority view' is the idea that a certain improvement has more value (or moral weight) if it befalls the worse-off: The worse someone's health is, the more important it is to improve his health. Health has diminishing marginal value, that is, a given increase in health is better (makes a larger contribution to population health) the further down the health scale it occurs. Every increase in health has value, however, for example, a large improvement for the healthy may well have more value than a small improvement for the unhealthy. (This idea is identical with (2) on page 28 above.)[23]

The view combines distributive concerns with aggregative concerns, and it thus partly avoids the problem of how the two concerns should be weighed against each other. In this view, it is not really possible to distinguish these two concerns from each other, but the problem is still there (internal to the view), since the shape of the value function partly depends on how the two concerns are weighed against each other. Once this problem is solved, the idea is that we should simply maximize people's weighed HALE-levels.[24] No further distributive considerations are necessary, for example, we need not be concerned with questions of justice. Is this a plausible view?

To reduce inequity

Those who think there is still something to be said for egalitarianism (that is, that relative levels matter) might consider the idea that not all inequalities matter, but only unjust or

---

[23] It is not easy to determine who should count as the worst off, for example, those with the worst health or those with the worst overall well-being. Moreover, we have to decide whether our concern for the worst off should focus on who is worst off at a certain point in time or on who is worst off over an extended period of time, such as a lifetime (Brock 2004). In my HALE view, public health should focus on who has the worst health over a lifetime, but in the case of health care, I tend to think that it is more appropriate to focus on who has the worst health at a certain point in time.

[24] It may not be possible to solve this problem in a principled way, however. In practice, it may well be necessary to use the PTO approach; see below.

immoral inequalities. In this view, public health should try to reduce health inequities, that is, those inequalities in health that are caused by unjust or morally unacceptable circumstances (Rogers, 2007). But what counts as an unjust inequality, that is, in virtue of what is an unequal distribution unjust or morally unacceptable?

In public heath contexts it seems rather common to regard an inequality as an inequity if it is due to the fact that the worse-off groups are poor, unemployed or discriminated against, or that they have less access to education or health care. This view seems to assume that all inequalities in health that are caused by social or economic inequalities should count as inequities. On this view, only those health inequalities that are caused by natural biological variations or freely chosen behaviours are morally acceptable (Rogers, 2007). But are all socio-economic inequalities really unjust or morally wrong, and if so why?[25] As far as I can tell, the idea that all or most socio-economic inequalities are unjust is often derived from the egalitarian idea that all inequalities are unjust *unless they can be justified* in terms of for example, need or desert (something which is rarely the case).[26] This view has been challenged by certain kinds of liberals, however, who argue that a distribution (equal or unequal) is morally acceptable if it has been caused by a process in which no negative rights have been violated, for example, if it is a result of agreements between free individuals. This is a substantive issue in political philosophy that should not be avoided, but there is no space to pursue it further in this chapter.

So, is it a good idea that public health should only concern itself with those inequalities that are unjust? This of course depends on what makes an inequality unjust, but I think the idea is practically useless in all its forms. In practice, it can be quite hard to distinguish those inequalities that are unjust from those inequalities that are, for example, caused by freely chosen behaviours. And even if this could be done, it would probably have no practical importance, since public health work is not concerned with targeting individuals. To the extent that egalitarianism and considerations of justice are relevant at all, public health should try to reduce the inequalities it can reduce, and not just some inequalities.

A critical level or a non-principled alternative?

The fourth distributive idea is another version of the general idea that we should give priority to the worst-off. On this view, there is a critical level analogous to the poverty line (for example, 'minimally acceptable health and life expectancy'), such that it should have high priority to move people from below this line to above the line. The percentage of the population above or below a certain level is a central measure when we measure the poverty in nations (the poverty line). The question is whether this idea can work in health contexts as well, and if so, how it can be incorporated into a plausible summary measure.

[25] And are naturally caused inequalities morally acceptable? Many political philosophers would argue that social justice *requires* that we compensate everyone who is worse off through no fault of her own, for example, because she is born with a handicap. On this rather widespread view, we act *unjustly* if we do not support these people, or more precisely: our *institutions* are unjust if they do not support these people.

[26] It is worth noting that on this line of reasoning, there is nothing special about socio-economic inequalities: naturally caused inequalities are even harder to justify. The idea that socio-economic inequalities are typically unjust may also be derived from the idea that everyone has a number of welfare rights, but only on assumption that these rights are rather extensive in scope, for example, that they entitle the right-holders to more than just a certain minimum.

The most promising way to justify the idea of a critical level (a cut-off point) is probably in terms of rights. It is not unreasonable to assume that we all have certain welfare rights, including a right to health. The human right to health is sometimes regarded as a right to 'the highest attainable standard of physical and mental health', but it is more plausible to regard it as a right to a certain minimum or adequate level of health care and other forms of health support, for example, the level of support needed to receive a fair chance in life, or why not 75 life years at a certain level of health (a 'fair innings' as it were, given that circumstances are normal)? But in my view, there is no need for any critical level. This level would be pretty arbitrary, it would depend on the amount of available resources (that is, vary from country to country), and it is doubtful whether there is any 'natural line' that is sharp enough to force us to modify the priority view.

There are also non-principled ways to evaluate different distributions. For example, it might be possible 'to develop a quantitative tool that measures the specific weight people give to equity concerns in comparing interventions that raise issues of distributive justice or benefit individuals differently' (Brock, 2004: 220). In Brock's view, the PTO approach may well be useful for this purpose. Let us assume that we have managed to assign utility values to different health states. We can then use PTO to determine the social value of whole distributions. For example, we might ask people how many patients treated with A (which will improve the value of their health state from 0.25 to 0.45) would be equivalent in social value to treating 1000 patients with B (which will improve them from 0.60 to 0.90). 'This will tell us in quantitative terms how much importance people give to treating the sickest when doing so conflicts with maximizing aggregate health benefits' (Brock, 2004: 220). If we do a similar thing in terms of HALE, it will help us construct the kind of function a prioritarian needs.

Conclusion: a summary measure of population health

To summarize the tentative suggestions I have made: The relevant individual outcome measure is a form of weighted HALE, where health is, roughly, regarded as a combination of (health-related) functioning and (health-related) well-being. We get this measure by creating a function that assigns a value to each health level-life expectancy pair (according to the priority view). In practice, it might be necessary to use some preference-based approach, such as TTO or PTO, to determine these values. To obtain a decent summary measure of population health, we simply have to aggregate these (weighted) HALE values. The higher the average level of this value is (in the relevant population), the better, that is, this is the value that public health should aim to maximize. It is possible that we can get an even better measure if we incorporate some further egalitarian (justice-based) considerations as well, but we must not forget that some egalitarian concerns are already embedded in the priority view. In short, the HALE version of the priority view may take us pretty far, and we may have less need for egalitarianism than we think.

References

Anand, S. and Hanson, K. (1997) Disability-adjusted life years: a critical review. *Journal of Health Economics*, **16**: 685–702.

Boorse, C. (1975) On the distinction between disease and illness. *Philosophy and Public Affairs*, **5**: 49–68.

Boorse, C. (1977) Health as a theoretical concept. *Philosophy of Science*, **44**: 542–73.

Brock, D. W. (2004) Ethical issues in the use of cost-effectiveness analysis for the prioritisation of health care resources. In *Public Health, Ethics, and Equity*, ed. S. Anand, P. Peter and A. Sen. New York: Oxford University Press, pp. 201–23.

Brülde, B. (2000a) On how to define the concept of health: a loose comparative approach. *Medicine, Health Care and Philosophy*, 3: 305–8.

Brülde, B. (2000b) More on the looser comparative approach to defining 'health': a reply to Nordenfelt's reply. *Medicine, Health Care and Philosophy*, 3: 313–15.

Brülde, B. (2001) The goals of medicine: towards a unified theory. *Health Care Analysis*, 9: 1–13.

Brülde, B. (2003) The concept of mental disorder. Web Series: No. 29. Gothenburg: University of Gothenburg.

Brülde, B. (2007a) Mental disorder and values. *Philosophy, Psychiatry, and Psychology*, 14: 93–102.

Brülde, B. (2007b) Happiness and the good life: introduction and conceptual framework. *Journal of Happiness Studies*, 8: 1–14.

Brülde, B. (2007c) Happiness theories of the good life. *Journal of Happiness Studies*, 8: 15–49.

Brülde, B. and Tengland, P.-A. (2003) *Hälsa och sjukdom – en begreppslig utredning [Health and Disease: A Conceptual Investigation]*. Lund: Studentlitteratur.

Buchanan, D. (2000) *An Ethic for Health Promotion*. Oxford: Oxford University Press.

Culver, C. M. and Gert, B. (1982) *Philosophy in Medicine: Conceptual and Ethical Issues in Medicine and Psychiatry*. Oxford: Oxford University Press.

Cummins, R. (1975) Functional analysis. *Journal of Philosophy*, 72: 741–65.

Kagan, S. (1992) The limits of well-being. In *The Good Life and the Human Good*, ed. E. F. Paul, F. D. Miller Jr and J. Paul. Cambridge: Cambridge University Press.

Karlsson, G. (1991) Värdering av hälsotillstånd och individuella preferenser [Valuation of health states and individual preferences]. In *Hälsa, sjukdom, livskvalitet [Health, Disease, Quality of Life]*, ed. P.-E. Liss and L. Nordenfelt. Linköping: Linköping University, pp. 159–66.

Kendell, R. E. (1975) The concept of disease and its implications for psychiatry. *British Journal of Psychiatry*, 127: 305–15.

Levin, L.-Å., Karlsson, G. and Carlsson P. (1991) Värdering av hälsotillstånd: en pilotstudie [Valuation of health states – a pilot study]. In *Hälsa, sjukdom, livskvalitet [Health, Disease, Quality of Life]*, ed. P.-E. Liss and L. Nordenfelt. Linköping: University of Linköping, pp. 167–81.

Lilienfeld, S. O. and Marino, L. (1995) Mental disorder as a Roschian concept: a critique of Wakefield's 'harmful dysfunction' analysis. *Journal of Abnormal Psychology*, 104: 411–20.

Munthe, C. (2008) The goals of public health: an integrated, multidimensional model. *Public Health Ethics*, 1: 39–52.

Murphy, D. and Woolfolk, R. L. (2000a) The harmful dysfunction analysis of mental disorder. *Philosophy, Psychiatry, and Psychology*, 7: 241–52.

Murphy, D. and Woolfolk, R. L. (2000b) Conceptual analysis versus scientific understanding: an assessment of Wakefield's folk psychiatry. *Philosophy, Psychiatry, and Psychology*, 7: 271–92.

Murray, C. J. L. (1996) Rethinking DALYs. In *The Global Burden of Disease*, ed. C. J. L. Murray and A. D. Lopez. Cambridge, MA: Harvard School of Public Health, on behalf of the WHO and the World Bank, pp. 1–98.

Murray, C. J. L. and Acharya, A. K. (1997) Understanding DALYs. *Journal of Health Economics*, 16: 703–30.

Nordenfelt, L. (1995) *On the Nature of Health. An Action-Theoretic Approach*, 2nd rev. edn. Dordrecht: Kluwer.

Nordenfelt, L. (2003) On the evolutionary concept of health: health as natural function. In *Dimensions of Health and Health Promotion*, ed. L. Nordenfelt and P.-E. Liss. Amsterdam: Rodopi Press.

O'Donoghue, M. F., Duncan, J. S. and Sander, J. W. (1998) The subjective handicap of epilepsy: a new approach to measuring treatment outcome. *Brain*, 121: 317–43.

Parfit, D. (1984) *Reasons and Persons*. New York: Oxford University Press.

Reznek, L. (1987) *The Nature of Disease*. London: Routledge.

Rogers, W. (2007) Health inequities and the social determinants of health. In *Principles of Health Care Ethics*, 2nd edn, ed. R. Ashcroft, A. Dawson, H. Draper and J. McMillan. Chichester: Wiley.

Rose, G. (1992) *The Structure of Preventive Medicine*. Oxford: Oxford University Press.

Rosser, R. and Kind, P. (1978) A scale of valuations of states or illness: is there a social consensus? *International Journal of Epidemiology*, **6–7**: 347–58.

Seedhouse, D. (1997) *Health Promotion: Philosophy, Prejudice and Practice*. Chichester: Wiley.

Selgelid, M. J. (2008) A full-pull program for the provision of pharmaceuticals: practical issues. *Public Health Ethics*, **1**(2): 134–45.

Sumner, L. W. (1996) *Welfare, Happiness, and Ethics*. Oxford: Clarendon Press.

Temkin, L. S. (1993) *Inequality*. Oxford: Oxford University Press.

Tengland, P.-A. (2006) The goals of health work: quality of life, health and welfare. *Medicine, Health Care and Philosophy*, **9**: 155–67.

Tengland, P.-A. (2007) Empowerment: a goal or a means for health promotion? *Medicine, Health Care and Philosophy*, **10**: 197–207.

Veenhoven, R. and Kalmijn, W. (2005) Inequality-adjusted happiness in nations: egalitarianism and utilitarianism married in a new index of societal performance. *Journal of Happiness Studies*, **6**: 421–55.

Verweij, M. and Dawson, A. (2007) The meaning of 'public' in 'public health'. In *Ethics, Prevention, and Public Health*, ed. A. Dawson and M. Verweij. Oxford: Oxford University Press, pp. 13–29.

Wakefield, J. C. (1992) The concept of mental disorder: on the boundary between biological facts and social values. *American Psychologist*, **47**: 373–88.

Wakefield, J. C. (2000) Aristotle as sociobiologist: the 'function of a human being' argument, black box essentialism, and the concept of mental disorder. *Philosophy, Psychiatry, and Psychology*, **7**: 17–44.

WHO (1948) *Official Records of the World Health Organization*, Vol. 2. Geneva: WHO.

Wilkinson, S. (2000) Is 'normal grief' a mental disorder? *The Philosophical Quarterly*, **50**: 289–304.

Williams, A. (1997) Intergenerational equity: an exploration of the fair innings argument. *Health Economics*, **6**: 117–32.

Chapter

3

Selective reproduction, eugenics and public health

Stephen Wilkinson

Introduction

In the wake of Nazi barbarities associated with eugenics, it has become impolitic to speak openly about improving population health and well-being by trying to influence the kinds of people who will be born. But is this goal in fact ethically unacceptable if dissociated with other immoral features of many historical eugenics programs?

(Wikler and Brock, 2007: 87)

This question, posed in a recent paper by Wikler and Brock, is the main concern of my chapter. Given recent and impending developments in reproductive and genetic technologies, it is likely that intervening before birth, before embryo-implantation, or even before conception, to alter the composition of future populations, will become an increasingly effective and cost-effective strategy for improving public health. In essence, ensuring that healthier future people are born, and conversely that unhealthier (possible) people are *not* born, may be a better way of delivering improved public health than the more usual biomedical and environment methods. Or even if it is not a better way, it may nonetheless be a useful addition to public health policy's 'toolbox'.

The first part of this chapter deals with a number of conceptual or definitional issues, all of which concern, in one way or another, the relationship between selective reproduction and public health. The second part of the chapter considers what I shall term *eugenics arguments* against using selection, ultimately concluding that worries about the 'spectre' of eugenics do not give us strong enough reasons to avoid using selective reproduction to achieve public health goals.

Selective reproduction

By 'selective reproduction' I mean the attempt to create one possible future child rather than another (Wilkinson, 2010). The reason for wanting to practise selective reproduction is usually that one possible future child is, in one way or another, more desirable than the alternatives. The kinds of desirability that people have in mind are many and varied, and the question of what counts as desirable is controversial. There is however one *relatively* uncontentious example: selection to avoid disease. If one possible future child would have a disabling, excruciating and life-shortening disease, while another would not, then many of us will think that ensuring that the disease-free child is created is the sensible thing to do. Disease-avoidance is the most prevalent and widely accepted rationale for selective reproduction, at least within 'Western' reproductive medicine and biomedical ethics.

Public Health Ethics, ed. Angus Dawson. Published by Cambridge University Press. © Cambridge University Press 2011.

Recent biotechnological developments (notably, the advent of preimplantation genetic diagnosis, the possibility of determining sex by sperm sorting and the ever increasing sophistication of prenatal tests) have made selective reproduction a pressing issue for regulators, academic bioethicists and the news media. However, selective reproduction need not be 'high tech' and has been around in technologically unsophisticated forms for many years. Perhaps the most obvious example of this is using contraception or sexual abstinence to delay conception. For instance, a (bioethically inclined) 15-year-old girl might think to herself:

> If I have a child now, then it will have a substantially lower quality of life than a different child conceived when I am 25. Therefore, I'll wait for a decade and create a better-off child instead.

This is an instance of selective reproduction: choosing an apparently better off possible future child over one that would be less well off. Interestingly, there is very widespread agreement that *this* sort of selective reproduction (avoiding teenage pregnancy through abstinence or contraception) is not merely morally unproblematic, but to be encouraged.

Another kind of 'low tech' selective reproduction is where a woman chooses a sperm donor with certain desirable characteristics (or indeed chooses to have sex with such a man) in the hope that his advantageous features will be passed on to her children. A good example of this is the renowned Repository for Germinal Choice. This was set up during the 1980s and dubbed the 'Nobel Prize Sperm Bank' because it was thought to contain several Nobel Prize winners' sperm. Similarly, in 1996, *The Times* reported that a sperm bank had been established for 'members of MENSA who wish to help create a master breed of super-intellectuals' (Rogers, 1996). Members of MENSA, 'The High IQ Society', are required to have 'an IQ in the top 2%' (MENSA, no date).

Same/different number scenarios and the non-identity problem

In this section, I briefly explain two important distinctions. First, 'selective reproduction' (as I use the term here) can cover both choices *between different possible future children* and *decisions about how many children to have (if any)*. Choices of the latter kind have been termed *different number* (because we are choosing between one number of children and another) while those of the former kind are called *same number* (because we are choosing not *how many* but rather *which* possible future children to create).[1] The same number versus different number distinction is often theoretically and ethically important but is rarely clear-cut when it comes to questions of policy. This is because many policy decisions affect both *who* comes to exist and *how many people* come to exist: both the constitution and the size of the future population. For instance, vigorously discouraging teenage pregnancy may well result in *different* children being born, but also in *fewer* children being born.

The second, more complicated, distinction is between choices that are *identity-affecting* and those that are not. Some choices *alter the characteristics of a determinate future person* (making someone more or less healthy, for example) whereas others amount to *choosing*

---

[1] This terminology originates in Parfit's seminal work, *Reasons and Persons*. He writes: 'Different Number Choices affect both the number and the identities of future people. Same Number Choices affect the identities of future people, but do not affect their number. Same People Choices affect neither' (Parfit, 1984: 356).

between the creation of distinct possible future persons (choosing a healthier one over one with a genetic disorder, for example). Selective reproduction (or at least the kind of selective reproduction that is the subject of this chapter) involves the latter rather than the former. The choices that we make when we practise selective reproduction are *identity-affecting*. They are also *existential*, causing people to exist who otherwise would not, or preventing the creation of (possible future) people. To make this distinction clearer, think about the following actions or policies:

> Vaccinating infants
> Encouraging breast feeding
> Discouraging smoking and drinking during pregnancy
> -----------
> Discouraging teenage pregnancy
> Preimplantation genetic diagnosis (PGD) and embryo selection
> Sperm sorting for sex selection
> Having 'unprotected' sex with numerous MENSA members (for reproductive purposes) rather than one's intellectually mediocre husband.

The first set of policies are not (or at least not directly or intentionally) identity-affecting. These policies, if successful, would lead not to the creation of different possible future people but rather to improvements in the health and longevity of people (or foetuses) who already exist, or whose future existence is not dependent on the action or policy in question. Of course, even these policies may have *indirect* effects that are identity-affecting or existential, affecting which (possible future) people come to exist and/or whether certain (possible future) people come to exist. Take the following case, for example:

> Grace, a young woman, smokes and drinks heavily during pregnancy. Tragically, as a result of this behaviour, Grace's baby, Olivia, dies during infancy. A year later Grace proceeds to have another child, Jack, who is in good health. Grace is certain that, had it not been for Olivia's death, she would not have had Jack.

If the population contains a number of women like Grace, it is safe to assume that implementing policies that discourage smoking during pregnancy will have identity-affecting side-effects. They will lead to the survival of babies like Olivia (which is not, considered in itself, identity-affecting) but also to the non-conception of (possible future) babies like Jack (an existential effect). But at least we can say of the policies in the first group that, while they may indirectly affect who comes to exist, this is not their main aim.

The actions and policies in the second group, conversely, are directly identity-affecting and altering the constitution of the future population is part of their aim (although those involved may not conceptualize it in quite these terms). These policies determine which (possible future) people will come to exist. For example, if we successfully encourage prospective teenage mothers to delay their pregnancies by ten years then we are getting them to have *different children* from the ones they would otherwise have had (and/or to have fewer children). When, following PGD, we choose between embryos for possible implantation we are choosing between one (possible future) child and others. When we separate X-chromosome sperm from Y-chromosome sperm and choose to use one or the other for sex selection, we are choosing between different (possible future) children and may, rather obviously, end up with a boy *instead* of a girl. And the same goes for a woman who is inseminated by MENSA members, rather than her husband: she is choosing to have a different (possible future) child.

Why do we generally regard such policies as identity-affecting? It may be because we accept what Parfit calls the *Time-Dependence Claim*:

> If any particular person had not been conceived within a month of the time when he was in fact conceived, he would in fact never have existed.
>
> (Parfit, 1984: 352)

However, this looks less credible than when his *Reasons and Persons* was first published because of the possibility of freezing and later using gametes. So perhaps what Parfit calls the *Origin View* is what underpins these intuitions about identity:

> . . . each person has this distinctive necessary property: that of having grown from the particular pair of cells from which this person in fact grew.
>
> (Parfit, 1984: 352)

According to the Origin View, coming from the particular sperm and the particular ovum from which I in fact originate is a *necessary condition* for something's being me. So, if those particular gametes had never existed, or if a different sperm had got to that egg first, then I would never have existed. A different (numerically distinct) person would have come to be instead.

In the case of preimplantation genetic diagnosis and embryo selection (and *a fortiori* in the case of selective abortion) there may be an additional reason for regarding selective reproduction as identity-affecting. In principle, each of the available embryos could be implanted and become a person (Embryo A would become Person A, Embryo B would become Person B, Embryo C would become Person C, etc.). And it seems to follow that, just as we could decide to implant them all and thereby create A, B and C, so we can *choose between* (possible future) Person A and Person C, by *choosing between* Embryo A and Embryo C. Perhaps one of the main underlying thoughts in the embryo selection case is simply that Embryo A and Embryo C are distinct organisms, spatially distinct physical objects. Thus Person C, *qua* Adult Body C, could not have been Embryo A because Embryo A and Adult Body C lack physical spatio-temporal continuity (whereas Adult Body C and Embryo C *are* spatio-temporally continuous). Two things (or 'thing-stages') are 'spatio-temporally continuous', in this sense, if they are connected by a continuous path through space-time; spatio-temporal continuity is widely regarded as being essential to the identity or persistence of physical objects over time.

Something like the Origin View (which we may also term *gametic essentialism*) appears to be the bioethics orthodoxy, but it is not entirely uncontroversial and has been questioned by some scholars (Wrigley, 2006). However, even if we were to eschew a fully fledged gametic essentialism (and to accept, for example, that there is a possible world in which I 'came from' a different spermatozoon) we could nonetheless retain the view that embryo selection (and *a fortiori* foetus selection) involve choosing between different numerically distinct (possible future) persons. This is because of the point just made: that in such cases we are choosing between existent spatio-temporally distinct physical objects. So since practices of this kind are my main concern in the rest of this chapter, it is safe to assume (for the present purposes) that selective reproduction is identity-affecting.

Table 3.1 Ruby and Emily: summary table of benefits and harms

	Who benefits?	Who is harmed?
Decide to create Ruby	Possibly Ruby, but only 'existential benefit'	Neither
Decide to create Emily	Possibly Emily, but only 'existential benefit'	Neither

The main reason for dwelling on the fact that selective reproduction is identity-affecting is that this has implications for the way in which the ideas of benefit and harm can be applied. For example, say we have a choice between bringing into existence:

RUBY: a (possible future) healthy child, and –

EMILY: a different (possible future) child with a genetic disorder, Z Syndrome; and that, according to existing people with Z Syndrome, it is extremely debilitating and painful but consistent with living a fulfilling and worthwhile life.

If we choose to create Ruby, who will have been benefited and who will have been harmed (leaving aside for the present the interests of third parties, such as parents and the National Health Service)? Arguably Ruby benefits, but the benefit for her is existential, the 'gift of existence'; crucially, it is not being born without Z Syndrome, because the choice facing us was not Ruby with or without Z Syndrome, rather it was Ruby or Emily. Of course, Ruby might feel glad not to have Z Syndrome and is better off than she would be if she had Z Syndrome, but this is true of all healthy children, not just selected ones. Turning now to Emily, she does not appear to benefit at all, both because she does not exist and because (even if we can make sense of non-existence being beneficial) her life, had it existed, would have been worth living and of some positive value to her. Has Emily been *harmed* by the decision to select Ruby? Probably we would say 'no' because of the problematic (arguably absurd) implications of allowing the idea that we harm a *merely possible* future person when we fail to bring her into existence.

What if we had chosen Emily instead? Similar considerations apply. If Emily has a worthwhile life overall we might say she had been benefited existentially (just as Ruby would have been if she had been chosen). And, while she would be better off without Z Syndrome (in that sense, it is a harmful *condition*), creating Emily has not harmed her because she would not be better off not existing. As for Ruby, we probably want to say (as we did of Emily in the previous scenario) that her non-existence neither benefits nor harms her (Table 3.1).

The relevance of this is that often, when practising selective reproduction, while there is an overall welfare gain (because of the absence of disease), there may be no particular individual who benefits (or is protected from harm) in any straightforward way because the welfare gain is distributed across different possible populations.

Selective reproduction and health

Is selective reproduction a public health issue? This question can be broken down into two parts. How does selective reproduction relate to *health*? And are those aspects of health to which it relates *public* health?

Selective reproduction does not necessarily have anything to do with health and it can be used for a variety of 'non-health' purposes. Sex selection (when not used to avoid sex-linked disorders) is an obvious example of this. However, as I mentioned at the outset, using selective reproduction to avoid disease, to bring about the birth of a healthy (or healthier) child is (at least in the UK and many other 'Western' countries) the most widely accepted rationale for selective reproduction. The link between selective reproduction and health is strongest (though still contingent) when we look at law and policy (and here my focus will be almost entirely on the UK). Two areas in particular stand out: the law on abortion, and the regulation of preimplantation genetic diagnosis (PGD).

Abortion

The Abortion Act 1967 allows for termination to be lawful where one of a number of conditions is met. One of these grounds, contained in section 1(1)(d), is that abortion may be authorized by two doctors who agree that there is a substantial risk that if the child were born it would be 'seriously handicapped'. Since 1990, there have been no time limits for terminations performed on this ground, a policy criticized both by 'pro-life' moral conservatives and by many activists and scholars from a 'disability rights' perspective (Sheldon and Wilkinson, 2001). Section 1(1)(d) of the Abortion Act thus enshrines in legislation the health rationale for selective reproduction (in this case, selective termination) by giving a 'privileged' status to abortions which are performed in order to avoid the birth of a child with a disability or disorder (a 'serious handicap').

The claim that this legislation is based upon the health rationale for selective reproduction does however require a couple of qualifications.

First, someone might object that the rationale for section 1(1)(d) is not obviously health (or not obviously *just* health). It may, for example, be concern for the welfare of prospective parents, or about the costs of health and social care. This may well be true and, in an earlier paper, Sally Sheldon and I explored some of the different possible justifications and motivations for this piece of legislation (Sheldon and Wilkinson, 2001). That said – even if the *fundamental* justification for section 1(1)(d) is saving the National Health Service money, or concern for the welfare of the prospective parents – health, or rather disease-avoidance, is nevertheless the intended means of delivering these more fundamental goods.

The second qualification is that some people, especially (though not exclusively) adherents of the 'social model' of disability, may want to say that the rationale for section 1(1)(d) cannot be health (or cannot *just* be health), because many of the characteristics selected against are not states of unhealth, but rather characteristics which are intrinsically neutral in health terms, but which cause people to suffer disadvantage and discrimination.[2]

We can distinguish three different critiques here.

The first, what we might term *social modelism*, says that none of the so-called 'serious handicaps' cited as grounds for abortion should be regarded as disorders; rather, they are all simply bases for social discrimination. On this view, being 'selected out' (aborted) for having a 'serious handicap' is morally exactly like being 'selected out' for being black, female or left-handed. This position seems implausible to me because at

---

[2] For exposition and critique of such views see, for example: Harris (2000), Oliver (1990; 1995), Shakespeare (2006) and Terzi (2004).

least some of the conditions labelled 'serious handicap' do involve serious physical impairment, including pain and/or premature death. For example, the *Abortion Statistics for England and Wales: 2006* (Department of Health, 2007a) tell us that section 1(1)(d) was used to justify 166 terminations for anencephaly (all before 24 weeks) and 44 for hydrocephalus (of which 10 were after 24 weeks). And, even if one accepts (as we probably should) that people with these conditions suffer from social discrimination, it is hard to deny that they are states of unhealth, given their very obvious effects on length and quality of life (effects that would, crucially, exist *even without* social discrimination).

The second critique concedes that some of the 'serious handicaps' are disorders but claims that, in practice, the line is drawn in the wrong place and that some things are misclassified as diseases. Claims of this kind received considerable attention when, in 2002, it was reported that a 'late' termination had taken place on the grounds that the aborted foetus had a cleft lip and cleft palate. Joanna Jepson, at the time studying to become an Anglican clergywoman, complained to the police about the case (which came to light in the official abortion statistics). Jepson is reported to have said:

> This is eugenics . . . I am not prepared to sit back and let it happen. I want people to know that this is the way society is going, and we need to do something about it.
>
> (Rogers, 2002: 13)

One issue was whether cleft palate is a health problem or whether it is merely a cosmetic state. Jepson, writing in the *Sunday Telegraph*, comments:

> It is as though such a child – though the cleft palate condition is trivial and easily corrected by surgery – somehow represents a threat to our society, increasingly obsessed as it is by a harsh, unattainable notion of cosmetic perfection.
>
> (Jepson, 2003)

Another example raising similar issues is Down's syndrome. This is a relatively common reason for abortion under section 1(1)(d), with 436 such terminations taking place in 2006 in England and Wales (but just 12 after 24 weeks) (Department of Health, 2007a). As with cleft palate, though, some people want to argue that Down's syndrome is more of a *difference* than a disease and that, as such, it does not justify abortion under section 1(1)(d).

Assessing the health status of cleft palate and of Down's syndrome is not the purpose of this chapter and there is not space here to consider the arguments on both sides (including the various different accounts of disability and disease that are in play). I simply note for the time being that both cleft palate and Down's syndrome do often involve features that we generally associate with disease, most conspicuously loss of mental and/or physical functioning. Also, as Rev Jepson herself concedes in the above quotation, cleft palate can be 'easily *corrected* by surgery' which suggests that it is a defect standing in need of a cure.

Third, and finally, it might be argued that although most of the so-called 'serious handicaps' used to justify abortion really are disorders, some of them (and, again, cleft palate and Down's syndrome will be leading examples) are not *sufficiently serious* to justify abortion. This view does not challenge the disease-status of these 'handicaps' but rather questions whether their impacts on (among other things) quality of life are sufficient to merit termination. I mention this view just for analytic completeness and will not attempt to assess it here. It is a view that will depend, for each condition, on the facts of the case (for example, to what extent, if any, does Down's syndrome reduce quality of life?).

Preimplantation genetic diagnosis (PGD)

Turning now to the regulation of preimplantation genetic diagnosis, the Human Fertilisation and Embryology Authority's (HFEA's) *Code of Practice* says:

> It is expected that PGD will be available only where there is a significant risk of a serious genetic condition being present in the embryo.
>
> (HFEA, 2003)

Hence, the view that the proper purpose of PGD (and selective reproduction generally) is to avoid genetic disorders is not merely part of established ethics and practice but is (in the UK at least) enforced by the regulator.

Interestingly, this view prevails (and is perhaps even slightly strengthened) in the Human Tissue and Embryos (Draft) Bill which, at the time of writing (2007), is being debated and scrutinized by the UK Parliament. The present version of the Bill would, if enacted, allow embryo testing to be licensed by the HFEA's successor-body only for specific purposes laid down in the draft legislation (Department of Health, 2007b: Schedule 2, 3, 1ZA(1)). In general terms, these are:

> to ascertain how likely a particular embryo is to 'result in a live birth' (and to enable the selection of embryos on these grounds);

> to enable the creation of a 'saviour sibling', in cases where the existing child (the one in need of salvation) 'suffers from a life-threatening medical condition which could be treated by umbilical core stem cells';

> where 'uncertainty has arisen', to test the embryo to find out whose gametes it came from;

> to test for 'gene, chromosome, or mitochondrion abnormality' *or* to sex select for the purposes of avoiding sex-linked genetic disorders.

So, with just one exception (testing to ascertain who the prospective parents are), all of the grounds for using PGD are health-oriented. PGD must aim either to increase the chances of a live birth (choosing a 'healthy embryo'), or at ensuring that the child born is free from genetic disorders, or at improving the health of an existing sibling.

Selective reproduction and public health

So, while selective reproduction is not *necessarily* a health-oriented activity, it is in practice often closely tied to health: in particular, to disease-avoidance. Indeed, when it comes to reproductive technologies like preimplantation genetic diagnosis, striving to create a healthy baby is (and is likely to remain) pretty much the *only* permitted kind of selection (with the small exceptions noted above). Selective reproduction then is closely associated with health, but is this *public* health? As with the link between selective reproduction and health, the answer here is that, while there is no necessary connection between selective reproduction and public health, there is a strong contingent connection and, in particular, many of the policy and regulatory issues raised by selective reproduction are public health issues.

My reasons for thinking this are based in part on Verweij and Dawson's (2007) useful discussion of defining public health. They draw our attention to two senses of 'public' in 'public health'. The first is *the health of the public*:

> . . . definitions and concepts of public health . . . almost all pick out interventions that aim at protecting and promoting the health of the public. Talking about the 'health of the public' obviously involves the health of more than one person (or even a few persons). Public health concerns the health of populations, or at least larger groups of persons.
>
> (Verweij and Dawson, 2007: 22)

Trying to improve 'the health of the public', as opposed to merely the health of individuals, has two distinctive features. First, as Verweij and Dawson put it:

> Public health interventions are expected to make a difference on a population level, and this seems to imply that they should affect the health of many.
>
> (2007: 22)

So there is a *quantitative threshold* for what counts as a *public* health intervention. Merely treating half a dozen patients in my own clinic will not normally be a public health intervention; although, of course, it could be if, for example, they were carriers of a highly infectious disease, or if these treatments were part of a wider systematic treatment *programme*. Public health actions then must impact substantially on the overall health status of a population: typically (though not necessarily) in ways that would show up in population-based statistical data (for example, about the prevalence of certain diseases). Verweij and Dawson also explore various complications concerning, among other things, what counts as a population, but I shall leave these to one side for the present.

The second relevant distinctive feature of public health actions is that they need not benefit identifiable individuals:

> It might be unclear, even with hindsight, which persons *in fact* benefited from the intervention. This is one of the salient dimensions of prevention: effective primary prevention results in things that do *not* happen (e.g. the onset of disease in persons). For example, as a result of an effective Hepatitis B vaccination programme fewer people will get Hepatitis, yet the 'persons' that benefit are not identifiable, and success exists only in a statistical sense . . .
>
> (Verweij and Dawson, 2007: 22)

Given Verweij and Dawson's remarks, it seems that the relationship between selective reproduction and public health is as follows.

Many individual decisions made by prospective parents (to go through PGD, or to have an abortion, for example) have nothing much to do with public health (even where the motivation is the desire to avoid the creation of a child with a disease or disability); and much the same can be said of the actions of individual clinicians. This is chiefly because such decisions, considered in isolation, do not meet the quantitative threshold for public health: essentially, they only affect (and are only meant to affect) one or a very small number of persons.

When however we move to the policy level then selective reproduction can, and often does, have a public health dimension. A fairly clear example of this is policies on prenatal testing and abortion. ('Policy' here could cover law, National Health Service policy, or professional practice.) Imagine, for example, that a government encourages all pregnant women to have their foetuses tested for *Condition X*, provides these tests for free, informs the pregnant women that *Condition X* is hideous (both for those with it and their carers), and ensures that abortion is both lawful and readily accessible (at least where the resultant child would have *Condition X*). This is a clear case of public health policy (although it may have non-health aims as well, such as ones to do with the autonomy of women).

Why is it a clear case of public health policy? First, because there is an obvious population health end in sight: reducing the prevalence of *Condition X*. Second, the policy would, I imagine, be above the quantitative threshold for public health interventions, given that all pregnant women are encouraged to have the test (and so the policy *applies to* them even if they decline the test, and even if the test result is negative). Finally, in common with many paradigm public health interventions, many of the benefits of the policy cannot be attached to determinate individuals in a straightforward way. Obviously, *some* of the benefits here can be attached to individuals. For instance, the testing programme will generate cases in which women abort foetuses with *Condition X* and go on to have other healthy children instead (or choose to remain childless). Given the dreadfulness of *Condition X*, probably many such women will live happier and healthier lives than they would have lived if they had been the mothers of children with *Condition X*. However, even for these women, there will be residual doubts about which ones have truly benefited, because we will not know for sure how well they would have coped with a *Condition X* child. The other benefits of reducing the prevalence of *Condition X* will be much harder to attach to any determinate individual. As Verweij and Dawson point out this is to a certain extent just a general feature of preventative measures. But one additional consideration here is that the policy is *identity-affecting*. Thus, if it is successful, many parents will in effect choose to 'replace' a (possible future) child without *Condition X* for one that would have had *Condition X*; in other words they will choose to abort the *Condition X* foetus and to have a different healthy child later. Who benefits from this? I have already mentioned possible third-party benefits to the parents and there may also (depending on how the health economics works out) be some savings for public service budgets. But what about direct benefits? The candidate direct beneficiaries seem to be the abovementioned 'substitute' children, those who would not exist were it not for the government's *Condition X* policy. If these children really are beneficiaries of the policy then the benefit involved is what I earlier termed *existential*. For these children have not been cured of, nor even prevented from having, *Condition X*. Rather, they have been created instead of someone else who would have had *Condition X*. So the benefit of which they are recipients (if any) is *existing-rather-than-not-existing*, not being free from *Condition X*. This of course raises various philosophical conundrums, ones that I will not get into here. For the present, it will suffice to say that it is difficult to assign some of the benefits of the policy to determinate individuals in a straightforward way, and that this is a typical characteristic of public health measures.

Policy concerning PGD can also be part of public health policy. For instance, the government could encourage couples at risk of having a *Condition X* child (or indeed *all* couples) to conceive using IVF and PGD. And, possible ethical differences notwithstanding, from a public health point of view, this would have essentially the same features as avoiding *Condition X* through prenatal testing and selective termination. In practice, PGD probably does not yet meet the quantitative threshold for being a *public* health measure since, as recently as 2004, there were only around 200 treatments per year in the UK (HFEA, 2005: 7). We can certainly envisage it and similar selection practices becoming more prevalent and eventually being viable public health interventions. As Wikler and Brock put it:

New reproductive methods present some choice among potential offspring, and more choices lie just over the horizon.

(2007: 87)

Eugenics

> . . . in activist literature, genetics becomes a coherent and consistent plot to eliminate disabled people.
>
> (Shakespeare, 2006: 85–6)

In their *direct* form, *eugenics arguments* say that using PGD (for example) to select out disability and/or disease is an instance of eugenics and so since (it is supposed) eugenics is wrong then so is this use of PGD. There are also several *indirect* eugenics arguments. One of these is the claim that, although using PGD may not itself be eugenic, it is likely to lead down the proverbial slippery slope to other practices that are. For reasons of space and focus, I shall concentrate for the present on a direct version of the eugenics argument, one which takes the following form.

1. Using PGD (and/or other selection techniques) to select out disability and/or disease is a case of eugenics.
2. Eugenics is morally wrong.
3. *Therefore*: using PGD (and similar techniques) to select out disability and/or disease is morally wrong.

This argument is logically valid: that is, (1) and (2) do jointly entail (3). However, questions can be raised about both of the premises: specifically, is PGD an instance of eugenics and is eugenics, in any case, wrong? Not surprisingly, both of these questions depend on what we *mean* by the word 'eugenics' and this is a contested issue with different sides in the debate using the term rather differently. I have dealt with some of the definitional complexities relating to 'eugenics' in more detail elsewhere (Wilkinson, 2007; Wilkinson, 2010). So for the present I shall offer a *working* definition before proceeding to tackle the substantive questions of whether premises (1) and (2) above are plausible.

The term 'eugenics' dates back to 1883, when it was coined by Francis Galton (Coutts and McCarrick, 1995: 163; *Oxford English Dictionary*). Galton defines 'eugenics' as the study of 'the conditions under which men of a high type are produced' and as 'the science which deals with all influences that improve the inborn qualities of a race' (*Oxford English Dictionary*; Galton, 1909: 35). Other definitions include those found in the *Oxford English Dictionary*, which defines 'eugenic' as 'pertaining or adapted to the production of fine offspring, *esp.* in the human race', and in the *Routledge Encyclopaedia of Philosophy*, which defines 'eugenics' as 'the attempt to improve the human gene pool' (Chadwick, 1998). This last definition is particularly relevant, since our primary concern is genetics and reproductive technologies, and it will therefore be adopted as my provisional definition. However, as I have stated, this is only a *working* definition and much more can be said about what eugenics is and about the different possible kinds of eugenics.

Eugenics is then an *attempt* to improve the human gene pool and thus has intention built into its definition (although we may also allow that *systems* are eugenic insofar as there are systemic aims that cannot readily be attached to individuals). However, as with public health programmes, the aims of the whole system (or the intentions of those running the system) may be quite different from those of individual actors. Thus, I suspect that very few individual parents (or prospective parents) could fairly be labelled 'eugenicist' even when they opt to terminate or 'select out' a (possible future) child with a genetic disorder. This is because such parents will usually have little interest in improving the gene pool as a whole. Rather their concern is with making sure that their (future) child has less pain and suffering in its life, or perhaps with their own inability to cope with looking after a severely disabled child. These prospective parents are not eugenicists; at most, they are colluding with or tolerating eugenics. Eugenics may nonetheless be a property of the complete system (of prenatal testing and termination) provided that improving the gene pool is one of the system's aims, or is intended by whoever designs or runs the system. Hence, it certainly makes sense to suggest, as some commentators have done, that eugenics may be an *emergent* property of contemporary prenatal screening and testing practices, even if individual doctors and patients at the 'coal face' do not have a eugenic intent. (Shakespeare, 1998: 667; Hampton, 2005: 553). (I do not claim that such commentators are correct – merely that their positions are coherent. Whether they are correct about any given system would be mainly an empirical matter.)

Authoritarian eugenics

It is also worth making a distinction, within eugenics, between what have been termed 'authoritarian' and 'laissez-faire' eugenics. This is best seen as a continuum, with some eugenic policies and practices being more or less authoritarian than others. At the authoritarian end of the range sit Nazi eugenics, compulsory sterilization programmes and the like. These are to be contrasted with what Nozick terms the 'genetic supermarket', in which children are produced according to 'the individual specifications (within certain moral limits) of prospective parents': a social setup which, for Nozick (1974: 315), 'has the great virtue that it involves no centralized decision fixing the future of human type(s)'.

Laissez-faire eugenics occurs when private individuals practice eugenics with no, or minimal, state involvement. Authoritarian eugenics is a little harder to characterize. Its main defining feature is that prospective parents are *compelled* to behave eugenically and are *forced* to reproduce, or to refrain from reproducing, or to reproduce in a particular way: normally, though not necessarily, by the state. A practice is authoritarian eugenics then only if *either* (1) prospective reproducers are physically forced to reproduce, or prevented from reproducing, in certain ways (for example, a woman might be kidnapped and forcibly inseminated or sterilized, or a pregnant woman might be subjected to prenatal testing and selective termination without her consent) *or* (2) prospective reproducers are allowed to decide for themselves whether or not to reproduce in particular ways, but their decisions are somehow *involuntary* (resulting, for example, from coercion or manipulation).

Whether a particular practice or policy falls into category (2) will often be a controversial and difficult question. One (putative) example of this relates to the levels of service offered to people with disabilities and their carers and an argument can be reconstructed along the following lines. Prospective parents (through prenatal testing and, to a lesser extent, PGD) are offered the choice of whether to have a disabled child or not. This decision could *in principle* be voluntary. However, prospective parents are on the receiving end of a systemic form of coercion. It works like this. The state (or society generally) ought to provide a certain level of support to people with disabilities and their carers. However, it in fact provides much less support than this and this position is unlikely to change in the foreseeable future. The state is then in effect coercing people into refraining from having children with disabilities by threatening them with poverty and social disadvantage – poverty and disadvantage that it has a moral responsibility to ameliorate, and for which it is therefore at least partly responsible. I have a great deal of sympathy with this *form* of argument, although whether it in fact applies to our present society is an open question that depends on two questions that I am unable to answer here. First, there is the thorny political question of what precisely the state owes its disabled citizens and their carers. Second, there is the equally tricky empirical question of whether this posited standard of care (whatever that is) is in fact met.

Another possible case of subtly authoritarian eugenics concerns the way in which prenatal tests are offered and presented to pregnant women. As Modra notes:

> Numerous commentators point to the conflict between the . . . system's commitment to promoting autonomous PNGD [prenatal genetic diagnosis] choices on the one hand, and its commitment to the prevention of genetic disability on the other. *They suggest that this leads to a covert yet decisive pressure on women to terminate affected pregnancies.*
>
> (2006: 259)

Thus if pregnant women offered PNGD were routinely *pressured* (perhaps subtly and/or unintentionally) into accepting the test and into going for a termination (if faced with an adverse result) then the prenatal testing system, considered as a whole, may be a sort of authoritarian eugenics (provided that the prevention of genetic disabilities and disorders is one of its aims). I should however reiterate that whether a practice is 'authoritarian' is a question of degree, and also note that this would be a relatively 'mild' form of authoritarianism compared to (for example) the compulsory sterilization of adults with disabilities. Nonetheless, other things being equal, it would be better if the fully voluntary (and sufficiently informed) consent of pregnant women could be obtained for prenatal testing and termination, and if similar outcomes could be achieved without anyone being pressured.

The significance of the preceding discussion for the eugenics argument is that many concerns about eugenics are really about *authoritarian* eugenics and so it is important to highlight the fact that eugenics is not *necessarily* authoritarian or coercive. As Caplan *et al.* tell us, while it is admittedly:

> . . . morally objectionable for governments or institutions or any third party to compel or coerce anyone's reproductive behavior . . . the goals of obtaining perfection, avoiding disease, or pursuing health with respect to individuals *need not involve coercion or force.*
>
> (1999: 1284, my emphasis)

Thus, in this respect at least, eugenics may be morally unproblematic. So when it comes to an assessment of eugenics' moral status we must be careful not to assume that it will be authoritarian. For, as Caplan *et al.* note, it is perfectly possible to support broadly eugenic aims while eschewing coercion and authoritarianism – just as one might support reducing the prevalence of obesity without thinking (for example) that the state has a right to micromanage people's eating or exercise behaviours.

The moral standing of eugenics

Ought we to *define* 'eugenics' such that being eugenic is always a wrong-making, or morally bad, property of actions or policies? Is 'eugenics' what Bernard Williams (1985: 129) terms a *thick moral concept* – one 'such as treachery and promise and brutality and courage, which seem to express a union of fact and value'.

The main reason for thinking of 'eugenics' as a negative moral term is that most people who use it in contemporary debates do so to express condemnation, and it is rare for people who support embryo selection to describe it as 'eugenic'. While, on the other side, those with 'pro-choice' or 'pro-biotechnology' views generally avoid the word. So nearly everyone agrees that 'eugenics' is hugely emotive and negative. As Raanon Gillon (1998: 219) puts it, 'Eugenics is widely regarded as a dirty word.' But while, for some, this is a reason to avoid it; for others, this makes the term 'eugenics' a good way of getting their message across. A useful comparator here is the expression 'unborn child'. Many people with 'pro-life' views use this to draw attention to (alleged) similarities between foetuses and children (or indeed to express the view that foetuses *are* children); while those with 'pro-choice' views generally avoid this expression since they have the opposite aims and views. The same goes for 'eugenics'. Those hostile to embryo selection often use 'eugenics' to draw attention to (alleged) similarities between practices such as PGD and historical atrocities associated with eugenics movements of the past; while those who support PGD generally avoid the word 'eugenics' in order to avoid drawing attention to these (alleged) similarities.

One implication of all this is that defining 'eugenics' is itself complex and controversial. In particular, the working definition suggested above was largely descriptive, 'the attempt to improve the human gene pool', so how can this be squared with the view that 'eugenics' is a negative moral term?

One option is to treat 'eugenics' as a moral term by defining it as '*wrongfully* attempting to improve the human gene pool'; on this view, permissible attempts to 'improve the gene pool' do not count as eugenic. Alternatively, we could insist that 'eugenics' be descriptively defined and therefore that there is at least a theoretical distinction, within eugenics, between permissible and wrongful eugenics. In this latter view, we could still take account of the point made earlier about linguistic politics, about 'eugenics' being a 'dirty word', and there still being good reasons not to *use* it except in cases of wrongful eugenics, but at least in principle permissible eugenics would be a possibility.

I have argued elsewhere that this definitional issue cannot be resolved prior to an assessment of the substantive moral arguments against eugenics (descriptively defined) (Wilkinson, 2008). And this is my next task: to look at one particular attempt to show that 'improving the human gene pool' is morally problematic. If this is successful then we will have some reason to view eugenics with distrust and there may also be reason to build wrongness into the meaning of the word 'eugenics'.

Is the very idea of 'genetic improvement' flawed?

As has been noted, some programmes that aim to improve the 'gene pool' are morally wrong because they use unacceptably authoritarian *means*. These however will be disregarded from henceforth and I shall focus now on whether there is something wrong with the *end* of genetic improvement.

Obviously, some things that are touted as genetic improvements are not really improvements. If someone suggested using selective reproduction to increase the incidence of tall blonds, we should be sceptical about whether this would be an improvement. Similarly, the history of eugenics is full of cases in which (for example) behavioural, cultural and racial differences are wrongly seen as defects (Kevles, 1999; Baker, 2002; Barnett, 2004). So we should approach 'improvement' claims with caution. However, it does not follow from the fact that many people have misused the idea of genetic improvement that it is necessarily flawed. We must though be clear in each case what kind of improvement we are talking about and demand *reasons why* the thing in question is not merely a change but an improvement, a change *for the better*.

The most obvious type of genetic improvement that we can make sense of, and one that is especially relevant to our present concern with public health, is health improvement: using selective reproduction to reduce the prevalence of disease and impairment in future populations. On the face of it, this looks like a kind of genetic improvement since most of us would agree that, other things being equal, a less diseased and disabled future population is preferable to a more diseased and disabled one – because of the positive effects that good health generally has on welfare.

So is reducing the prevalence of genetic disease and impairment through selective reproduction a genuine instance of improving the 'gene pool'? (Gillott, 2001; Human Genetics Alert Newsletter, 2001; Savalescu, 2001: 413; Holland, 2003: 402). It seems that it is, on account of the strong connection that exists between disease and disability and reduced welfare. However, this view is challenged by what I have elsewhere termed the Equal Value Principle (Wilkinson, 2006: 26–51).

Shortly after its creation in 2000, the Disability Rights Commission (DRC, n.d.) was asked by LIFE for its view on section 1(1)(d) of the Abortion Act 1967 (as amended by the Human Fertilisation and Embryology Act 1990) which, as we saw earlier, permits (without any time limit) termination on the ground that 'there is a substantial risk that if the child were born it would suffer from such physical or mental abnormalities as to be seriously handicapped'. In response, the DRC said that while 'Section 1(1)(d) is not inconsistent with the Disability Discrimination Act' it is nonetheless:

> . . . offensive to many people; it reinforces negative stereotypes of disability; and there is substantial support for the view that to permit terminations at any point during a pregnancy on the ground of risk of disability, while time limits apply to other grounds set out in the Abortion Act, *is incompatible with valuing disability and non-disability equally.*
>
> (DRC, n.d., my emphasis)[3]

In the same statement, the DRC informs us that:

> Throughout its programme of work on ethical issues, the DRC will be guided by two principles: *valuing disability and non-disability equally*, and the right of individuals to make informed, autonomous choices.
>
> (DRC, n.d., my emphasis)

It is the first of these principles, the Equal Value Principle, that I shall focus on here. For it seems as if this principle could underpin an ethical argument against any reproductive practice that selects against disability. After all, if disability and non-disability were valued equally then why would anyone have reason to select the latter and deselect the former? Furthermore, if disability and non-disability were valued equally then we could not regard reducing the prevalence of genetically-based disability and impairment as an *improvement*, since improvement means moving from something less valuable to something more valuable. It may be argued then that using PGD (and similar techniques) to select out disability is wrong because it is not consistent with the Equal Value Principle.

Two questions are raised by the Equal Value Principle. First, does 'screening out' disability necessarily involve failing to value disability and non-disability equally? And second, how plausible is the Equal Value Principle itself?

---

[3] For a more detailed discussion of this issue see Sheldon and Wilkinson (2001).

Taking the first question first, one view is that clinicians who offer embryo testing and selective implantation to prospective parents are not themselves making value judgements about disability. Rather, they are offering *choice* to the parents. So, as far as the ethics of clinical practice is concerned (as opposed to the personal morality of the prospective parents) the doctors have not acted badly because they are merely facilitating choice.

This *could* be true in *some* possible cases. However, there are reasons to doubt whether this degree of neutrality exists in many actual cases, and whether the general policy context within which clinical practice takes place can support such a neutral stance. One such reason is that clinicians offering specific preimplantation genetic tests usually know what the prospective parents' preferences and values are and, more often than not, are only carrying out the tests because they know that the parents wish to select against a particular genetic disorder. This does not of course *entail* that the clinicians involved do not value disability and non-disability equally. Nonetheless, it does at least raise the question of whether a clinician who subscribes to the Equal Value Principle should really support and collaborate with parents' attempts to avoid disability or disease.

Another more policy-oriented reason is that, as we have seen, the HFEA only licenses PGD for certain purposes. In nearly all cases, the aim of these licensed procedures is to prevent the birth of a child with a disease or disability and, as we have already seen, the HFEA's *Code of Practice* tells us that 'it is expected that PGD will be available only where there is a significant risk of a serious genetic condition being present in the embryo' (HFEA, 2003: 24. s. 14.22). (One notable exception to this is PGD with tissue typing where the aim, or one of the aims, is to save an existing child's life [HFEA, 2004].) It cannot therefore be argued convincingly that the aim of the overall system of PGD is *merely choice*, because the system is so clearly oriented towards disease-avoidance and disability-avoidance (which presumably stem from valuing non-disability more highly than disability, and health more highly than disease). So, rightly or wrongly, the general policy context in which selective reproduction occurs is very much shaped by the medical goals of disease-avoidance and disability-avoidance and it is hard to see why someone would have such goals unless she valued non-disability and the absence of disease more highly than disability and disease.

Turning now to the second question, how plausible is the Equal Value Principle? It seems to me that the principle is not as compelling as the DRC has suggested, mainly because its proponents neglect an important distinction between valuing disability and non-disability equally, and valuing disabled and non-disabled *people* equally. Clearly, we should value disabled and non-disabled *people* equally and give them equal respect and rights as human beings, but it does not follow from this that we must value disability and non-disability equally.

This is clearest when the disability in question involves a straightforward physical injury. Take, for example, people with injured and permanently non-functional legs. Obviously, we should value people with and people without functioning legs equally and grant them equal respect; indeed, we should go further and grant people without functioning legs additional resources to compensate for their reduced mobility, and (where practicable) modify built environments to facilitate access. None of this however requires us to value functioning and non-functioning legs equally. On the contrary, most of us have a strong and rational preference for functioning legs. So it is tempting to say that, while people with and people without disabilities should be treated as equals in terms of their moral status, given a choice, non-disability is usually preferable to disability.

This point is bolstered by another argument against the Equal Value Principle, which claims that the principle has absurd, or at least unpalatable, consequences. For commitment to this principle entails that we should not seek to cure people when they acquire disabilities, and certainly should not use public resources to do so, because this would suggest that disability is less valuable than non-disability. Indeed, if we do not value non-disability more highly than disability then (with the exception of non-curative interventions such as pain relief) it is hard to see what rationale there could be for having a medical profession and for making people pay taxes to fund the National Health Service (Edwards, 2004). So the Equal Value Principle appears to have unacceptable implications and should be rejected.

So is the very idea of improving the 'gene pool' fundamentally flawed? It seems to me that, with some qualifications, the answer is *no*. There have of course been many versions of 'eugenics' that have incorporated dangerously flawed ideological and pseudo-scientific beliefs, such as Nazi racial 'science'. However, there is no need to assume that *all* attempts to improve the 'gene pool' will be similarly flawed, and we can imagine versions of 'gene pool' improvement, such as the attempt to create healthier future populations, that would and should attract very widespread support. So perhaps (for example) improving the 'gene pool' in ways that improve future public health would be morally acceptable (and even desirable). Against this, some people (notably proponents of the Equal Value Principle) have argued that even the attempt to improve population genetic health is unethical because it is premised on valuing non-disability more highly than disability. However, it seems to me that this argument (along with the Equal Value Principle itself) is unsound and should be rejected. There is nothing wrong with assigning a negative value to the functional impairment aspects of disability and disease and this negative valuation of impairment does not entail and need not be accompanied by any negative valuation of the *person* with the impairment.

Conclusion

Given recent developments in reproductive and genetic technologies, it is likely that intervening before birth or before embryo-implantation to alter the composition of future populations, will become an effective strategy for improving public health. The ethics of selective reproduction is thus a part of public health ethics, insofar as selection is practised, promoted or regulated with a view to achieving public health goals. In the first part of this chapter, I suggested that selective reproduction is already being treated in this way, citing abortion law and the regulation of preimplantation genetic diagnosis as leading examples.

One objection to using selective reproduction as a means of achieving better public health is that doing so is eugenic. How should we respond to such claims? The view that I have argued for here (and at greater length elsewhere) is that we should concede, *though with some important caveats*, that public health-oriented selective reproduction may be eugenic, although perhaps the *term* 'eugenics' is best avoided (especially outside academic work) because of its extremely negative connotations and historical associations (Wilkinson, 2008; 2010).

So what are these important caveats? First, it must be noted that the term 'eugenics' is being used here non-morally to mean 'improving the gene pool'; and while clearly there is a sense in which even this definition is evaluative (for we are talking about *improving* genetic health, not merely changing it) the evaluation appealed to is not a moral one as such, but one concerning either physiological functionality or welfare, or both. Second, it has to be conceded that *certain sorts of* eugenics are generally wrong. In particular, *authoritarian* eugenics is usually objectionable because of the harms and violation of autonomy that it entails. Similarly, eugenics (*pseudo*-eugenics perhaps) that passes off mere differences (such as real or perceived racial differences) as defects and then attempts to eliminate them is morally objectionable. Having made these qualifications then, we can assert that *some* forms of eugenics may be acceptable, particularly those that genuinely aim at public health and which are robustly *non*-authoritarian, requiring the valid consent of any individuals concerned (especially prospective parents). Hence, using selective reproduction to achieve public health goals may (under certain circumstances) be permissible *even if* this is eugenic.

Finally, though, I should add that there are of course many other arguments against selective reproduction that I have not had chance to consider here. Hence, insofar as this is not a comprehensive survey of *all possible* arguments against using selective reproduction as a public health policy instrument, any conclusions must remain somewhat provisional.[4]

References

Baker, B. (2002) The hunt for disability: the new eugenics and the normalization of school children. *Teachers College Record*, **104**(4): 663–703.

Barnett, R. (2004) Keywords in the history of medicine: eugenics. *The Lancet*, **363**: 1742.

Caplan, A., McGee, G. and Magnus, D. (1999) What is immoral about eugenics? *British Medical Journal*, **319**: 1284.

Chadwick, R. (1998) Genetics and ethics. In *Routledge Encyclopaedia of Philosophy*, ed. E. Craig. London: Routledge.

Coutts, M. and McCarrick, P. (1995) Eugenics. *Kennedy Institute of Ethics Journal*, **5**(2): 163–78.

Department of Health (2007a) *Abortion Statistics for England and Wales: 2006*. London: Department of Health. Available at: http://www.dh.gov.uk/en/ Publicationsandstatistics/Publications/ PublicationsStatistics/DH_075697 (accessed: 19/7/08).

Department of Health (2007b) *Human Tissues Embryos (Draft) Bill 2007*. London: Department of Health.

Disability Rights Commission (n.d.) *DRC Statement on Section 1(1)(d) of the Abortion Act 1967*. Manchester: DRC.

Edwards, S. (2004) Disability, identity, and the 'expressionist objection'. *Journal of Medical Ethics*, **30**: 418–30.

Galton, F. (1909) *Essays in Eugenics*. Honolulu, HI: University Press of the Pacific.

Gillon, R. (1998) Eugenics, contraception, abortion and ethics. *Journal of Medical Ethics*, **24**(4): 219–20.

Gillott, J. (2001) Screening for disability: a eugenic pursuit? *Journal of Medical Ethics*, **27**(Suppl. II): 21–3.

Hampton, S. J. (2005) Family eugenics. *Disability and Society*, **20**: 553–61.

Harris, J. (2000) Is there a coherent social conception of disability? *Journal of Medical Ethics*, **26**: 95–100.

Holland, S. (2003) Selecting against difference: assisted reproduction, disability, and regulation. *Florida State University Law Review*, **30**(Winter): 401–10.

Human Fertilisation and Embryology Authority (HFEA) (2003) *Code of Practice*, 6th edn. Available at: http://www.hfea.gov.uk (accessed: 19/7/08).

Human Fertilisation and Embryology Authority (HFEA) (2004) HFEA agrees to extend policy on tissue typing. Press release, 21 July. Available at: http://www.hfea.gov.uk (accessed: 19/7/08).

---

[4] Many of these other arguments are reviewed in Wilkinson (2010).

Human Fertilisation and Embryology Authority (HFEA) (2005) *Choices and Boundaries.* Available at: http://www.hfea.gov.uk/docs/Choices_Boundaries.pdf (accessed: 19/7/08).

Human Genetics Alert (2001) Newsletter. Issue 1, December.

Jepson, J. (2003) Herod is not alone in his fear of the helpless. *Sunday Telegraph,* 21 December.

Kevles, D. (1999) Eugenics and human rights. *British Medical Journal,* **319**: 435–8.

MENSA (n.d.) Mensa information. Available at: http://www.mensa.org/index0.php?page=10 (accessed: 19/7/08).

Modra, L. (2006) Prenatal genetic testing kits sold at your local pharmacy: promoting autonomy or promoting confusion? *Bioethics,* **20**: 254–65.

Nozick, R. (1974) *Anarchy, State and Utopia.* Oxford: Blackwell.

Oliver, M. (1990) *The Politics of Disablement.* Basingstoke: Palgrave Macmillan.

Oliver, M. (1995) *Understanding Disability: From Theory to Practice.* Basingstoke: Palgrave Macmillan.

Oxford English Dictionary. Oxford: Oxford University Press.

Parfit, D. (1984) *Reasons and Persons.* Oxford: Oxford University Press.

Rogers, L. (1996) Mensa sperm bank set up to create 'super humans'. *The Times (London),* 11 February: 1.

Rogers, L. (2002) Police to probe late abortion of harelip baby. *Sunday Times (London),* 27 October: 13.

Savalescu, J. (2001) Procreative beneficence: why we should select the best children. *Bioethics,* **15**(5–6): 413–26.

Shakespeare, T. (1998) Choices and rights: eugenics, genetics and disability equality. *Disability and Society,* **13**: 665–81.

Shakespeare, T. (2006) *Disability Rights and Wrongs.* London: Routledge.

Sheldon, S. and Wilkinson, S. (2001) Termination of pregnancy for reason of foetal disability: are there grounds for a special exception in law? *Medical Law Review,* **9**: 85–109.

Terzi, L. (2004) The social model of disability: a philosophical critique. *Journal of Applied Philosophy,* **21**(2): 141–57.

Verweij, M. and Dawson, A. (2007) The meaning of 'public' in 'public health'. In *Ethics, Prevention, and Public Health,* ed. A. Dawson and M. Verweij. Oxford: Oxford University Press, pp. 13–29.

Wikler, D. and Brock, D. W. (2007) Population-level bioethics: mapping a new agenda. In *Ethics, Prevention, and Public Health,* ed. A. Dawson and M. Verweij. Oxford: Oxford University Press, pp. 78–94.

Wilkinson, S. (2006) Eugenics, embryo selection, and the equal value principle. *Clinical Ethics,* **1**: 26–51.

Wilkinson, S. (2007) On the distinction between positive and negative eugenics. In *Arguments and Analysis in Bioethics,* ed. M. Hayry, T. Takala and P. Herissone-Kelly. Amsterdam: Rodopi.

Wilkinson, S. (2008) 'Eugenics talk' and the language of bioethics. *Journal of Medical Ethics,* **34**: 467–71.

Wilkinson, S. (2010) *Choosing Tomorrow's Children: The Ethics of Selective Reproduction.* Oxford: Oxford University Press.

Williams, B. (1985) *Ethics and the Limits of Philosophy.* London: Fontana.

Wrigley, A. (2006) Genetic selection and modal harms. *The Monist,* **89**(4): 505–25.

Chapter

4

Risk and precaution

Stephen John

Introduction

The concepts of risk and precaution are central to public health policy, and therefore to philosophical and ethical reflection on such policy. A wide range of public health activities – such as health and safety legislation, food standards monitoring and the emerging field of public health genomics – are explicitly framed in terms of risk-reduction and risk-management. Furthermore, we can use the concept of 'risk' to understand public health policies that are not normally framed in these terms. For example, draining a malarial swamp can be understood as eliminating health-risks, as can a policy of compulsory vaccination. The control, minimization or elimination of health-risks can, then, be seen as the shared concern of the heterogeneous activities that comprise public health policy.

Normally, we understand the reduction of risk as instrumentally valuable. That is to say, we view it as a tool for ensuring a particular distribution of health-outcomes (or, perhaps, a distribution of opportunities for health). Arguably, we might also view the reduction of risk as directly valuable, because living in an environment where risks of serious physical harm or suffering have been reduced is a constituent of what Amartya Sen (1992) calls our 'capabilities', our 'real freedoms' to achieve valuable functionings. Someone who lives in an environment in which malaria has been eradicated, for example, is not only less likely to suffer ill-health than someone who lives in a malarial environment, but may also be said to enjoy greater 'positive freedom'; the range of activities she may reasonably choose to pursue is greater than the range of activities her counterpart can reasonably choose to pursue.[1] A narrow focus on the health-outcomes that follow risk-reduction can, perhaps, hide from us the more general benefits that follow from creating risk-free environments, pointing towards an important, if little-explored, distinction between the value of prevention and of cure.

Just as we can frame an account of the means and the ends of public health policy in terms of 'risk', we can also pose the challenges of 'public health ethics' in these terms. Examples of such problems include the following. How ought we to choose between public health policies that will have different effects on the overall distribution of health-risks in the population? For example, should we focus on alleviating the plight of the most vulnerable or on minimizing expected overall mortality and morbidity? How ought we to decide when the risks associated with some activity are 'tolerable'? Is there an important

---

[1] See Olsaretti (2005) for a complex argument for these kinds of claims.

Public Health Ethics, ed. Angus Dawson. Published by Cambridge University Press. © Cambridge University Press 2011.

difference between policies that *impose* risks on individuals and policies which merely *fail to reduce* the risks individuals suffer? For example, if we must decide whether or not to allow a drug, with known benefits for many but potential side effects for *ex-ante* unidentifiable others, onto the market, is there a morally significant distinction between not allowing the drug onto the market, leaving some at risk, and allowing the drug onto the market, placing some at risk? Is there a difference between 'voluntary' and 'involuntary' risk? If so, is regulating risky activities performed by consenting adults unacceptably paternalistic?

Unfortunately, developing an ethics of risk is no easy task. In the literature, we find battle-lines drawn between a 'scientific' or 'statistical' account of risk associated with the policy tool of 'risk cost-benefit analysis' (RCBA) – described by Adams (1995) as the 'Royal Society' view of risk – and a 'constructivist' or 'sociological' account of risk, often associated with the 'precautionary principle'.[2] Proponents of the first 'approach' accuse proponents of the second of being un- or anti-scientific; proponents of the second 'approach' accuse proponents of the first of 'technocracy'.[3] Those who combine aspects of both approaches are attacked from all sides. These debates are both heated and theoretically complicated because they involve four issues that cross the empirical/normative boundary: how we ought to define risk; how members of the public actually think about risk; how people ought to think about risk; and how we ought to handle risks in a democratic society.

On the one hand, it seems clear that an ethics of risk is necessary for ethical debate of much public health policy, and may have wider ramifications for 'public health ethics' as a whole. On the other hand, the ferocity and complexity of the debates mentioned above make the task of constructing an ethics of risk – indeed, even understanding what 'risk' is – extremely difficult. In this chapter, I will set out one way in which we might understand these problems, by looking at the arguments of those who promote the 'precautionary principle' as an approach to both risk-assessment and to risk-management. In the first section, I set out the standard view of risk, which the 'precautionary principle' is often claimed to challenge. In the second and third sections, I set out ways in which we might understand a 'precautionary approach' to public health policy, and in the fourth section, I show how these claims relate to the debate between 'technocratic' and 'constructivist' accounts of risk. In the fifth section, I suggest that perhaps the most interesting feature of the precautionary principle is that it leads us to rethink the relationship between ethical norms and scientific testing. It should be stressed that this paper is not intended to provide a substantive account of the ethics of risk for purposes of public health policy. Rather, the aim is to provide the reader with a guide through a complex debate, and, in so doing, to outline some of the key issues for and constraints on any substantive theory of the ethics of risk. In the sixth section, I do, however, show how the arguments sketched in this chapter might help us to construct a new ethics of risk.

---

[2] See, also, Ling and Raven (2006) for a standard account of these disputes. The standard text for a social-constructivist account of risks is Beck (1992). See Douglas and Wildavsky (1980) for an altogether more interesting anthropological approach to these debates, which might seem to suggest that both sides of the dispute can be explained from an anthropological perspective.

[3] See Sunstein (2002) for an example of the first sort of charge, and Jasanoff (1999) for an example of the second. These debates are well summarized in Lewens (2007).

The precautionary principle and RCBA

A precautionary approach to policy is often understood to be opposed to the standard model of risk identification and risk-management, identified with the tools of RCBA.[4] In this section, I shall outline this approach. To understand the concept of 'risk' and the methodology of RCBA, it is useful to consider the model of rational choice theory from which RCBA derives. Imagine that I want to buy a sandwich. I can either go to Shop A next door, which makes awful sandwiches, or to Shop B on the other side of town, which makes delicious sandwiches. These two courses-of-action have different benefits associated with them – an awful sandwich or a delicious sandwich – and they have different costs associated with them, a short walk or a long walk. The alternative courses-of-action might also be associated with different probabilities of suffering harm: going to Shop B involves crossing a busy road, thereby running a small probability of serious injury, whereas popping next door does not. The term 'risk', as used in its 'Royal Society' sense, is typically used to denote such possibilities of suffering harm: we say that there is a risk associated with going to the far-off shop, and no risk (or comparatively low) risk associated with popping next door.[5]

Sometimes we say that we would not be willing to run a risk of serious harm for any potential benefit. However, our behaviour often runs contrary to this platitude. I, for one, regularly run all sorts of risks of serious harm for the sake of minor benefits, although I would not run much higher risks of harm for the same benefits. I regularly run a small risk of being run over in return for a tasty sandwich, but would not run a much higher risk of harm for the same sandwich. So doing does not seem irrational. Indeed, not to do so would be to lead to a dreadfully impoverished life. One way in which to model these kinds of everyday decisions is to say that I act (or ought to act) in accordance with the goal of maximizing my overall expected utility. For example, we can model my decision thus:

> Expected utility of going to Shop B = (value of tasty sandwich) plus (negative value of walking so far) plus (probability of being hit by a car multiplied by negative value of being hit by a car).

The greater the probability of serious injury attached to my walk to the shop, the lower my expected utility, and the more attractive the option of popping next door instead (where the expected utility of doing so is simply value of awful sandwich minus cost of walking a short distance).[6]

RCBA applies a version of this model at the social level as a guide to policy. We choose between different policies by asking what the certain costs and benefits and risks associated with each of those policies are. Our choice, then, is guided by asking which action has the best expected outcomes. Of course, the use of RCBA in policy-making is not straightforward. However, very roughly, the idea is simple: first, we construct a single scale along

---

[4] For useful introductions to RCBA see Shrader-Frechette (1980) and Sunstein (2002). Note that, strictly, there are differences between the claims made by proponents of RCBA, by proponents of cost benefit analysis and by proponents of risk-trade-off-analysis. For our purposes, however, these differences are relatively unimportant.

[5] Although we should note that the term 'risk' can be used in other ways, leading to some confusion. For a useful overview, see Hansson (2007).

[6] This is a very simplified model of the kind of theory proposed by such writers as Luce and Raiffa (1958). For a useful history of the relevant arguments (which makes clear the link between developments in the theory of risk and the collection of epidemiological statistics) see Hacking (1975) and Hacking (1990).

which we can compare all possible benefits and costs of potential outcomes of action (normally, a monetary scale is used for these purposes). We can then compare different policies by comparing the expected costs and benefits of those actions (by multiplying the probability of those outcomes by their magnitude). It is important to recognize here that many people find the idea of constructing a single scale along which we might compare all outcomes of action to be morally suspect. I will return to these issues below. However, before going further, it is important to note that treating disparate outcomes as commensurable seems to be consistent with everyday life: someone who regularly refused to trade-off risks of death against even such minor pleasures as a tasty sandwich would seem very strange.

I have identified two substantive aspects of RCBA. First, there is a claim about how we ought to reason: we ought to aim to maximize our expected utility. Second, a claim that we can place all costs, benefits and risks on a unitary scale, such that we can rank risks from most to least serious by multiplying the extent of harm associated with some event by the probability of that event. This way of thinking about policy-making is extremely powerful as a tool for thinking about public health policy, most notably health-and-safety policy. After all, we do think that there are limits on which public health policies we ought to pursue; even if obtainable, 'safety at any cost' would not necessarily be reasonable: RCBA seems to provide us with a way in which to quantify such judgments.[7]

There are two necessary conditions for any philosophical defence of some government policy tool: a condition of practicability and a condition of justifiability. By 'practicability', I mean that it should be clear how we ought to apply any proposed tool for policy-making. Although sometimes fraught in practice, as noted above, it is clear how RCBA should be applied in practical contexts. However, a defence of any policy tool should also meet a justifiability constraint. This task is particularly difficult in societies such as ours where there is widespread ethical disagreement. Therefore, I suggest that a defence of a policy tool should show how that tool relates to the political principles which constitute what Rawls calls a 'free-standing module', on which there can be an 'overlapping consensus'. That is, we should be able to defend use of a policy tool in such a way that different members of our community can agree to use of this tool for policy-making, regardless of their own views of the good life (Rawls, 1993). One key advantage of standard models of RCBA is that they are supposed to be 'ethically neutral', and, thus, to meet this publicity condition.

This may appear puzzling. After all, RCBA obviously involves placing some kind of valuation on different outcomes, and the justification of such valuations – say, treating a human life as 'costing' £x million – may seem extremely difficult. However, typically, the value-inputs into RCBA are supposed to be generated by adopting citizens' own valuations of different outcomes. The value claims necessary for comparing risks are generated either by looking at individuals' behaviour or by a process whereby their preferences between different outcomes are elicited. In effect, then, by assuming that everyone always reasons so as to maximize expected utility, in the way set out in the sandwich case, we generate an account of what people do value, and base policy on such valuations. RCBA is supposed to be ethically neutral in that (at least in its pure form) it does not rest on an objectivist account of good and bad, but generates claims about value on the basis of what people

---

[7] For a useful analysis of these tools as they apply in the context of railway safety, see Wolff (2002; 2006).

actually do value. This process leads Cass Sunstein (2005a) to suggest that such procedures are justifiable because they promote citizens' well-being – use of such tools avoids forcing individuals to 'pay more' for some good such as risk-reduction than they would be willing to pay – and respect citizens' autonomy – by respecting their valuations of outcomes.

The precautionary principle and value

Having identified some of the key aspects of RCBA, I will now turn to the precautionary principle. It is common to distinguish two forms of 'bioethics': 'environmental ethics' and 'medical ethics', and to note that these are very distinct areas of applied philosophy (O'Neill, 2002). An interesting feature of 'public health ethics', however, is that, although it is clearly related to 'medical ethics', insofar as both focus on normative problems related to individuals' health, it also shares concerns with 'environmental ethics'. The pursuit of public health policy often resembles environmental policy – both involve structuring features of a shared environment with the end of preserving certain sorts of goods – and similar normative problems, most notably problems of 'free-riding', occur in both contexts. Therefore, it is no surprise that the 'precautionary principle', much debated in recent environmental ethics, has increasingly been appealed to in public health ethics (Martuzzi and Tickner, 2004).

The canonical version of the precautionary principle states that 'where there are threats of serious or irreversible damage, lack of full scientific certainty shall not be used as a reason for postponing cost-effective measures to prevent environmental degradation' (United Nations, 1992). It is clear that, in and of itself, this principle is not directly relevant to public health policy (unless there is always some link between 'serious or irreversible environmental degradation' and public health). However, proponents of a 'precautionary approach' to public health claim that, by replacing 'serious environmental damage' with some set of outcomes such as 'serious negative public health problems', we can generate a 'precautionary principle', which ought to guide public health policy.[8]

'Precautionary thinking' has had an impact on UK public health policy, most notably in the 2000 'Stewart Report' which recommended on 'precautionary grounds' that mobile-phone masts should not be placed near schools (Burgess, 2004). Furthermore, the importance of adopting 'precautionary approaches' to public health policy has been stressed by EU directives (European Commission, 2000). There is much disagreement over what precisely is involved in adopting a 'precautionary approach' to public health policy. However, at least in the environmental context, it is assumed that there is a tension between the use of RCBA as a guide to policy and a more 'precautionary' approach. Therefore, we can expect that an interesting 'public health' version of the precautionary principle would also be in tension with the tools of RCBA.

What is implied by the claim that we ought to adopt an alternative 'precautionary approach' to policy? It might seem as if a precautionary approach to policy involves denial of the first aspect of RCBA: the claim that we ought always to seek to maximize expected outcomes. Within the literature on rational-choice-theory, some have argued that in

---

[8] Indeed, an alternative influential version of the principle, the 'Wingspread formulation', explicitly focuses on health issues: 'when an activity raises threats of harm to human health of the environment, precautionary measures should be taken even if some cause and effect relationships are not fully established scientifically' (see http://www.sehn.org/wing.html). For purposes of exposition, I shall, however, focus on the UN formulation.

circumstances where there is uncertainty over the likelihood of certain sorts of outcomes, we ought to adopt a strategy of 'maxi-min': we should adopt the policy with the least bad outcomes. In turn, some defenders of the precautionary principle have claimed that it can best be understood as a formulation of a maxi-min principle: that is, where there is good reason to believe that there is some risk of serious harm associated with some policy, then we should not adopt that policy, even if, for some reason, we cannot establish the risk precisely.[9]

However, I suggest that this way of reading the precautionary principle is orthogonal to many of the concerns expressed by proponents of 'precautionary reasoning'. Claims that we ought to adopt maxi-min strategies normally assume a framework where all harms and benefits are, ultimately, to be viewed as commensurable. Interesting versions of the precautionary principle, by contrast, seem to involve a more general claim: that the assumption of commensurability implicit in RCBA is suspect.

In light of these comments, one interpretation of the precautionary principle is that we (rightly) possess a tripartite division of the outcomes of action. Unlike 'normal bad outcomes' (ugly mobile-phone masts), which might be outweighed by 'good outcomes' (greater ease of communication), we ought to treat certain outcomes (the avoidable death of innocent children) as 'special bad outcomes'. In some sense, risks of such outcomes are not subject to the standard tools of RCBA, and, for some related reason, claims about such risks ought to be given credence even when they have not been established with 'scientific certainty'. Before deciding precisely *how* to interpret these claims – that is, answering the practicality worry above – we need to answer a prior question, related to the 'publicity' condition: are there non-controversial reasons to think that certain sorts of bad outcomes ought to be treated as 'special'?

I shall distinguish two kinds of argument for such a tripartite distinction of outcomes: standard-consequentialist and non-standard-consequentialist. I use 'standard-consequentialist' here to mean ethical theories which assess actions in terms of the states-of-affairs produced by those actions, and which assume that there is commensurability between different states-of-affairs. It looks as though it is precisely the assumption of commensurability underlying RCBA to which proponents of the precautionary principle object. However, it is possible to argue from a standard-consequentialist standpoint, which views all outcomes as ultimately commensurable, to a view that certain sorts of outcomes ought to be treated with particular care. To do so, we must show that a policy which does not treat those outcomes as special is, over time, likely to lead to worse outcomes than is a policy which treated that class of outcomes as special. We might, as it were, treat certain outcomes as outside the purview of standard RCBA not because those outcomes *are* 'really' special, but because we have good long-term reason to treat those outcomes *as if they were* special.

Such an argument might, in turn, be motivated by inductive evidence. Some of the worst public health crises of the twentieth century would have been avoided had we treated the threat of certain sorts of 'serious or irreversible damages' as special, and, therefore, we ought now to treat such threats as special. Perhaps the most famous examples of such catastrophes born of misplaced certainty are DDT in the USA and

---

[9] For a version of this kind of account of the precautionary principle in the environmental context see Gardiner (2006). Arguments for maxi-min strategies are, of course, famous in political philosophy because of their use in Rawls (1999).

thalidomide in the UK. This form of argument seems to be in-line with repeated arguments for adoption of the precautionary principle in an environmental context, where inductive evidence of past failures of science policy is used to cast doubt on contemporary risk-analysis (Harremoes *et al.*, 2002).

Does a standard-consequentialist argument meet the 'publicity condition'? Defenders of precautionary reasoning might respond to this question in a hypothetical mode: if you think that risk-cost-benefit-analysis, the methodology to which precautionary reasoning is normally opposed, meets the publicity condition, then precautionary reasoning also meets the publicity constraint as it is grounded on RCBA. The two approaches stand or fall together.

Even if we think that the 'standard consequentialist' argument for treating certain outcomes as 'special' fails, we might simply adopt a non-standard-consequentialism which denies the commensurability of outcomes. We might argue that certain sorts of outcomes cannot be traded-off against other sorts of outcomes. The deaths of innocent children, for example, might be thought simply to fall into a different category of outcome than the annoyance felt by many people at being unable to get mobile-phone reception. In turn, we might think that such incommensurability implies we ought to accord the avoidance of the relevant 'special' bad outcomes some kind of 'priority' over all other consequences in our moral reasoning. Whenever there is a possibility of 'special bad outcomes', we ought to seek to avoid those outcomes irrespective of 'normal' costs and benefits. (A similar sort of argument is sometimes used in the environmental context, where it is claimed that the 'intrinsic value' of nature is such that it is a mistake to think that we can ever trade-off environmental degradation against other kinds of harms and benefits [see, for example, Elliot, 1997].)

Deontological defences of the precautionary principle and the argument over lay-rationality

I shall discuss one way in which we might defend 'non-standard consequentialism' in the next section. First, however, I shall outline a more interesting route for defending the precautionary principle, by appeal to 'deontological' considerations. What is a deontological approach to the precautionary principle? One common complaint against the precautionary principle is that it seems to tell us to regulate against new technologies or innovations, when those technologies or innovations pose some threat of serious or irreversible damage, even when we have good evidence that those technologies will probably help many. Defenders of the precautionary principle are accused of a peculiar form of myopia (Sunstein, 2002, 2003, 2005b).

However, we might claim that the precautionary principle's focus on avoiding harm, rather than alleviating suffering, can be justified by appeal to the distinction between 'doings' and 'allowings'. For example, in the environmental context, Marion Hourdequin (2007) has argued that the precautionary principle represents or incorporates a distinction between 'doing' environmental damage and merely 'allowing' environmental damage to occur (Hughes, 2006). Of course, this way of reading the principle poses a new challenge, as some past harms may have been the result of 'human' actions: taking seriously a doing/ allowing distinction is not the same as the conservative principle that action always requires more justification than inaction. However, Hourdequin's key point is simple and compelling: in everyday thought and political discussion, we distinguish between human-caused environmental damage and environmental damage which occurs 'naturally'. This distinction, which we overlook if we think of policy solely in terms of outcomes, is one which the precautionary principle aims to respect. If we take seriously some kind of deontological intuition, then, we are likely to think that RCBA is a deeply flawed methodology, because it treats the risks which would, in some sense, be imposed by action as equivalent to the risks which action might aim at relieving. Of course, we need not deny that there is *some* perspective from which we might say that the risks associated with action and inaction are 'equal'. However, we might deny that all we do, or ought to, care about is this kind of information. Rather, when considering action, we need to ask whether any resultant risks of harm would arise as a result of our actions or as a result of our inactions.

The deontological sense of a distinction between doings and allowings is, arguably, one which is reflected not only in environmental contexts, but in contexts of health-and-safety regulation. Consider, for example, whether we ought to allow a drug onto the market. We know that the drug will save many lives, but we are worried that it *might* have 'special' bad effects for a small (but *ex-ante* unidentifiable) sector of the population. What does the precautionary principle tell us to do in such cases? It seems to tells us that we ought not to allow the drug onto the market because there is a small chance that so doing will lead to 'serious or irreversible damage' (as a result of the possible side-effects). However, it also seems to tell us that we ought to allow the drug onto the market, as not to do so also involves running a risk of 'serious or irreversible damage' (that is, the deaths of many people whose lives would have been saved had the drug been put on the market). Such arguments against the precautionary principle seem strong. However, a deontological account of the principle can show why they may be mistaken. The key difference between allowing the drug onto the market and not allowing the drug onto the market is that, in the first case but not in the second, the deaths of some people would be a result of our actions, whereas, in the second case, the deaths would be something we allow, rather than do. Conservatism might not be a form of indifference or myopia, but, rather, an expression of a certain conception of the extent of (and limits to) our obligations.

I have suggested, then, that we might want to base a defence of the precautionary principle on the deontological distinction between doings and allowings. This claim may seem vulnerable to a familiar worry – already hinted at above – that the doing/allowing distinction is extremely difficult to defend; deciding precisely when health-and-safety regulation would prevent risk-imposition (and, thus, is demanded to stop a social 'doing') and when such regulation would merely reduce 'natural' risks seems likely to be an impossible task. It is worth noting here, then, that a strong doing/allowing distinction need not be the only way in which we could incorporate deontological concerns into discussions of the regulation of risk. In recent work, for example, Thomas Pogge (2004) has argued that accounts of justice and health have systematically overlooked the important differences between different ways in which the 'same' health problem might have been generated (for example, through deliberate discrimination, through lax implementation of laws, through the results of natural processes, through individuals' behaviour, and so on). In turn, he has suggested that the strength of the demand that we prevent or cure illness turns, in part, on these kinds of considerations. This is not the place to develop or to defend Pogge's claims. However, there is some plausibility in the claim that the strength of the demand that we do something to prevent individuals falling ill (that is, the strength of the demand that we reduce the risks they face) turns, in part, on the source of the risks they face. To the extent that a version of this claim can be defended, then it might serve to explain not only why the precautionary principle seems to focus on a particular class of outcomes, but also why it seems to pay particular attention to ensuring that human agencies are not (causally) responsible for those outcomes, even if avoiding such (causal) responsibility is, in other ways, 'costly'.

Scientific and constructivist views of risk

It is one thing to say that we can distinguish between different kinds of outcomes or different kinds of obligations, either of which views might underlie 'precautionary' approaches to policy, another to say that either of these distinctions is conceptually sound, and yet another to say that such a distinction can be part of a 'free-standing module' on which there might be an overlapping consensus. How might the very general claims about how we might understand the philosophical urges behind some formulations of the precautionary principle be defended in a pluralist society?

To understand our options here, it is useful to turn to some of the issues that arise in the heated controversy over risk. There often seem to be differences between how experts and members of the public talk and reason about 'risk': risks which the experts claim are 'intolerable' are tolerated by the public, whereas risks which the experts think the public should, if they are to be consistent, tolerate are not tolerated (Slovic, 2000; House of Commons Science and Technology Committee, 2006). I shall focus on a distinction between two ways in which we might make sense of the apparent 'gap' between 'expert' and 'public' views of risk (these two approaches do not jointly exhaust the sociological approaches to risk, but are the most interesting accounts for our purposes).

One approach is to suggest that 'public' views of risk are, quite simply, misguided. For example, it is clear that some public views about risk – say, the risks associated with genetic technologies – are based on scientific misunderstanding. Furthermore, there are experiments which seem to show that people often have difficulty with understanding probability, and that their reasoning is influenced by misfiring 'cognitive heuristics'. These factors can, then, be appealed to in an attempt to explain how the public, who are assumed to think about risks and how to deal with risks in terms of maximizing their expected utility, are often led astray (Sunstein, 2002). This approach to thinking about 'lay views' of risk is, of course, consistent with the project of RCBA: RCBA provides a way in which to overcome the cognitive failings inherent in public discourse about and understanding of risk-based policy. (Although it should also be noted that such results also warn us that if we want to gauge what people's preferences are as the basis for RCBA, we need to be extremely careful how we do so, as both what people do and what they say may not be a good guide to what they really value.)

However, there is a second way of understanding 'public' reasoning about risk. Rather than say that the public are simply 'confused' about risks, some theorists have argued that 'lay' reasoning about risk displays an 'alternative', 'lay' or 'thick' rationality, which differs fundamentally from the kind of consequentialism implicit in much risk-assessment.[10] According to these views, when members of the public say that some Risk A is far worse than a second Risk B (although both represent the same probability of similar harm), then, their fears *may* simply reflect a cognitive failure, but it may also be the case that they are expressing a view about the moral status of these different risks. Arguments to the effect

---

[10] Versions of the view suggested here maybe found in Slovic (2000); Wolff (2006) and, in a very different form, Irwin (1995).

that 'lay' reasoning about risk is not irrational, but in fact grounded on complex (if perhaps inchoate) ethical theories, have been mounted in a range of different public health policy debates, most notably in debates over the BSE crisis, and in debates over health-and-safety, such as railway safety (Irwin, 1995; Wolff, 2006). Sometimes such accounts of 'lay' reasoning about risk are described as 'social constructivist'. However, this is slightly misleading insofar as to say that some concept is 'socially constructed' is normally understood to debunk that concept (Hacking, 2000). Furthermore, this appellation may be confusing as there are some 'social constructivist' writers who seem to suggest that there is no distinction between the public perception of risk and what risks there are (Beck, 1992). Arguments that 'lay' risk-assessment is value-laden, by comparison, do not necessarily deny any distinction between 'risks' and 'risk-perception', but, rather, they suggest that what might appear from the viewpoint of RCBA to be a cognitive confusion is often better understood in terms of evaluative disagreement.

A better way in which to understand these approaches, then, might be to say that they argue that identification of and reasoning about risks is highly 'ethically loaded'. Whereas the 'standard' view of risk associated with RCBA assumes that we can rank all risks from most to least severe by multiplying the probability of outcomes against the badness of those outcomes, 'lay' reasoning involves a far more complex process, where risks are ranked not merely in terms of expected harm, but in terms of their 'wrongness', or in terms which deny that all harms are commensurable.

In turn, we can use such claims to argue against the acceptability of standard RCBA in two different ways. First, the fact that 'public' attitudes towards risk seem to incorporate such concerns can help to strengthen an argument that RCBA rests on a particular moral theory, and a moral theory that requires further defence (Cranor, 2007). That is to say, we can treat public views about risk as reminding us that what appears to be an ethically neutral way in which to guide health-and-safety policy – by assessing policies in terms of expected outcomes – actually rests on assumptions, such as that all outcomes are commensurable or that doings and allowings are morally symmetrical, which reasonable individuals can (and, in fact, do) dispute.

Second, we might adopt a kind of democratic approach to argue against the use of RCBA in policy contexts. Rather than defending the correctness of 'non-standard-consequentialism' or some 'deontological' view of risk, which we claim to be implicit in everyday thought, we might instead argue that members of the public hold such views, the views are not clearly false, and, as such, they ought to be respected in the decision-making process. Just as the proponent of RCBA claims simply to be 'reflecting' social values when she constructs an account of value, the proponent of some kind of precautionary approaches to policy might claim simply to be 'reflecting' social values when she denies the legitimacy of RCBA.

Precaution in practice: questioning the ethical/epistemic divide

In the previous sections, I argued for two ways in which we might interpret the motivations behind 'precautionary' thought: either as reflecting the view that a certain class of outcomes are (or should be viewed as) special, and thus outside the ambit of RCBA, or, more interestingly, as reflecting a deontological distinction between the wrongness of different sorts of risks. It should at this point be stressed that many of the writers I have cited throughout my discussion of the precautionary principle would not normally be thought of as defenders of the precautionary principle. My aim has not been so much to provide an exposition of standard precautionary thought, but to provide an exposition of alternatives to RCBA, paying particular attention to the question of justifiability.

I have suggested that a second constraint on any account of the precautionary principle is that it ought to show us how and when we are to adopt the principle. This 'practicality' constraint is particularly important as it has seemed to many that the precautionary principle is too vague to be of any real use in policy-making (Sandin et al., 2002). This might explain why even those who deny RCBA do not necessarily commit themselves to the precautionary principle.

The precautionary principle faces multiple problems as a guide to action. Showing that a tripartite distinction of outcomes is defensible is not the same as specifying precisely how the importance of certain outcomes ought to be treated as 'special'. Similarly, claiming that the avoidance of imposing certain sorts of risks ought to have priority over allowing similar risks to continue 'naturally' does not tell us how to choose between policies. However, rather than focus on all of these questions here, for purposes of exposition, I will focus on a rather puzzling feature of the standard formulation of the precautionary principle; the claim that we ought to act to forestall the risk of certain kinds of harms even when we lack 'full scientific certainty' that there is a link between some policy and a risk of such harm. This widens the informational bases on which our choices are to be made. However, so doing seems to leave the principle open to charges of being, at best, irrational, obscurantist and anti-scientific, and, at worst, of being impracticable.

To see why, let us return to the case of placing mobile-phone masts next to schools. Imagine that all agree that childhood cancer is incommensurably worse than other outcomes, such that if an official policy, say allowing masts to be placed anywhere, poses a risk of such an outcome, then we have strong precautionary health-and-safety reasons not to adopt that policy. Even if we can agree with the claim, we might be reluctant to reject a *laissez-faire* policy regarding mobile-phone masts, thus potentially foregoing many benefits, when there is no scientific certainty over whether there is such a risk *at all*. The Stewart report's recommendations seem, then, to rest on two dubitable premises: first, *any* risk of childhood cancer associated with locating mobile-phone masts next to schools would make it illegitimate to locate masts next to schools; second, we should act as if there is some risk of such harm even when there is no scientific certainty that there is any such risk. Opponents of the principle object that it seems to allow 'hunches', rather than 'knowledge', to guide policy.[11]

Furthermore, opponents of the precautionary principle note that allowing 'hunches' or 'mere possibilities' to guide our reasoning reopens the possibility that the principle will lead to paralysis. Just as there is no 'scientific certainty' that mobile-phone masts pose a potential risk to children, so there is no 'scientific certainty' that mobile-phone masts do not promote good health. If so, the non-standard-consequentialist defender of the precautionary principle seems to have the following choice: allow masts to be placed next to schools or do not allow masts to be placed next to schools. Adopting the first course-of-action is associated with a non-ascertained risk of harm, but so, if we are to base policy on any old claims, is the second course-of-action. Even if we have a principle for choosing between

---

[11] Resnik (2003) provides a useful overview of many of these debates, paying particular attention to the context of environmental policy.

courses-of-action in situations where both are associated with some risk of 'special harm', our principle will be inapplicable in this situation, as we have no risk-data on the basis of which to choose, as there is no scientific certainty that *either* option poses any risk at all. Admittedly, a deontological reading of the precautionary principle, one which stresses the idea that there are certain sorts of actions we ought not to perform might not be vulnerable to the 'paralysis' problem. However, it will certainly seem vulnerable to attack on the grounds that a policy of never being involved in the imposition of risk, regardless of how certain we are that there are such risks, seems to threaten extreme conservatism in action.

Of course, a proponent of the precautionary principle could say that it 'makes sense' to think that there is a possibility that mobile-phone masts pose a risk and no reason to think that there is a possibility that they might potentially benefit children, even if science has not shown either claim to be true (or false). However, we need some way in which to distinguish those claims that have not been proven with 'scientific certainty', which we should take seriously, from claims not thus proven, which we should not take seriously. As stated, the principle does not help with this task.

This 'epistemic' objection to the precautionary principle is extremely strong. One option would be to give up on the aspect of precautionary thought which seems to set extremely low epistemic thresholds on when precaution is warranted.[12] However, in the rest of this section, I shall suggest one way in which a defender of the principle might motivate the claim that we ought to act *as if* courses-of-action pose some threat even in the absence of 'full scientific certainty' that they do so, and suggest one way in which this general claim could lead to a practicable principle. In the arguments above, I implicitly assumed – as do many contributors to this debate – that, when generating the 'factive inputs' into policy-making, our choices are either to rely on those risk-claims we have established with 'scientific certainty' or to rely on 'hunches' and 'guesswork'.

However, matters are not as simple as this sharp dichotomy suggests. To see why, consider what happens in epidemiological testing. In standard scientific statistical testing, we wish to discover, on the basis of the evidence available, whether we ought to say that there is some connection between some kind of event and some kind of outcome (the relevant connection may be expressed in probabilistic terms: the epidemiological evidence does not show that if you smoke, then you are bound to develop lung cancer, but that if you smoke, then there is a higher-than-normal chance that you will develop lung cancer). In standard scientific testing, we choose a 'null hypothesis' – that there is no connection between two events, for example, smoking and developing lung cancer – and an 'alternative hypothesis' – that there is some connection (perhaps a probabilistic connection) between the two events, for example that smokers are at greater risk of developing lung cancer than are (comparable) non-smokers.[13]

---

[12] Note that the problem raised here is not unique to the interpretation of the precautionary principle as involving either a tripartite distinction between outcomes or a focus on deontological concerns. Even defenders of the precautionary principle who make it a version of maxi-min thought need to be able to distinguish those cases where we ought to worry about some threat, the probability of which is not established with scientific certainty, from cases where a non-established threat is not worth worrying about (see Gardiner, 2006).

[13] Note that I leave to one side the metaphysics of risk – regardless of whether we think of risk as epistemic or as ontological, we can be more or less accurate in terms either of how the world is or what we ought to believe about the world. For more discussion of these topics, see Mellor (2006).

A statistical test can produce one of two results: either, it tells us that we ought to reject the 'null hypothesis' (that there is no link) and accept the 'alternative hypothesis', or it tells us that there is insufficient evidence to reject the 'null hypothesis'. In testing, however, we can make two kinds of errors: we can generate 'false positives' (we accept the alternative hypothesis when it is false) and 'false negatives' (we do not accept the alternative hypothesis when it is true). It is impossible to minimize both of these kinds of errors simultaneously (Levi, 1962). In standard scientific testing, it is thought that 'false positives' are a more serious kind of error than are 'false negatives'. Therefore, investigators routinely set very high p-values for their statistical tests, thus minimizing their chances of generating 'false positives' (asserting there is some significant connection when there is no connection), but also running a risk of generating 'false negatives' (failing to assert that there is some connection when there is, in fact, a connection (Levi, 1964).[14] Setting a high p-value means that if we claim that there is some connection between two events, we are warranted in an extremely high degree of certainty that we are right in our positive claim, as the chance that we have (falsely) made such a claim has been minimized. As the term 'confidence level' suggests, the higher the p-value we adopt for statistical testing, the more confident we can be that a positive result is correct.

A failure to show that the 'alternative hypothesis' is true is not the same as showing that the 'null hypothesis' is true. Rather, the proper conclusion to be drawn when we fail to prove the 'alternative hypothesis' is that there is insufficient evidence to reject the 'null hypothesis'. After all, as we have seen, with a high p-value, it is possible that we will often generate 'false negatives', that is, we will not say that there is a link when there is a link between the relevant events. There is, then, an important distinction, perhaps elided by our choice of symmetrical terms, between 'false positives' and 'false negatives'. To generate a 'false positive' is to make a claim that is a false, whereas to generate a 'false negative' is, strictly, merely to fail to assert a claim that is, in fact, true.

However, it is clear that when scientific results are transferred from journals and laboratories to the context of policy and decision-making, failure to show a link is often treated as proof of no link. This is a simple epistemological error – the claim that we have insufficient reason to believe some proposition p ('there is insufficient reason to believe that there is a link between X and Y') is confused with the claim that we have reason to believe not-p ('there is no link between X and Y').

Such confusion can have grave consequences for action, because acting as if it is the case that not-p, when all that we can reasonably say is that p is not proven, can lead us to act on false beliefs. This can have disastrous results. For example, return to the question of whether or not we ought to allow mobile-phone masts to be placed next to schools. Imagine that we cannot show, with 'scientific certainty', that the location of masts is linked to childhood cancer. Therefore, we go ahead with placing masts next to schools, something that we would not have done had we thought that so doing poses an excess risk – however small – that children might, as a result, develop cancer. However, also imagine that there is *in fact* a link between the location of mobile-phone masts and schools: our claim that there was no link was a 'false negative'. In this case, a policy of

---

[14] Indeed, these standards are often set in computer programmes as default.

epistemic caution – only acting on those claims about probabilistic relations which we have very good reason to believe are true – might lead us to a course-of-action which, had we been less epistemically cautious, we would have rejected.[15]

These facts help us to understand what may be at stake in (at least some, but not all) discussions of the precautionary principle. Many proponents of the precautionary principle list examples of cases where scientific evidence that some activity was safe turned out to be wrong, thus leading to catastrophic effects for the environment or for human life (Harremoes *et al.*, 2004). Of course, we can claim that there are many different kinds of lessons that we ought to learn from such past mistakes. For example, at least in the environmentalist context, it is often claimed that we have overwhelming evidence that we misunderstand the complexity and underestimate the fragility of nature (Carson, 1962). However, a more modest lesson we might draw from the past record is that we ought to think more about the 'burden of proof'; we ought to change our standard testing methodologies – at least in some cases – to minimize our risk of 'false negatives' even at the cost of generating many 'false positives'. Of course, setting out which *p*-values we ought to adopt, and how such asymmetric testing methods might work is no easy task. However, philosophers of science, most notably Carl Cranor (1993), have worked on alternative testing methodologies which incorporate such concerns.

We can, then, generate a sympathetic reconstruction of the precautionary principle as a complex combination of a decision principle with an epistemic rule. The non-standard-consequentialist proponent of the precautionary principle can be interpreted as claiming that certain sorts of outcomes represent 'special bad outcomes', and, as such, avoidance of these outcomes has lexical priority (of some kind) over other sorts of considerations (such as the expected sum-total of normal harms and benefits associated with some potential action). However, as well as this decision rule, she also suggests an epistemic rule for the generation of inputs into policy-making. Even if standard statistical testing procedures ought to be used to ascertain the possible connections between various courses-of-action and 'normal' good or bad outcomes, special 'bad outcomes' are somehow importantly different, such that we ought to lower our normal scientific standard of proof – we ought to lower our *p*-values – when investigating the possible connections between some course-of-action and these outcomes. In effect, 'special' bad outcomes are doubly special: first, avoiding such outcomes has lexical priority when choosing between different courses-of-action; second, the 'factive' claim that there are such possibilities can legitimately be asserted in policy-making contexts even when such a claim has not been demonstrated to the level of certainty we normally require of scientific claims.[16]

---

[15] Similar points were raised in the epidemiological context by Austin Bradford Hill, one of the founders of modern epidemiology. See Hill (1965), especially the final section.

[16] How do these claims relate to the 'deontological' version of the precautionary principle? I cannot answer this question fully here, but it is interesting to note that we do often seem to vary our standards-of-proof in proportion to what seems natural to call the 'moral costs' of acting wrongly: consider, for example, the difference between the standards of proof in the criminal and in the civil law. Therefore, it seems reasonable to assume that the deontologist defender of the precautionary principle might reach a similar conclusion.

Risk, tolerability and action: the way forward for an ethics of risk?

The arguments in the preceding sections suggest that there are serious challenges to an unthinking use of the tools of RCBA to risk-assessment and risk-management. One way in which to frame these challenges would be to say that RCBA overlooks at least two important issues: first, it assumes that all outcomes are ultimately commensurable, thus ignoring important ethical distinctions between different kinds of outcomes; second, it fails to recognize the complex web of obligations which might relate to the pursuit of public health policy. Furthermore, although strictly a reliance on standard statistical testing procedures is not an essential feature of RCBA, a proponent of the precautionary principle might suggest that most RCBA rests on an implausibly idealized view of the value of normal models of scientific inquiry. However, this view of science ignores the fact that the values of scientific caution may be in conflict with our other ethical norms and worries.

There are serious ethical challenges to both our standard way of assessing risk and our standard way of managing risk. However, RCBA has one extremely important feature, arguably missing from many accounts of the precautionary principle: It recognizes the unavoidability of trade-offs between the ends of public health policy and other kinds of social goods. We might find something distasteful about placing a monetary value on human life, but it is unclear that we always think that the fact that some policy or human activity poses some risk that lives will be lost is a decisive argument in favour of ending that policy or banning that activity. Rather, sometimes we do think that some system or policy is 'safe enough', because the costs of making that system any safer would be excessive. An advantage of RCBA is that at least it makes such judgments explicit. As I have already indicated, it is unclear quite which 'public health outcomes' are relevant to precautionary thought, but there seems a danger that a precautionary approach involves commitment either to the claim that no level of safety is ever 'safe enough' or to the claim that we can always avoid trade-offs. Neither of these claims seems at all plausible.

Therefore, constructing an ethics of risk for public health policy is no easy task. I do, however, suggest that the arguments above provide us with one way in which we might construct a plausible account of how we ought to deal with risks. The key claim of RCBA is that we can legitimately impose risks on individuals or allow them to suffer certain sorts of risks because of the social costs of not imposing or allowing those risks. An ethics of risk for public health policy should, of course, allow that some risks are 'tolerable' because those risks are somehow necessarily related to the pursuit of other goods (Cranor, 2007). Of course, RCBA sometimes seems to miss the complexity of such trade-offs. It would seem odd, for example, to think that a trade-off between limiting liberty and reducing health risks should be framed in monetary terms. However, at least, RCBA seems to provide a framework for trading-off risks, costs and benefits of policies in a way in which the claims that we should treat certain bad outcomes as 'special' or that we should avoid 'doing' certain sorts of harm, even at the cost of 'allowing' similar harms to occur, do not.

It seems, then, that RCBA's great advantage as an account of risk tolerability is that it recognizes the unavoidability of trade-offs, whereas evocations of the precautionary principle do not. However, reflection on some of the arguments for the precautionary principle discussed in the third and fourth sections above can show a fact that proponents of RCBA often overlook: what makes risks 'tolerable' or 'intolerable' is extremely context-sensitive, and related to complex ethical considerations. To make this point vivid, let us return to an example where RCBA may seem at its strongest. Let us imagine, for example, that mobile-phone masts do pose a risk of childhood cancer.[17] However, we also know that increased ease of communication might save lives (for example, because if it is easier to use mobile phones, then people will find it easier to telephone the emergency services). In this situation, a proponent of RCBA would say that a reasonable policy with regard to the regulation of mobile-phone masts would have to balance the risks that children will develop cancer against the risks that some people will be unable to phone the emergency services when considering legislation on the location of mobile-phone masts.

However, this seems far too simplistic a way to view this decision. After all, if we place mobile-phone masts next to schools, then we are placing children at risk, through our adoption of a policy, and, furthermore, we are placing them at risk in an environment which is one which they are legally compelled to attend. If we fail to place mobile-phone masts next to schools, then we are leaving some at risk (that is, those who would, otherwise, be able to contact emergency services using a mobile phone). Of course, all things considered, it is normally a good thing to save lives. However, we might think that, in this case, there is an important distinction, overlooked by RCBA, between imposing risks on some and merely failing to reduce the risks some suffer. This sense might be strengthened if we discover that most of those who need to use mobile phones to call emergency services end up in this situation because of their own actions. Of course, the issues here might get even more complex again, but my point is simple: reasoning about this case (and, I suggest, any case which involves risk reduction) requires not only that we balance outcomes, but that we balance an extremely complex set of moral judgments, concerning both magnitudes of harm and the causation of harm.

The key point that emerges from discussion of the precautionary principle, then, is that the tolerability of risk may be extremely context-sensitive, and that this context-sensitivity might relate to ethical considerations in a manner which cannot necessarily be captured in monetary terms. Furthermore, an advantage of this context-sensitive view of risk tolerability is that it allows us to make sense of, at least some, features of how the public seem to view and think about risk. When the public express fears over some risk which RCBA tells us is not a serious risk, their fears may not be cognitively confused, but, rather, might reflect a genuine ethical worry. Note, however, that this is not to say that the public cannot be wrong about what the risks are. Rather, it is to say that public claims over risks can be a useful *guide* to ethical considerations for risk policy.

The idea that we can use 'public attitudes' towards risk as a guide to the ethical issues in risk-management is also related to the issues discussed above, concerning the relationship between ethical and epistemic norms in the identification of risks. Public scepticism about scientific claims that some policy is 'safe enough' need not be understood as expressing an unwarranted anti-scientific world view. Rather, in at least some cases, they may be understood as pointing us towards an important question: whether the costs of acting on a false-negative in some particular case are so great that we ought to change our standard statistical norms in this context.

These comments on risk-tolerability are sketchy. However, I hope that they help the reader to understand how we might hope to construct an ethics of risk which takes account

---

[17] I should stress at this point that there seems to be very little evidence of any possible link between mobile-phone masts and childhood cancer. The example here is chosen purely for expository purposes.

of the fact that risk policy cannot be isolated, either from the pursuit of other important social goods (as the precautionary principle would seem to suggest) or from complex webs of obligation (as RCBA would seem to suggest). Rather, to identify and to manage risks requires us to construct an account of when risks are 'tolerable', a highly contextual affair. Furthermore, as the fifth section suggests, there may be reasons to be suspicious of using standard statistical tools for the purposes of finding out what risks there are. Therefore, an ethics of risk – which still requires a complete articulation – might provide a useful guide not only to public health ethics but to the ethics of epidemiology.

References

Adams, J. (1995) *Risk*. London: UCL Press.

Beck, U. (1992) *Risk Society: Towards a New Modernity*. London: SAGE.

Burgess, A. (2004) *Cellular Phones, Public Fears and a Culture of Precaution*. Cambridge: Cambridge University Press.

Carson, R. (1962) *Silent Spring*. Boston, MA: Houghton Mifflin.

Cranor, C. (1993) *Regulating Toxic Substances: A Philosophy of Science and the Law*. Oxford: Oxford University Press.

Cranor, C. (2007) Towards a non-consequentialist approach to acceptable risks. In *Risk: Philosophical Perspectives*, ed. T. Lewens. London: Routledge.

Douglas, M. and Wildavsky, A. (1980) *Risk and Culture*. Berkeley, CA: University of California Press.

Elliott, R. (1997) *Faking Nature*. London: Taylor & Francis.

European Commission (2000) *Communication from the Commission on the Precautionary Principle*. Brussels: European Commission. Available at: http://eurlex.europa.eu/LexUriServ/LexUriServ.do?uri=COM:2000:0001:FIN:EN: PDF (accessed: 10/1/08).

Gardiner, S. (2006) A core precautionary principle. *Journal of Political Philosophy*, **14** (4): 33–60.

Hacking, I. (1975) *The Emergence of Probability*. Cambridge: Cambridge University Press.

Hacking, I. (1990) *The Taming of Chance*. Cambridge: Cambridge University Press.

Hacking, I. (2000) *The Social Construction of What?* Boston, MA: Harvard University Press.

Hansson, S.-O. (2007) *Risk*. In *Stanford Encyclopaedia of Philosophy*. Available at: http://plato.stanford.edu/entries/risk/ (accessed: 10/1/08).

Harremoes, J., Gee, D., Macgarvin, M., Stirling, A., Keys, J., Wynne, B. and Vaz, S. G., eds (2002) *The Precautionary Principle in the Twentieth Century*. London: Earthscan.

Hill, A. B. (1965) The environment and disease: association or causation? *Proceedings of the Royal Society of Medicine*, **58**(5): 295–300.

Hourdequin, M. (2007) Doing, allowing and precaution. *Environmental Ethics*, **29**(4): 339–58.

House of Commons Science and Technology Committee (2006) *Scientific Advice, Risk and Evidence Based Policy Making*. London: The Stationery Office.

Hughes, J. (2006) How not to criticize the precautionary principle. *Journal of Medicine and Philosophy*, **27**(3): 355–68.

Irwin, A. (1995) *Citizen Science*. London: Routledge and Kegan Paul.

Jasanoff, S. (1999) The songlines of risk. *Environmental Values*, **8**(2): 135–49.

Lewens, T. (2007) Introduction: risk and philosophy. In *Risk: Philosophical Perspectives*, ed. T. Lewens. London: Routledge, pp. 1–20.

Levi, I. (1962) On the seriousness of mistakes. *Philosophy of Science*, **29**(2): 47–65.

Ling, T. and Raven, A. (2006) Pharmacogenetics and uncertainty: implications for policy makers. *Studies in the History and Philosophy of the Biological and Biomedical Sciences*, **37** (3): 533–49.

Luce, R. D. and Raiffa, H. (1957) *Games and Decisions*. New York: Wiley.

Martuzzi, M. and Tickner, J., eds (2004) *The Precautionary Principle: Protecting Public Health, the Environment and the Future of Our Children*. Copenhagen: WHO.

Mellor, D. H. (2005) *Probability: A Philosophical Introduction*. London: Routledge.

Olsaretti, S. (2005) Endorsement and freedom in Amartya Sen's capability approach. *Economics and Philosophy*, **21**: 89–108.

O'Neill, O. (2002) *Autonomy and Trust in Bioethics*. Cambridge: Cambridge University Press.

Pogge, T. (2004) Relational conceptions of justice. In *Public health, Ethics and Equity*, ed. F. Anand, F. Peter and A. K. Sen. Oxford: Oxford University Press, pp. 135–62.

Rawls, J. (1993) *Political Liberalism*. New York: Columbia University Press.

Rawls, J. (1999) *A Theory of Justice*, rev. edn. Oxford: Oxford University Press.

Resnik, D. B. (2003) Is the precautionary principle unscientific? *Studies in the History and Philosophy of the Biological and Biomedical Sciences*, **34**(2): 329–44.

Sandin, P., Peterson, M., Hansson, S. O., Ruden, C. and Juthe, A. (2002) Five charges against the precautionary principle. *Journal of Risk Research*, **5**(4): 287–99.

Sen, A. K. (1992) *Inequality Reexamined*. Oxford: Oxford University Press.

Shrader-Frechette, K. (1980) *Nuclear Power and Public Policy: The Social and Ethical Problems of Fission Technology*. Dordrect: D. Reidel.

Shrader-Frechette, K. (1991) *Risk and Rationality: Philosophical Foundations for Populist Reforms*. Berkeley, CA: University of California Press.

Slovic, P. (1987) Perception of risk. *Science*, **236** (4799): 280–5.

Slovic, P. (2000) *The Perception of Risk*. London: Earthscan.

Sunstein, C. (2002) *Risk and Reason*. Cambridge: Cambridge University Press.

Sunstein, C. (2003) Beyond the precautionary principle. *University of Pennsylvania Law Review*, **151**(3): 1003–58.

Sunstein, C. (2005a) Environmental protection and cost-benefit analysis. *Ethics*, **115**(2): 351–85.

Sunstein, C. (2005b) *Laws of Fear: Beyond the Precautionary Principle*. Cambridge: Cambridge University Press.

United Nations (1992) *Rio Declaration on Environment and Development. Report of the United Nations Conference on Environment and Development, Rio de Janeiro, June 3–14*. New York: United Nations.

Wolff, J. (2002) *Railway Safety and the Ethics of the Tolerability of Risk*. London: Railways Safety Research Programme. Available at: http://www.rssb.co.uk/pdf/policy_risk.pdf (accessed: 10/1/08).

Wolff, J. (2006) Risk, fear, blame, shame and the regulation of public safety. *Economics and Philosophy*, **22**(3): 409–27.

Smoking, health and ethics

5

Richard Ashcroft

Introduction

The moral status of smoking is much disputed. Because smoking is known to be harmful to the health of the smoker, and to those exposed to their smoke, and because smoking is addictive, it is natural for public health practitioners and policy makers to consider smoking to be a public health problem, and to seek ways to eradicate it, or at least bring it under control (Boyle *et al.*, 2004). Because smoking is for many smokers a pleasure, and an activity rich in social and cultural meaning, it is natural for such smokers (and some non-smokers) to resist these attempts to control smoking. For those smokers for whom their smoking is no longer a pleasure, or for whom it may be a pleasure but who accept that it is a pleasure they wished they could forego, attempts to control smoking can be both aid and irritant. And even unrepentant smokers would concede that encouraging young children to take up smoking would be discreditable at least, immoral at worst.

In many respects, then, smoking provokes as complex social, moral and legal reactions as those other risky, scandalous and usually pleasurable activities sex and drinking. We can begin to get an understanding of the moral issues by distinguishing those moral issues that arise in connection with the smoker's self-regarding behaviour, and those which arise in connection with her other-regarding behaviour. Another way to approach the issues would be to look at the manufacture, supply and marketing of tobacco products, and to consider the ethical aspects of regulating the tobacco market. From a public health practitioner's point of view this might actually be the more logical approach, since it uses a kind of population perspective. Yet this would be to neglect the crucial feature of tobacco regulation (as distinct from say environmental pollutant regulation), which is that there is a buoyant market of tobacco users who for various reasons want to consume the regulated product. We need to understand the nature of that want, and its moral standing, if we are to understand the grounds for regulating the product and its markets. For this reason, I will proceed from the tobacco smoker up, rather than from the market down.

The morality of smoking itself

The painter David Hockney has been widely interviewed on his opposition to banning smoking in public places. In a letter published in the *Guardian* newspaper on 1 June 2004 he wrote:

Public Health Ethics, ed. Angus Dawson. Published by Cambridge University Press. © Cambridge University Press 2011.

[. . .] Smoking is a great pleasure. If it knocks some time off your life, it's only at the end of it. So what!

I admit people might not like smoky places, but you have to accept that some people don't mind them, it's a price you pay for some excitement, but the dreary don't want anybody near smoke.
I loathe the view of life that thinks some people have so much more knowledge of life that their advice must be listened to. I'm the expert on my life, not the doctor. He can advise, make suggestions, but ultimately I decide what will give me the excitement I want from life.

I take exercise. I walk in Holland Park, here in west London, every morning. One morning I was watching a peacock strut around with two rabbits scampering about, and then a black-and-white bird arrived. The scene was magical to me. I smoked a cigarette.

Three girls came by, jogging. One looked at me, shaking a finger and tut-tutting at me for smoking. OK, but they didn't see the peacock or the rabbits or the bird – they were so obsessed with their own bodies, and they thought their activity was healthier than mine. I do not think it was, but I don't want to ban jogging in Holland Park.

(Hockney, 2004)

In an open letter published in the *Guardian* on 25 February 2006, he wrote:

[. . .] Gordon Brown is a prig P.R.I.G., a dreary atheistic Calvinistic prig, who I'm sure will never be elected in England. He goes along with a 'health lobby' whose view of life itself I detest.

I have utter contempt for it. I feel I am entitled to my opinion. I don't mind prigs but when they want to take my little corner as well, I have a right to argue against their dreary view of life contaminating mine.

(Hockney, 2006)

On 15 May in the following year, he said in a further article in the same newspaper 'I smoke for my mental health. I think it's good for it, and I certainly prefer its calming effects to the pharmaceutical ones (side effects unknown)', going on to identify the motives behind the smoking ban as being 'anti-smoker', being led by 'mean-spirited and dreary people' and 'a political and media elite'. In particular, he sees this as part of the loss of 'a sense of messiness'. Both the ban, and the signs required in shops and offices to proclaim it, are signs of 'the uglification of England' (Hockney, 2007).

None of Hockney's interventions were distinguished by much in the way of careful argumentation, but he highlights an important concern about the regulation of smoking. While proponents of smoking regulation see this as regulation in the interests of health, Hockney suggests that it is more properly understood as the regulation of pleasure. He thinks that one's pleasures are no one else's business, and that the interference of the state in his pleasures is illegitimate. Its illegitimacy lies both in the extension of the reach of government outside its proper sphere, and in the transfer of personal dislikes into public policy by prigs with power, and in the colonization of the messy but beautiful world by bureaucratic tidiness in all its (unintended?) ugliness. I will return to the question of the proper reach of government later, but here I want to concentrate on the charge of priggishness.

Smoking, virtue and vice

Consider the activity of smoking itself. Is there anything we can say about it, morally, insofar as it affects only the smoker himself? Set aside for the time being the questions about possible harms to others. Conceivably, one could argue that smoking is morally praiseworthy. This would fit most naturally into a virtue ethics framework. Hockney would no doubt like us to see him as a genial fellow, who takes his pleasures where he finds them, does not impose his views or himself on others, and has sympathy for the underdog and an appreciation of the ramshackle. The opposite of a prig, in fact. And his smoking could be understood in relation to his character as a genial fellow.

The difficult part here would be in establishing whether the activity of smoking was intrinsic to his character as genial fellow, or accidental. If intrinsic, this would presumably mean that he would be less genial without his smoking, and one could inquire as to why this would be so. Most likely, it would be because he would be tenser, or more irritable, or less tolerant of the failings of others and their own particular foibles and habits. Disentangling this from the consequences of dependency on nicotine, either chemical or psychological or both, would be difficult. Evaluating the moral significance of this from a virtue ethical point of view would also require us to consider the interdependence of the virtues his smoking enables him to actuate with other virtues (such as virtues of moderation and self-denial, even-temperedness and so on). If a consequence of stopping smoking was to become less genial, then we might say that the smoking was a necessary condition for the geniality; equally, we might say that while we value the geniality, we disapprove of the irritability displayed when he is deprived of his tobacco. And this would connect the tobacco as much to a vice as to a virtue. In other words, it is not that smoking is morally praiseworthy as such, but rather that it points us to particular moral features of Hockney (and people generally) underlying the habit and practice of smoking. The same would apply to other activities, such as eating good food or drinking fine wine.

Conversely, if we take features of tobacco smoking that are intrinsic to the substance and the practice of smoking it, we do know that it is both harmful to health and addictive. It is also the case that, unlike alcohol or most foods, it is harmful even in small quantities. So we might say that smoking is morally blameworthy in itself, because it involves deliberate harm to self. While most harms to self are regarded as beyond the proper reach of law and government, at least where these harms are inflicted knowingly and voluntarily, virtue ethics and most varieties of natural law theory would hold that self-harm is immoral. However, this is also difficult to cash out in detail. Many – most? – pleasures and indeed many morally obligatory activities involve a degree of taking risk to one's own welfare. It would be difficult to distinguish consistently between smoking and other risky pleasures. Moreover, if we frame the issue in terms of self-harm, it is not clear that the argument goes through. Hockney (2007) claims that he smokes for his mental health, and if so, we could see the choice to smoke as an example of a 'health-health trade-off' (Sunstein, 1997: ch. 12). And even if it were a trading off of health against some other personal good (such as pleasure), it would not be easy to say why an adult cannot or should not choose to make this trade-off.

The addiction issue is different. From a virtue ethics point of view, it is questionable whether a self-harming behaviour that is addictive could be virtuous, even if it was contingently a condition for the exercise of some virtue in this individual, since as an addiction it would interfere with virtues of self-possession and self-control. Nonetheless, this is a fiddly argument to make out, since the connection between virtue and habit, and virtue and character trait, is complex.

Are voluntary, self-inflicted harms to health special?

One factor that may confuse us here is the connection between smoking and health. If smoking were not hazardous to health, but simply something that was pleasurable while attracting some other kind of cost – for instance, making the smoker smelly, or look ridiculous – there would be no question of paternalistic regulation. There is of course a question of ensuring that people make choices that are both genuine choices and adequately informed, especially since smoking is addictive. It may be that this is purely a question of ensuring that choice is autonomous; once that is done – if it can be – is there anything else to say? There is an interesting question to be asked about why it is health that attracts special attention in terms of (attempted) paternalistic regulation. Another way to think of this comes from the observation, frequently made, that if tobacco were to be introduced to the market today, no government would allow it to be sold. This would be because it is addictive and harmful to health, even in small quantities, and, in addition, causes harm to third parties exposed to second-hand smoke. Again, we will return to the harm to third parties arguments later. The observation we are considering here suggests that governments are keen to regulate hazards to health, including hazardous consumer goods. But this does not explain why hazards to health are particularly important to governments, nor the source of the normativity of health concerns for government. Moreover, the observation points out a feature of public policy that matters: it does not have to be consistent. We might, with hindsight, regret the introduction of tobacco smoking. But that regret does not provide a strong basis for removing tobacco smoking, if we set it against the other interests relevant in this case, in terms of the interests smokers have in smoking. The same goes for alcohol, gambling and so on. Unless there is something about health that justifies paternalistic intervention to protect it, the basis of the paternalist regulation of smoking would seem to be mere disapproval. And this would be precisely the kind of 'tyranny of the majority', which classical liberalism tried to control. As we shall see below, health hazards to third parties, considered as involuntarily incurred harms, are a justification for the regulation of smoking, but this is, if paternalistic, of a different kind to the paternalistic regulation of first-party harm–pleasure trade-offs.

Moral uncertainty and moralism

Given these difficulties in sorting out the morality of smoking insofar as it bears on the agent's own self-regarding behavior, it is reasonable to decide to set the issue aside. We might set it aside on one of the following grounds. First, we might hold that in a situation of moral uncertainty, we should withhold judgement. Second, we might decide that while there may be a moral question involved, it is not our place to decide on it as it applies to the conduct of another. Or rather, third, we may think what we like, but it would be rude to express our view when the behavior has no impact on us. To do so would be to be priggish or moralistic (Fullinwider, 2005). I feel some sympathy with Hockney confronted by the joggers in Holland Park.

None of what I have sketched here necessarily involves an appeal to respect for autonomy, first person privileged access to her preferences, or similar liberal premises. In starting off by considering the moral standing of smoking from a self-regarding point of view, I eschewed the assumption that the autonomous choices of the individual cannot be evaluated, or that personal preferences are not subject to rational or moral correction. The argument so far has led us to the point where we have a qualified defence of an autonomy principle, to the effect that taking the agent as an integrated person, and his projects and preferences in the round, we cannot form a settled judgement on the morality of smoking from a self-regarding point of view. We should leave the smoker to work out for herself whether she thinks of her smoking as a moral issue at all and, if she does, what she makes of it.

Suppose then, with Hockney, we see the citizens of England as being oppressed by a moralistic elite intent on denying them a pleasure of which there is no convincing moral ground for disapproval – so far as it affects the smoker alone. We might well think of activities such as banning smoking in enclosed public places, imposing steep taxes on tobacco products, and so on as the means by which an elite dislike or disapproval of smoking is imposed on individuals who like smoking, and groups of individuals who like smoking together, and on individuals with non-smoking friends and relatives who do not object to being in the presence of smoking. Absent good moral reason for regulating the behavior of individuals, this would be the imposition of elite preferences without justification. Even if there were good moral reason for disapproving of the conduct of smokers from a self-regarding point of view, this might not be sufficient to warrant public policy or legislation to regulate their behavior (Hart, 1963). Even if one took the view that some moralistic legislation is proper if it secures the commonly shared values in a community (Devlin, 1965), one could argue, with Hockney, that the relevant values requiring protection are those of toleration and un-priggishness.

Harms to self, the 'undeserving patient' and taxation

The public health practitioner is by now probably very impatient. The public health practitioner does not see the regulation of smoking as a matter of moral regulation, but simply as a matter of health promotion. And more importantly, even if the individual is free to go 'to hell in his own way', as Robert Frost put it, we are entitled to regulate the impact his choices have on others. We will come to the latter part of the argument in due course. But there is a residual area of concern with the conduct of the individual which would bear on the public health practitioner's interests.

We can argue that our health is our own, and that while we have a legitimate interest in controlling actions and policies of others which threaten that health, what we do to our own health is our business. Some religious believers do not accept this, holding that our lives, bodies and health are gifts from God, which we are to safeguard. Similarly, some communitarians would argue that care of our health is part of our general collection of obligations to each other in a moral community: only by maintaining ourselves in good health, so far as this lies within our power, are we able to discharge our responsibilities to the weaker members of society and to promote the common good. Neither of these lines of argument are especially widely shared at present. But it is commonly argued that someone who deliberately damages his health is less deserving of health care that could fully or partially remedy that damage to his health. The smoker is often argued to be a good illustration of this principle. Let us consider the arguments briefly.

Imagine a smoker of 60 years of age, who has advanced heart disease and would be a candidate for a heart transplant, other things being equal. One clinical approach would be to consider her for a transplant without regard to the smoking. She might be listed, or not, purely on the basis of likely chances of success and expected survival post-transplant, in the same way as any other transplant candidate. Another would be to distinguish between the smoking-related cause of the illness and the impact post-transplant smoking would have on the success of the transplant. She could be asked to agree to stop smoking as a condition of the transplant. This might be understood as a moral requirement (damaging one's donated heart or one's health could be seen as wilful self-harm or as damaging a scarce resource someone else could have benefited from), or simply as an evaluation of likely effectiveness of a transplant. She could be assigned to the transplant list with a lower priority than an equivalent non-smoker. Or she could be refused access to the list. Setting aside general issues of distributive justice in health care which concern duties to rescue, allocation by need or allocation by expected outcome, and so on, we can distinguish two claims about desert and access to treatment in this situation. The first claim is that past health behavior can affect the degree to which one deserves treatment for ill health resulting from that behavior. The second claim is that future health behavior can affect the degree to which one deserves treatment for ill health relating to that behavior. The first claim involves a claim that the behavior itself is discreditable. Most clinicians would express some discomfort about applying a retrospective judgement, perhaps because they believe it to be moralistic, or perhaps because they see it as involving a double jeopardy (you smoked, so you are ill, but because you smoked, we will not treat your illness). The second claim involves a judgement of relative desert between candidates for transplant which can be affected by the fact of smoking. This may be defensible, if the fact of continued smoking is taken on good evidence as a sign that compliance with other necessary treatment will be less likely.

Although there are some arguments which might explain offering a transplant to a smoker on conditions, or not at all, which do not depend on moral judgement of their past or present smoking, it is more plausible to say that we do judge smokers, and to consider whether this is justified. Consider two people, one our smoker just described, another a lifelong non-smoker of similar age and ill health. Both need a heart transplant and there is just one heart available. If we think the non-smoker should have the heart because he is a non-smoker, rather than because of likely success or greater life expectancy or some other more general principle of distributive justice in health care, then why is this? It may be that the smoker is somehow responsible for doing the non-smoker out of the heart, if she gets it. How would this be? It may be because we think the non-smoker would be ill anyway, whereas but for her smoking, the smoker would not be. If so, we are considering that the smoker has caused her ill health, and also that by claiming a scarce resource to restore that health, she is denying someone else that resource. So she is displacing the consequence of her behavior onto another, blameless, person. Thus, her smoking cannot be considered a purely self-regarding behavior in this context, even neglecting (as we have so far) the third party effects of smoking. This is hard to defend, however. Any allocation of a scarce resource between parties with a claim on it will involve winners and losers. The losers suffer no wrong at the hand of the winners, other things being equal. If we admit desert into our allocation scheme for health care resources, we have three problems. First, we have little settled agreement on the conception of desert that we ought to use, or what its scope may be. Second, people rarely come to allocation decisions 'clean', in the sense that everyone has some health-related habit which undermines our health to some extent, be it smoking, drinking, physical idleness, excess workplace stress, or even jogging. Adjudicating between the claims of differently 'compromised' individuals is at least difficult to do objectively. Third, we may be happy to transfer technical and professional responsibility to doctors. We are much less happy to see them as moral experts who can adjudicate between patients' differing degrees of desert.

In passing, another issue arises in connection with publicly funded health care. It is sometimes observed that the proceeds of taxation on tobacco products exceeds the costs to the National Health Service of smoking-related illness. This would require some justification. Imagine, however, that these two figures were more or less in balance. Then we could see this tax as a kind of insurance against eventual tobacco-related illness. In that case, we would have no 'scarce resource' argument for non-treatment of smokers, save as regards those resources which are scarce on non-financial grounds (such as organs for transplant). Imagine, next, that the taxation income does not cover the costs to the NHS of smoking-related illness. Then we might say that smokers deserve lesser treatment because they have not paid their way. The basis of the NHS is solidary coverage of the nation's health care costs; some pay more than they take out, others take out far more than they can contribute. What could be objected to in the case of the smoker is deliberate 'over-drawing'. Of course, the answer here would likely be to increase the duty on tobacco products, rather than to restrict smokers' access to health services. So, if smokers are 'over-contributing', does this give them special claim to health resources? This possibility becomes even more probable if one considers not only the contribution made by smokers through taxation but also the way that smokers by dying earlier than average draw less than their expected entitlement from the pensions system over their post-retirement lifetime, given that that section of their life may well be shorter than average. The main reason for taxation is not to insure smokers against the risks of their smoking, but to raise revenue for the State, to fund the NHS, and to discourage smoking. The solidary basis of NHS funding through income taxation and national insurance does not allow for special claims related to level of contribution. So as a matter of public policy smokers are not entitled to priority treatment merely because they have paid more in. What the taxation issue points out is partly that there is indeed a degree of State moralism regarding smoking, but also that the State has other reasons for wishing to discourage smoking than the regulation of individuals' self-regarding behavior (Wilkinson, 1999).

Other aspects of smoking and its regulation

The classical liberal approach to the regulation of personal behavior is to avoid doing so unless that behavior imposes harm on others without their consent. This is a superficially simple criterion, but its subtleties are quite deep. For instance, we need to know whether any harm at all should be prevented through regulation, or whether a threshold approach is needed. Some harms may be trivial in intensity or duration. Second, we need to know whether harms caused by omission or inaction are as significant as harms caused by action. Can people be obliged to act so as to prevent a harm? Third, we need to know whether the burden of regulation itself is proportionate to the harm prevented or controlled. Fourth, we need to know whether the harm prevented can be characterized objectively. For instance, liberals try to distinguish harms from nuisances or irritations; the former may well elicit a legal response, while the latter will do so only in relatively extreme circumstances. Finally, we need to know whether consent by the injured party is enough to remove government interest.

The regulation of information about smoking

Until the evidence for the impact of 'passive smoking' became conclusive, smoking could be conceived as purely a matter of harm to self, combined with potential nuisance to others. Harm to self would not normally be grounds for paternalistic intervention, as we have seen, *unless* it could be shown that this harm was unwitting in some way. Perhaps from this point of view it is the addictiveness of smoking which is more important than the harm of the activity of smoking itself – harmful though each cigarette is, it is the accumulation of harms and the difficulty of stopping which creates the most serious problems. Thus the earliest stages of smoking regulation concentrated on measures to improve or regulate information to smokers. For instance, tobacco advertising is tightly regulated or even banned. Where it is permitted, the attractive images used in advertising and branding are supplemented by striking warnings of health hazards; and information about the nicotine and tar content of tobacco products are also closely supervised. Aggressive public information campaigns about the dangers of smoking are pursued, and in many countries this negative advertising may now be the only mass media advertising of tobacco products which is permitted. This way of regulating the tobacco market achieves a number of functions. It ensures that smokers (or would-be smokers) have access to accurate information about the risks and benefits of the product they are using. It provides a constant stimulus to smokers to inspire thoughts of giving up smoking or to reinforce the will to quit among those who are trying not to take smoking up again. It provides a discouragement to those who would see smoking as something worth trying. The essential function of this information regulation is to improve the quality of consent to tobacco consumption (or its refusal), but it also seeks to make that choice less attractive, and to alter the cultural presumption in the direction of the disapproval of smoking – its de-normalization.

Now against a backdrop of a long period in which smoking was normal and acceptable, arguably because people were unaware of how dangerous smoking was to their health and that of others, this is understandable. But it is at least debatable whether actively discouraging people from smoking, and focusing messages on 'smoking is bad' rather than choices between different kinds of tobacco product or different brands of cigarette, is justifiably paternalistic. The natural response to this argument is to point out two features of tobacco marketing: first, that until tobacco advertising was regulated, people were given sometimes extremely favourable and misleading information about cigarettes and their health benefits, and that there was no debate about the paternalism in pro-advertising. Second, because smoking is addictive, the impact of addiction on the will is to undermine autonomy, so that paternalistic intervention in terms of countervailing messages is justifiable as a proportionate response to autonomy compromised by addiction (Hansson, 2005).

What cannot easily be defended is the use of informational measures to alter the context of smoking by promoting a dislike or intolerance of smoking by third parties as a means to altering the behavior of smokers. And yet it is a known feature of behavior modification that altering the climate of acceptance of a given behavior is an effective method for changing that behavior. A good example of this is in teenage health education. We can try to discourage teenagers from taking up smoking directly, through the restriction of sales and through health education. But an important means for discouraging teenage smoking is to get teenagers themselves to despise their smoking peers, for whatever reason. Questions of teenage autonomy aside, persuading a teenager that smoking is uncool affects both the self-regarding behavior of the teenager but also their other-regarding behavior. The former is presumably acceptable, the latter more difficult to justify. Of course, it may well be justified as a desirable but unintended consequence of the promotion of positive self-regarding health behaviors. But there is something questionable about using teenagers' clique-forming behavior to ostracize smokers as a method of making smoking unattractive. All of this must be taken in the context of very powerful cultural and social psychological factors disposing teenagers to smoke, from their tendency to seek risks and identify behavior disapproved of by authority figures as attractive, to the associations of smoking with other forms of teenage social life (such as attendance at performances of popular music and discotheques). What may be hard to justify on its own merits in terms of direct attempts to modify behavior and cultural attitudes needs to be seen against the background of other, no less direct, means by which behavior and culture are continually shaped with very little consideration of ethics.

Regulating smoking as a nuisance

In the period before passive smoking became a major focus of smoking regulation, a regulatory approach focused on smoking as a nuisance to others was also developed. This would include the establishment of non-smoking carriages on trains, non-smoking sections of restaurants or non-smoking rooms in hotels, and, more subtly, the gradually rising social unacceptability of 'lighting up' without asking permission and thence the gradually rising social acceptability of refusing permission. But notice that all these measures arise out of more or less explicit 'contracts' between parties, rather than formally imposed state regulation of nuisance.

Regulating smoking as a harm to others

Taking the various approaches to tobacco control we have examined so far, we see that *if* we exclude harm to others, tobacco regulation largely turns on smoking being seen as a social problem. It may be a nuisance to others, and we may be concerned about the quality of information available to those who in smoking may be more or less unwittingly harming themselves or becoming addicted, especially where the most vulnerable are those who for other reasons are imperfect decision-makers. But the appropriate response to these features of tobacco use would be better information and regulation of the marketing of tobacco, rather than regulation of its consumption. And we might retain, with David Hockney, a sense that many of the initiatives in this area do tend to present smoking as a nuisance to third parties, rather than as a pleasure to first parties, and further, to regulate that nuisance in a paternalistic way.

However, just as we could not examine smoking regulation for long without recognizing its third party effects, neither can we consider those third party effects without considering those which amount to substantial harms. Three cases are of particular importance. The first case is that of smoking in enclosed public places. The second case is that of smoking in the home. The third case is that of the impact of smoking on the unborn child.

Smoking in the workplace and in public

Smoking in enclosed public places has received a lot of attention recently as national and regional governments across the world have begun to implement bans. There are two broad kinds of justification offered. The first is harm-related; the second is public good-related. The harm-related argument focuses on harms to third parties exposed to 'second hand smoke' involuntarily. The public good-related argument focuses on the way in which smoking may degrade a public good, clean breathable air. We will return to this argument later.

Other things being equal, if person A smokes, and person B consents to being in the presence of that smoke, this releases person A from any responsibility for the harm caused to person B by that smoke. Obviously, if person B's consent is uninformed, or not truly voluntary, this would potentially invalidate the consent. It need not matter whether person B comes into contact with person A directly. If person B enters a bar, say, knowing that this is likely to be a place where smoking is permitted, then that may be sufficient to count as consent. Until recently, it may have been accepted that the most efficient way to achieve a reduction in smoking in public places was via consent. Places wishing to attract non-smokers would bar smoking, or try to restrict it to separate rooms with strong extractor fans, for instance. Places wishing to attract smokers would make no such efforts. As more people favoured smokeless environments, the market would work its magic, and gradually a pattern of facilities, shops and offices would emerge in which a small number of places would cater specifically for smokers and their friends, and while most places would exclude smoking. Some (particularly in the tobacco industry) hoped for technological innovation which would allow environments to be virtually smoke free without the noise or drafts associated with extractor fans. For whatever reason, this seems not to be a possibility at present.

This market based approach continues to attract support, but in the United Kingdom and elsewhere a more direct approach is now favoured (Royal College of Physicians, 2005). This is to impose a ban on smoking in public places. A weak argument for this might be that where one's consent is presumed upon too freely and generally, then it is not consent. Imagine a society where people are casually rude to each other in a way which is not directly and deliberately offensive, but merely betokens a sort of mild incivility. Suppose that a generation before, people were generally civil (if somewhat formal) with each other. A survivor from that generation might well mark and regret this difference. Nonetheless, they go about their business in the new world, *faute de mieux*. We can hardly say that they *consent* to this general incivility. It is more that they put up with it. Perhaps 'consent' is ambiguous here, meaning both a weak sense of agreement ('putting up with', 'going along with, possibly under protest') and a strong sense of endorsement.

A stronger argument for smoke-free public places points us to the individuals who are least likely to be giving voluntary consent to smoke exposure, who are the workforce in smoky environments, rather than the consumers who can come and go as they please. Labour markets being what they are, workforce members are relatively weak in bargaining over their conditions of employment, especially where they are in a service industry where consumer preferences are thought to be crucial. Unlike most consumers in bars, bar workers (a typical example) will be exposed to smoke all day, every day, without much say in the matter, and without control over how much they 'smoke'. It could be suggested that they could change employment, but many bar workers take this sort of work in circumstances where suitable alternative work is hard to find. Under these circumstances, one could argue that exposure to second-hand smoke is not free, and thus not consented to. And thus, the harm argument for regulating smoking to protect non-consenting third parties is able to get off the ground.

Two objections might arise here. First, one might question the level of risk being regulated. If we could, by use of fans or equivalent, lower, without eliminating, the risk to workers, would we not reach a situation in which the exposure to the hazard of smoking is analogous to other, less regulated workplace hazards? Why should we adopt a zero tolerance approach to exposure to workplace smoke, but not to other hazards? Second, one could argue about the proportionality of the regulatory response. While some smoky dive bars are definitely hazardous to health, a large well-ventilated modern office block does not present the same exposure, given the relatively small number of office workers who now smoke. It is accepted that some workplaces (such as prisons and psychiatric hospitals) are exceptions to regulations, since their inmates are not free to move around. But surely the workers in these workplaces are just as deserving of protection as bar workers?

Objections like these, which have some merit on the face of it, direct us to two features of public policy. The first is that public policy will be framed partly with an eye to simplicity and enforceability. A simple ban with limited exceptions is much easier to enforce (and much fairer, since clear to all regulated under it) than a complex ban. The second is that consistency is not a necessary component of public policy. That there may be other less well regulated workplace hazards does not justify regulating workplace smoke exposure more loosely – it just means that they may well be subject to different balancing exercises, or be candidates for further regulation in their turn in future. Of course, it may well be that there are wider objectives behind a ban than simply regulating harm to third parties. For public health minded policy makers, reducing smoking in the name of protecting non-smokers has the likely useful consequence of reducing smoking by smokers. It is probably accepted that this is not an appropriate goal of non-paternalistic anti-smoking policy, but no public health policy maker is going to regret this 'unintended consequence'.

Smoking in the home and during pregnancy

From the point of view of protecting the vulnerable third party, it is possible to argue that regulating the smoky workplace is a less important task than that of protecting young children in the home. While spouses and partners of smokers can have their own ways of persuading smokers to quit, or to regulate their behavior, or can be considered to consent, children may have relatively little influence, and can be particularly vulnerable both to the health effects of passive smoking and to taking up smoking. However, what measures could be applied to regulate smoking in the home? A range of methods could be used at the draconian end of the spectrum: it is not true, as is sometimes thought, that the home is a sacrosanct place, where the reach of the law does not run. One could criminalize smoking, and then carry out raids on homes where smoking was suspected; one could take children of recalcitrant smokers into care or make smoking into grounds for assignment of custody in divorce cases to the non-smoking parent. However, we have to ask whether these methods are proportionate in their response to the risks of smoking, respect other important principles such as the human right to a private and family life, and are in any event effective in reducing smoking in the home. Similar arguments apply, with even more force, to the case of smoking during pregnancy (by the expectant mother or by her co-resident family members). There is a strong moral appeal that can be made not to risk harm to vulnerable others, but given other ethical and policy arguments in support of women's autonomy and bodily privacy, it is unlikely that an argument for compelling smoking-cessation (through criminal or civil law remedies) could be successfully mounted.

New directions in the debates on ethics and smoking

Three recent debates are of particular note. The first, mentioned above, is a new approach to arguing for the control of smoking which focuses not on harm but on the protection of a public good (Smith et al., 2003). A public good may be defined as a good which is non-excludable (that is, anyone can use it) and non-rival in consumption (that is, my use of it does not diminish its quantity or availability to you). The standard example is clean, breathable air. Public goods may be destroyed, however. Again, consider clean air. A release of toxic gas into the atmosphere would significantly degrade the air quality. Public goods have interesting properties for the economist. In particular, because anyone can use them, it is in no one's personal interest to pay for them, or to preserve them. Hence there is a need for state action to provide or secure them as public. If we consider tobacco smoke as a noxious degrading of clean air, harmful to all, but not consented to by all, then we can mount an argument for the regulation of smoking that is not based on unconsented harm to identifiable third parties. Recently public health practitioners have suggested that not only is smoke-free air a public good, so is tobacco control itself (Smith *et al.*, 2003). Whatever the merits of the clean air argument, this seems to go too far in confusing means and end. We do not 'enjoy' tobacco control the way we enjoy clean air or an environment relatively hazardless to health.

An alternative public good approach would be to say that the good is not the smoke-free environment, but rather an environment free from inducements to harm oneself or others. Given that smoking is addictive, we would enjoy an environment that lacks both inducements to smoke and signals that smoking is possible or even desirable (thus protecting non-smokers from the hazard that they may take it up) and triggers that would provoke recidivism among 'recovering' smokers. Similarly, we might say that the good we enjoy is public health itself – as we all benefit indirectly from the health of others as well as directly from our own health. These proposals are more plausible than the 'clean air as public good' proposal, but it seems to me to be a straining of language to consider this a 'good', even a 'public good'. Rather, we might say that we value this sort of environment, and that we assent to the sort of soft paternalism it involves.

In any case, public good arguments are difficult to apply in practice, partly because we cannot easily perform trade-offs between public goods, or between public and private goods. For example, Hockney would perhaps agree to see toleration (of smoking) as a public good. How do we decide which public good is more important to us? A consequentialist argument would presumably be relatively easy to construct, either on general welfare principles, or more narrowly on health-related welfare principles, but consequentialist arguments are relatively difficult to dovetail with rights-respecting liberalism. And even on strict consequentialist grounds, it is far from clear that a Hockney-type utility function could not be constructed that traded present pleasure against future ill health and shortened life span in a way which favoured present pleasure. Psychologists of risk have indeed shown how people do seem to carry out this trade-off in respect of their smoking behaviours (Slovic, 2001).

A second debate of importance concerns the availability of tobacco products that are primarily aimed at making stopping smoking easier. There has been a long-standing debate over the tobacco industry's proposals to market 'safer' products, from lower tar cigarettes, to smokeless cigarettes, to alternative ways to consume tobacco (such as Swedish snus). There has been a tendency in the tobacco control movement to argue that there is no such thing as a 'safe' tobacco product, although this is not uniformly agreed internal to that movement (Kozlowski and Edwards, 2005). Recently, new tobacco-derived products designed as medically supervised substitutes for smoking have been widely adopted, such as nicotine patches. The current debate concerns whether these should be much more widely available, as over-the-counter pharmacy products, or subject to lighter taxation than smoking tobacco. The ethical issues here largely turn on standard concerns in the ethics of harm reduction: do 'safer' products provide a gateway to riskier products, or slow down smokers attempts to move to complete cessation, or communicate that message that safe smoking may be possible? One approach, which may be feasible, is to regulate the market in tobacco products in a more comprehensive way, in the name of public health and safety

(Royal College of Physicians, 2002). This approach would need to be underpinned by an ethical framework that would justify both the continued manufacture and sale of a harmful and addictive product range, and the concentration on tobacco in contrast to other similar harmful products, such as alcohol (Fox, 2005). This is a consistent problem for advocates of harm reduction: while harm reduction proponents see what they propose as ethically necessary, they are consistently attacked by tougher minded public health and public policy people for 'condoning' the vice or wrong they are nominally trying to alleviate and remove (Royal College of Physicians, 2007).

The third current debate concerns health inequalities. It is well known that smoking prevalence is higher in poorer socio-economic groups, and that there is a linear relationship between economic wealth or income and life expectancy and health status, and an inverse linear relationship between economic wealth or income and smoking prevalence. If we are concerned not only with individual liberty and harm prevention or reduction, but also with equality, then the liberal approach I have broadly supported in this chapter is inadequate unless supplemented with egalitarian principles. This is even more obvious when one notes the role of direct taxation in tobacco control and the further fact about the 'inverse care law' in access to health care by poorer people. Whole access to health care can be improved by committing resources to reversing or removing inequalities in access to health care, the measures that could be taken to reduce smoking rates in poorer socio-economic groups will, on the one hand, perhaps diminish inequalities in health but, on the other hand, impose more severe burdens on just those people as they make (or fail to make) the transition to being non-smokers. This is an area that merits detailed investigation by ethicists and policy makers.

Conclusion

As we have seen, tobacco smoking provokes heated and complex debates, and in part this is because while there is a public health consensus about the need to control tobacco use, and prevent the very large number of preventable deaths and illness related to its use, there is not a wider social consensus about seeing tobacco use as *primarily* a public health problem. While many democratic states are willing to construct a political and legislative consensus around controlling smoking in public places, especially as the prevalence of smoking continues to decline, there is a residual concern, even among non-smokers, about the moralism that sometimes accompanies tobacco control efforts. While this chapter has done little more than sketch the main issues, I hope the overall message – that smoking is an important hazard to health, and that controlling it in the interests of the unconsenting and vulnerable is important – is clear. One topic has been given what I accept is quite inadequate discussion, viz. the nature of smoking as addictive. In my defence, I have tried to concentrate on what is distinctive to smoking, and the arguments presented here should be complemented with more general arguments about the regulation of addictive products and practices (including gambling, drinking, overeating, taking addictive psychoactive substances, and perhaps other activities including the use of pornography, abuse of consumer credit and so on). What is not clear is the wider issue of how we reconcile the public health's laudable concern with health with other social interests. And this is a problem that will reappear again and again as problems such as obesity, teenage pregnancy and workplace stress are framed as health problems (Cribb, 2005; Rose, 2007).

References

Boyle, P., Gray, N., Henningfield, J., Seffrin J. and Zatonski, W. (eds) (2004) *Tobacco: Science, Policy and Public Health*. Oxford: Oxford University Press.

Cribb, A. (2005) *Health and the Good Society: Setting Healthcare Ethics in Social Context*. Oxford: Oxford University Press.

Devlin, P. (1965) *The Enforcement of Morals*. Oxford: Oxford University Press.

Fox, B. J. (2005) Framing tobacco control efforts within an ethical context. *Tobacco Control*, 14(Suppl. 2), 38–44.

Fullinwider, R. K. (2005) On moralism. *Journal of Applied Philosophy*, 22(2): 105–20.

Hansson, S. O. (2005) Extended antipaternalism. *Journal of Medical Ethics*, **31**: 97–100.

Hart, H. L. A. (1963) *Law, Liberty and Morality*. Oxford: Oxford University Press.

Hockney, D. (2004) Smoking is my choice. *Guardian*, 1 June.

Hockney, D. (2006) A letter from David Hockney. *Guardian*, 25 February.

Hockney, D. (2007) I smoke for my mental health. *Guardian*, 15 May.

Kozlowski, L. T. and Edwards, B. Q. (2005) 'Not safe' is not enough: smokers have a right to know more than that there is no safe tobacco product. *Tobacco Control*, 14(Suppl. 2), 3–7.

Rose, N. (2007) *The Politics of Life Itself: Biomedicine, Power and Subjectivity in the Twenty-First Century*. Princeton, NJ: Princeton University Press.

Royal College of Physicians (2002) *Protecting Smokers, Saving Lives: The Case for a Tobacco and Nicotine Regulatory Authority*. London: Royal College of Physicians.

Royal College of Physicians (2005) *Going Smoke-Free: The Medical Case for Clean Air in the Home, at Work, and in Public Places*. London: Royal College of Physicians.

Royal College of Physicians (2007) *Harm Reduction in Nicotine Addiction: Helping People Who Can't Quit*. London: Royal College of Physicians.

Slovic, P. (ed.) (2001) *Smoking: Risk, Perception and Public Policy*. Thousand Oaks, CA: Sage.

Smith, R., Beaglehole, R., Woodward, D. and Drager, N. (eds) (2003) *Global Public Goods for Health: Health Economic and Public Health Perspectives*. New York: Oxford University Press.

Sunstein, C. R. (1997) *Free Markets and Social Justice*. New York: Oxford University Press.

Wilkinson, S. (1999) Smokers' rights to health care: why the 'restoration argument' is a moralising wolf in a liberal sheep's clothing. *Journal of Applied Philosophy*, **16**: 275–89.

Further relevant literature

Caan, W. and De Belleroche, J. (eds) (2002) *Drink, Drugs and Dependence: From Science to Clinical Practice*. London: Routledge.

Elster, J. and Skog, O.-J. (eds) (1999) *Getting Hooked: Rationality and Addiction*. Cambridge: Cambridge University Press.

Feinberg, J. (1984–1988) *The Moral Limits of the Criminal Law* (4 vols) New York: Oxford University Press.

Feinberg, J. (1991) Review of Robert Goodin: *No Smoking. Bioethics*, **5**: 150–7.

Fox, B. J. and Katz, J. E. (eds) (2005) Individual and human rights in tobacco control. *Tobacco Control*, 14(Suppl. 2): 1–49.

Goodin, R. E. (1989) *No Smoking: The Ethical Issues*. Chicago, IL: University of Chicago Press.

Hall, W., Carter, L. and Morley, K. I. (2004) Neuroscience research on the addictions: a prospectus for future ethical and policy analysis. *Addiction*, **29**: 1481–95.

House of Commons Health Committee (2006) *Smoking in Public Places; First Report of Session 2005–2006* (3 vols). London: The Stationery Office.

Husak, D. N. (1992) *Drugs and Rights*. Cambridge: Cambridge University Press.

Mill, J. S. (1989) *On Liberty and Other Writings*, ed. S. Collini. Cambridge: Cambridge University Press.

Pope, T. M. (2000) Balancing public health against individual liberty: the ethics of smoking regulations. *University of Pittsburgh Law Review*, **61**: 419–98.

Royal College of Physicians (2000) *Nicotine Addiction in Britain*. London: Royal College of Physicians.

Scruton, R. (2000) *WHO, What and Why? Transnational Government, Legitimacy and the World Health Organization*. London: Institute of Economic Affairs.

Skrabanek, P. (1994) *The Death of Humane Medicine and the Rise of Coercive Healthism*. London: Social Affairs Unit.

Verweij, M. (2000) *Preventive Medicine: Between Obligation and Aspiration*. Amsterdam: Kluwer Academic.

Verweij, M. (2007) Tobacco discouragement: a non-paternalistic argument. In *Ethics, Prevention and Public Health*, ed. A. Dawson and M. Verweij. Oxford: Oxford University Press, pp. 179–97.

Wilson, N. and Thomson, G. (2005) Tobacco taxation and public health: ethical problems, policy responses. *Social Science and Medicine*, **61**: 649–59.

Chapter

6

Infectious disease control

Marcel Verweij

Introduction

Infectious diseases have been one of the major factors affecting public health in the past, and will probably remain so in the future. There was a time that physicians thought that, at some point in the future, the perils of infectious diseases would have been overcome. In the middle part of the twentieth century, progress was made in controlling diseases such as smallpox, measles, typhoid and plague. Better diet and hygiene, improved living conditions and vaccinations all helped to strengthen people's immunity against several diseases. Patients who got ill could be treated effectively with antibiotics. Morbidity and mortality due to several infectious diseases decreased significantly. However, this success story has had its limits: advances in medicine and public health have mainly benefited the developed world, whereas infectious diseases in the developing world have remained high; new viruses such as HIV and SARS have created new problems in both high- and low-income contexts; extreme multi-drug resistant forms of tuberculosis are spreading, especially among people living with HIV and AIDS; and, lastly, at the beginning of the twenty-first century, many countries and the World Health Organization started preparations for an influenza pandemic that could in the future be reminiscent of the 1918 Spanish Flu.

Medical treatment of patients with clinical symptoms is only one and probably not the most important way to control infectious diseases. The spread of disease can be reduced most effectively by controlling infection, for example by improving hygiene, by social distancing or quarantine, by raising immunity, etc. Many of these interventions require collaborative 'public' action (Verweij and Dawson, 2007). If human contact is a source for infection, then preventive measures must aim at reducing or even prohibiting such contacts. However, such measures can have negative if not detrimental consequences for some. Measures of control may involve excluding some individuals or groups *from* public life. This chapter discusses various examples of measures to protect public health against infectious diseases. The focus will be on contagious disease that spreads from human to human, because controlling measures against such diseases can have a deep impact on personal life and well-being. Moreover, such controlling measures are often compulsory and set constraints on the liberties of individuals or groups. The largest part of the ethical discussion in this chapter will focus on the justifications for such compulsory interventions.

Protection against animal diseases (including avian influenza), food-borne diseases (for example, salmonella) and non-contagious diseases (for example, tetanus) also raise moral questions but these will not be discussed.

Historic examples

The phrase 'social distancing' as a measure to prevent infection is a relatively new term, but it has been practised throughout history; as long as it has been known that certain diseases are contagious. People have always tried to protect themselves and others by setting patients with particular diseases 'apart', and excluding them from the rest of society. People with suspected symptoms of a disease could be treated as outcasts or outlaws, or sent to a closed institution, such as a leprosarium. History provides numerous examples that illustrate how such measures could be harmful and unjust to the victims of disease. Saul Brody describes how in the Middle Ages, leprosy patients – or at least persons who were thought to have this disease – were cast out of society. The first step would be to detect suspected lepers. They were then presented to special committees of 'experts' with the job of making a diagnosis. This physical examination might be carried out by doctors and surgeons, or often certain laypersons, such as gate porters, policemen, priests, monks or even other lepers (Brody, 1974: 63–4).

There must have been a considerable risk that diseases were misclassified: any skin disease or abnormality could be seen as a form of leprosy. If a person was judged to be a leper, the victim was told that he would be separated from the healthy population. The law could be very hostile to lepers, and for many, the leprosarium might even be a relatively save haven:

> In brief, the law could place a person outside of society by depriving him of his rights to marry or to stay married, and to own and transmit property. It could simply and effectively deprive the leper of the right to have a home, and that being so, it could compel him to depend upon the very society which, out of loathing and fear, wrote those laws. Under such circumstances, the best the leper could do would be to turn from the world and enter the closed society of the leprosarium. There, at least, he would have a bed and food. The prison could also be a refuge.
>
> (Brody, 1974: 86)

This may sound like ending the social life of a person, and actually it was meant to be so: the diagnosis of leprosy could be a reason for authorities to officially declare that the victim was now judged socially dead. The church played an important role, providing symbols and rituals that were similar to those of a funeral. A mass was held for the leper, who at some places was required to stand in a grave in a cemetery. The officiating priest would throw some earth from the grave over the victim's head, explaining that this symbolized the death of the leper to the world. As harsh as this may sound, the fear of leprosy sometimes led some to enact even more drastic measures. For example, Henry II of England, as well as Philip V of France,

> . . . chose to replace the religious service with a simple civil ceremony. It consisted of strapping the leper to a post and setting him afire. [Edward I of England] adhered a trifle more closely to the letter of the ecumenical decree. Lepers, during his reign, were permitted the comforts of a Christian funeral. They were led down to the cemetery and buried alive.
>
> (Roueché, 1953: 117)

Leprosy is a devastating and mutilating disease, which explains the phobia-like responses to lepers throughout history. However, despite this fear, leprosy was not a disease that disrupted cities or the whole of society like some epidemics of other infectious diseases. For example, the various pandemics of bubonic plague could easily destroy city life in a short time, as the panic accompanying such disasters must have been immense. The Great Plague of 1665 killed almost one-third of the inhabitants of London who did not flee

(Moote and Moote, 2004). Whole families passed away. People would become ill and die on the same day. Inevitably, such panic could lead to drastic measures. Houses of patients could be sealed until the victims either recovered or died. Guards were posted at the door to see that no one got out. The guard had to be bribed to allow any food to pass to the inmates. If patients were not isolated at home but sent to a plague house, they did not only face the dangers of the plague itself, as unconscious patients were easily confused for those who were deceased and taken to the cemetery. Although some authorities advised against burying corpses for 24 hours after death, the fear of infection stimulated caregivers to bury victims as soon as possible (Noordegraaf and Valk, 1988: 104). If a patient recovered from the disease, he or she could still be considered dangerous. Like other suspected persons, they were often required to walk with a white stick, thus motivating others to avoid them (Noordegraaf and Valk, 1988: 103).

In order to prevent spread of the plague in 1347, the city of Venice and other cities proclaimed quarantine measures for ships coming from infected areas. Such ships and their crew were isolated initially for 30, later for 40 days (*quaranti giorni*). People who did not develop symptoms of the disease were released after this period and allowed to enter the city (Biraben, 1976: 173–5). The quarantine rules thus went beyond isolating patients from healthy persons: all persons on a ship coming from a suspect area were sent to quarantine. In theory, these measures could protect cities against incoming disease, but they involved clear risks for those held in quarantine: if someone among them became ill, all ran the risk of being infected. Some may have tried to escape from quarantine, but they would then face other risks: violations of the quarantine orders could be punished with the death penalty.

Another classic example of isolation and restriction of liberties is the story of 'Typhoid Mary' (Porter, 1997: 424–5; Wald, 1997). Between 1900 and 1907 Mary Mallon was a cook in New York. Twenty-two people for whom she cooked or cared for developed typhoid fever. Mallon remained healthy, but she was suspected and later identified to be a carrier of the disease. Understandably, she could not grasp that she had caused all the cases of disease, not having been ill herself. Mary Mallon was isolated against her will in a hospital on North Brother Island in 1907. In 1910 the public health authorities released her, on condition that she would refrain from taking up her job as a cook. Unfortunately, in 1915 she did return to cooking, accepting a job in the Sloane Hospital for Women. Twenty-five people developed typhoid fever and two of them died. Again Mallon was identified as the vector, and this time she was sent into quarantine for life. She died in 1938, after having been quarantined for 26 years of her life.

Mary Mallon's case is especially interesting from an ethical perspective, because she was not only restricted in her liberties (apparently for good reasons) but also held personally responsible for the spread of disease. Public health officials possibly contributed to this accusation, naming her 'Typhoid Mary' in their medical publications. Later newspaper articles showed cartoons of Mallon adding small skulls in a frying pan (*The New York American*, 20 June 1909). For the public it might have been difficult not to see her as an evil cook who poisoned her employers and clients.

Measures of infectious disease control

The life of Mary Mallon illustrates how public health authorities can have the power to restrict people's individual liberties. Effective infectious disease control may require a large number of coordinated measures, from surveillance to notification, restricting traffic to mandatory isolation or even compulsory medical treatment. Let me review various measures briefly, with an eye on the values and rights that are at stake. As will become clear, the impact of such public health interventions on individual well being and freedom can be immense. After this brief inventory of various measures and their implications, I will discuss the moral justification of restrictions to freedom in more detail.

Surveillance, screening and notification

Most preventive measures will only be effective if enacted in a timely manner. A good surveillance mechanism is therefore indispensable. This involves acquiring data about infectious diseases – including personal information about individual human beings. In most, if not all countries, physicians and medical laboratories are legally required to notify public health authorities if they find cases of specific infectious diseases. For several diseases an anonymous report may be sufficient, but for many others it will be necessary to mention the diagnosis together with the patient's name and address. This is in contrast to the general requirement to maintain confidentiality, central to Hippocratic as well as modern medicine.

However, such notification procedures for identified and diagnosed cases will not be sufficient as a means of surveillance within a population context. Surveillance and control of infection may be more effective if healthy people are tested on a large scale. For example, in the Netherlands and many other countries, pregnant women are tested for HIV and Hepatitis B on a routine basis. Similar practices exist for other diseases, including tuberculosis. In some contexts people may have the right to 'opt out' if they do not want to be tested, but in other contexts or countries it may be practically difficult or even legally impossible to refuse a test. Hence such interventions result in restrictions to the rights to autonomy and bodily integrity, and moral rules that govern normal medical practice, such as voluntary informed consent, on the grounds of protecting the public health. Other ethical issues arise if these tests and their results can have negative effects on the well-being of the persons involved. For example, a positive HIV-test might make it difficult for someone to acquire health care insurance or life insurance; it could lead to stigmatization or even social rejection. These disadvantages may sometimes outweigh possible benefits of the test result, such as timely access to antiviral treatment. Routine test policies especially raise ethical issues in low-income contexts, where there may be insufficient access to health care. In such a case, test subjects may be informed that they have a disease, but left without the treatment they need. This may for example happen in countries in which HIV is endemic: routine testing for HIV exists, but antiretroviral treatment may not be available for those who test positive (Rennie and Behets, 2006). If there are many reasons for individuals to forego testing, then routine tests in a health care setting may also have drawbacks from a public health perspective. People who feel ill may decide to abstain from seeking medical care or postpone their visit to a clinic. This is not only undesirable for the person herself: if the person is pregnant, or if she suffers from an infectious disease, then it might be harmful to others if she does not seek medical care in time.

Screening procedures can also be applied at airports, seaports or other places open to international traffic. During the SARS outbreak in 2003, countries required inbound and outbound airport passengers to have their bodily temperature taken, with the aim of detecting those infected and so stop further spread of the disease. One of the problems for any screening programme is that tests and procedures can be imprecise. Test results can therefore be unreliable as an indication of disease. Where there is a case of an alarming outbreak of a highly infectious disease, screening of travellers should not 'miss' cases. However, if tests are made very sensitive – hence minimizing the risk that cases are missed (false-negatives) – this will inevitably lead to large numbers of false-positive test results. Consequently, many passengers will need to undergo further examination and tests before they can be allowed to continue on their journey.

Measures after cases have been found: contact-tracing and further testing

If a case of a contagious disease has been confirmed there may be reason to trace people who have been in contact with the index-patient. The necessity and urgency of contact-tracing, as well as the way to do it, will differ for various diseases. A disease like tuberculosis spreads easily in the right conditions. Contact-tracing may involve mobilizing whole communities to test family members, neighbours, colleagues or classmates; or, alternatively, warning the public that everyone who has been at a specific place at a specific time (for example, a shopping centre or cinema) should report to the health authorities and have themselves tested. One problem with such a strategy is that it may raise panic and fear. In some cases however, the commotion and concerns, or even fear, that are part of panic, may be justified. More important moral issues occur if such panic arises where the name of the index-patient is known to the public. If they are in fear of infection, people may easily confuse natural causes and transmission with culpability and responsibility, thereby stigmatizing and possibly harming the initial victim of the disease. Contact-tracing and screening programmes should therefore protect privacy where possible.

Somewhat different problems of privacy and confidentiality arise if public health professionals try to trace and notify contacts of people with a sexually transmitted disease. The natural way to do this is to ask the index-patient to contact his or her sex partners, as it will be difficult for public health nurses to trace contacts without the index-patient's cooperation. However, for most people, sex is a private matter, and if a patient does not want to cooperate, or contact the partners him/herself, further attempts to trace contacts will be futile. In some cases however, a physician or public health professional may have good reason to consider traceable individuals to be at risk. One typical example is where a physician is treating a person with syphilis and knows that the patient's spouse is not aware of the diagnosis. On the one hand, the physician could protect the spouse by warning them about the patient's condition, but, on the other hand, the physician has an obligation of confidentiality towards their patient. Some would argue that a patient who deceives their spouse and refuses to warn them about the risk they run, forfeits all rights to confidentiality. However, for public health physicians working on sexually transmitted diseases, the importance of confidentiality goes beyond the right of the individual patient. For infectious disease control to be effective, the public should be able to trust public health authorities to keep their personal health information confidential. This holds especially for prevention and treatment of sexually transmitted diseases. STD clinics will be most effective if patients can trust that their private details and stories are held confidential. If confidentiality is not respected in public health, many patients with infectious diseases may postpone or even forego visiting a STD clinic. Confidentiality has its limits, but partner notification without consent, as a measure of infectious disease control, may only be justified in exceptional cases.[1]

Public health measures: reducing contacts, quarantine and isolation

An important part of infectious disease control is to prevent further spread of disease during an outbreak. This is especially true for respiratory infections like influenza, where coughing, sneezing or talking are important means of transmission, as it makes sense to limit the number of contacts between healthy people, and to avoid large group meetings or other risk situations. In an outbreak, public health authorities may decide to cancel fairs, football matches, to close schools, crèches, companies or shops. Again this will be a clear – but sometimes necessary – restriction of liberties for many people, but moreover, these measures will have significant impact on their daily life, as well as on their financial resources or their property. For example, the closing of factories, offices and shops and cancelling of mass-events will involve financial burdens for companies and citizens. Employees may run the risk of losing their job if their place of work is closed for a long time. Such burdens will be faced particularly severely by vulnerable groups who are social-economically worse-off, for example employees with temporary jobs or no contracts at all. If certain groups of people run risks and bear significant extra costs due to public health measures, the question arises whether they would have a justified claim to receiving compensation for their losses. Government-based compensation schemes can be considered as an expression of solidarity: if there is a public health threat then all citizens should be willing to share in the costs of protective measures – after all, if such measures are effective then everyone will benefit.

Compensation schemes are also an important issue for containment of animal diseases such as avian influenza. Livestock have, throughout time, played an important role in the spread and transmission of many human infectious diseases. Nowadays, outbreaks in livestock are often countered by mass culling of all animals that have either been exposed to the disease or even all animals within a particular distance of confirmed cases. Compensation schemes may not only be a matter of justice and solidarity; they can also serve a pragmatic role in maintaining surveillance. Few farmers may be willing to report disease in their livestock early on in an outbreak, if they face having their animals culled without compensation. Compensation schemes may thus support surveillance programmes, which are essential to any timely and effective response to an outbreak of infectious diseases.

From an ethical point of view, the most appalling public health measures are quarantine and isolation of persons. Both concepts are used for the same sort of measures, but it makes sense to distinguish them in a way that is morally relevant. Gostin defines isolation as the physical separation and confinement of an individual or group of individuals who are known to be infected with a contagious disease from non-isolated individuals, to prevent or

---

[1] Such a breach of confidentiality may be justified more often in the practice of individual health care. One such case would be where a health care provider, for example, a family physician, is caring for a patient who has a sexually transmitted disease and who refuses to tell their spouse, and where the physician also has a caring relationship with the spouse. The patient's refusal would make it impossible for the physician to sustain a fiduciary relationship with their other client.

limit the transmission of the disease to non-isolated individuals (Gostin, 2000: 210). Quarantine also involves separation, but this applies to *healthy* individuals or groups who may have been exposed to a contagious or possibly contagious disease. Both isolation and quarantine measures can be applied to large groups. As was illustrated in the historical examples given above, extreme forms of isolation or quarantine may be similar to putting individuals in jail, excluding them from public life completely – possibly for the rest of their lives. Even if the means of separations are less severe, the impact on personal life may be overwhelming, as it combines most of the adverse events that arise in all other public health measures. Isolation and quarantine effectively make it impossible for individuals to continue their lives as planned, to fulfil their jobs and responsibilities, to earn their living, to see and care for their loved ones. The separation of persons also has an important symbolic dimension. Individuals or groups are labelled as dangerous, which could undermine their sense of being part of a community. Being separated from the community, there is a risk that isolated and quarantined groups will not have sufficient access to such basic needs as food or health care. In short, all quarantined and isolated individuals are deprived of at least some essential sources for well-being. Moreover, quarantine measures may mean that all suspected persons are held together: this includes persons who are in fact exposed to the disease and may get ill in the short term, as well as those who are only believed to be exposed but are in fact not infected. The non-infected persons may be detained with people who may infect them. In this way, quarantine procedures, while intended to reduce the risks of contagion within the larger population, may actually increase the risk for (at least part of) the quarantined population.

It is clear that isolation and quarantine procedures can have extremely adverse implications for individuals and that procedures should be applied with due care. In the last few decades, much work has been done to develop procedures and regulations in such a way that risks for quarantined persons are minimized, and that they at least have rights to due process that protect citizens from arbitrary detention. However, even if these measures are applied with due care, they remain morally problematic and require a strong moral justification. Before turning to this issue, let me briefly discuss a last category of measures of infectious disease control.

Mandatory medical treatment

Surveillance, routine testing and quarantine procedures may only have limited effects if infected patients are not treated against their disease. Medical treatment of infectious diseases is not only beneficial (if not necessary) for the patient himself, it will also be essential to prevent further infections of others. Hence, the availability of, and compliance with, antibiotic or antiviral treatment is not only an issue of individual health care but of public health. One of the most frequent contexts for compulsory treatment is tuberculosis control. Antibiotic treatment for tuberculosis may take up to 6 months in 'normal' cases, and 24 months in cases of multi-drug resistant forms of tuberculosis. Completion of therapy is not only necessary to result in a cure, and to take away the risk of infection, but also to prevent the development of drug resistant forms of tuberculosis. However, many patients may decide to stop treatment as soon as they feel better. Adherence to therapy may be particularly difficult for persons who belong to marginalized groups such as the homeless or drug abusers. Hence, various strategies have been developed to promote adherence to therapy. Apart from voluntary schemes, there are also compulsory options.

A common approach to ensure adherence to treatment is directly observed therapy (DOT): patients are monitored to ensure they take their drugs, at least for a certain period. DOT as such may not be compulsory, although it does impose restrictions upon a patient's freedom. Yet if this approach is not successful, for example, because a patient does not come to the physician to receive treatment, public health officials may consider compulsory detention for the duration of the treatment (Lerner, 1999). The combination of detention with compulsory treatment is a step further than 'just' isolation of patients, as it involves a violation of bodily integrity and the right to refuse treatment – rights that are central in modern health care practices in Western societies. However, the right to refuse treatment and the rules of informed consent may be primarily relevant for medical decisions about patient care, where the benefits and harms of treatment and non-treatment primarily concern the patient herself. If patients with infectious diseases neglect the treatment they need, this could have harmful implications for others, and that may be reason to overrule the requirements of informed consent.

Just as in the case of isolation and quarantine, it is reasonable to install requirements of due process, in order to protect patients from unnecessary restriction upon their freedom. Diseases like tuberculosis are often most prevalent among the marginalized in society, and detention (sometimes even in gaol) may reflect social prejudice rather than just public health concerns. Public health officials should not simply assume that patients who belong to certain risk groups (for example, intravenous drug abusers) can only be treated if they are detained.

Well-being and freedom

All these measures for infectious disease control involve a tension between the importance of protecting public health, and the liberty and interests of individual people (patients, infected persons, possibly infected persons) whose freedom may be curtailed in the name of public health. Let me review in more detail the main values at stake, well-being and freedom, before discussing possible ways to justify compulsory measures.

First of all, most interventions, especially when compulsory, curtail the freedom to move, to travel, to meet persons one wants to meet, etc. Although such liberties are of intrinsic value themselves, restrictions will especially be problematic where they deprive people of certain important sources of well-being. For example, restrictions upon travelling may effectively make it impossible for people to go to work, to earn their living, or to sustain their business. The financial burdens of such forms of control on individuals and companies may be immense. The losses due to public health constraints, however, go far beyond economical and financial burdens. Quarantine measures and travel restrictions may prevent people from seeing their loved ones, or caring for their children, parents or friends. Many people who are less independent may face significant risks to their health if caregivers cannot come and help them. The possibly infected people held in quarantine with others may run a significantly higher risk of becoming a victim of the disease because they are held together with others who are in fact infectious. Moreover, if certain groups of people are 'set aside' because they are considered to be a (potential) risk to the rest of the community, this may have an enormous impact on how they are viewed by that community. From a moral point of view these groups are innocent; from a medical point of view they may be a source of infection – hence potentially dangerous. In the process of stigmatization that goes with outbreaks of contagious diseases, medical and moral judgments may get easily confused. As a result, diagnosed patients or suspected persons may be systematically avoided and have their interests neglected. In short, while public health measures, from screening to quarantine, are aimed at protecting the health and welfare of the public, such measures inevitably will have negative if not detrimental effects on the well-being of certain sub-groups.

Second, even apart from the impact on human well-being, the constraints on liberty and individual rights are morally controversial as such. Measures of infectious disease control may force people to behave in specific ways, hence curtailing their freedom of choice and movement. Surveillance and notification policies may be considered a violation of rights to privacy and confidentiality; and compulsory vaccinations and treatment violate moral rights to bodily integrity. A central idea behind these values is that individual persons are capable of reasoning, making choices and determining the course of their lives – and that these capacities are grounds for respecting persons and the choices they make. In a liberal society where individual rights are considered of utmost importance, the possibilities to curtail or overrule those rights should therefore be limited. One should treat persons with respect: that is, treat them as ends in themselves, and not *merely* as means to or obstructing factors for the realization of other ends – however worthwhile aims such as the protection of health might be. They are autonomous beings, that is, beings with practical reason, who can and do set their own ends. Rules of informed consent – as common as they are in individual health care – are often seen as especially important in protecting autonomy. The ideal route for infectious diseases control is therefore to inform persons about necessary precautions (to have themselves screened, to isolate themselves, to accept treatment, etc.) and to trust that they will act accordingly. However, the circumstances of infectious diseases control, and especially outbreak management, are far from ideal. Infectious diseases may raise panic, and people may distrust government institutions, and therefore refuse to cooperate. Moreover, while measures of infectious disease control are aiming at protecting the health of the many, they will often impose risks on individual persons. Hence, for these individuals it could be most rational to refuse to cooperate, and to avoid tests, quarantine or vaccination. In such circumstances, compulsory measures may be inevitable to prevent spread of disease. Which moral grounds could provide justification for such infringements on individual rights and freedom?

The harm principle

Even ethical theories that see individual rights and especially liberty rights as the strongest possible moral claims – as trumps vis-à-vis other moral considerations such as the common good – will necessarily acknowledge limits to those rights. If people use their freedom to harm others or otherwise impose their will on another person, then the freedom of the aggressor is undermining the freedom of others. Any liberal framework that endorses freedom or autonomy as an important value will therefore accept that someone's freedom must be curtailed if this is necessary to protect the freedom of other persons. Ideally every individual enjoys maximum freedom that is still consistent with the equal liberties of her fellow citizens. According to John Stuart Mill (1859: 22) the only purpose for which someone's freedom can be constrained is to protect other individuals. One should not compel persons to act in specific ways for their own good, but it is justified to limit their freedom in order to prevent evil to third parties. This idea is normally referred to as the *harm principle*:

HP_1: It is justified to restrict the liberty of person A in order to prevent A from causing harm to person B.[2]

Moreover, according to Mill, this is the *only* justification of liberty-limiting actions and policies. Even the strongest libertarian will agree with liberty-limiting interventions that protect against harm, and HP_1 is therefore relatively uncontroversial. Moreover, the application of the principle to protection against the harms of infection may seem rather straightforward. The principle and its application however do raise important questions. First, the concept of 'causing harm' is not as clear as one might hope – certainly not in relation to the harmful nature of contagion. Second, the harm principle as understood in HP_1 can be given a very strong justification as it is in a sense a necessary condition to freedom as such, but this is a rather narrow interpretation of Mill's harm principle. Although HP_1 may apply to certain measures of infectious diseases control, many forms of infection (hence policies to prevent infection) fall outside the scope of HP_1. Many authors in fact endorse a broader interpretation of the harm principle, but such an expanded principle HP_2 (see below) may require other sources of justification.

'Causing harm'

A paradigmatic case of harm, where the harm principle would obviously apply, is one where someone deliberately intends to infect another with a dangerous disease. A recent example is the Groningen case in the Netherlands. In 2007, three people in Groningen were arrested because they had injected others with HIV-infected blood. The culprits – all HIV seroposi-tive themselves – contacted their victims through internet chat boxes, and invited them to homosexual sex parties at home. During these meetings they first intoxicated their victims, and then administered intravenous injections with HIV-infected blood. They also injected blood in each other's veins, 'just for the kick' as they confessed after their arrest.

Although persons with HIV can be treated relatively well (at least in high income countries), the infection does severely undermine their health. Adequate medical treatment involves a complex regimen of drugs that negatively affect their quality of life. A deliberate and malevolent act to infect someone else with HIV is a clear case of harm. State interven-tions to prevent such harms and to punish evildoers are justified on the basis of the harm principle.

The Groningen case may be a paradigmatic case of inflicting harm, but it is not a paradigm case of infectious disease control. Public health measures to control contagious diseases do not focus on active malevolent behaviour, but on more common means of infection. For example, even though persons may be aware that they are a carrier of a virus or other infectious agent, they may simply forget to take precautions, or otherwise act negligently and spread disease. The story of 'Typhoid Mary' Mallon is a case in point. At some point she was told she carried a disease that could be easily transmitted if she worked in a kitchen, but she decided to take up her job after all, hence infecting more persons. As discussed before, public health measures that demand people isolate themselves, or refrain from certain activities, or otherwise take precautions, may be detrimental to their own well-being, and this may well motivate them to be non-compliant or negligent. The reason why such measures as compulsory isolation are used is because such behaviour, even though

---

[2] It is not necessary for the principle that B is a specific person. It could be a non-assignable member of the public.

normally not malevolent, can be dangerous to others. If there is a clear risk that infected persons will harm others, even though the harm is caused by negligent rather than malevolent behaviour, then the harm principle may justify compulsory measures.

So far we have focused on cases where people have negligently or malevolently imposed risk on others. Again, these cases cover only part of all current possibilities for compulsory measures. Infectious diseases may spread where no one is yet aware of the infection. A disease could have an incubation period where an asymptomatic person is already infectious. Or persons may have certain symptoms, but not realize that they are infectious. Many policies – including compulsory measures – aim to prevent spread of disease in such contexts: mandatory screening at borders, routine HIV-tests for pregnant persons in risk groups, prohibition of mass events, closing of schools, etc. Can the concept of harm and the scope of the harm principle be stretched much further, and justify such measures as well? It is often assumed in public health law and ethics that the principle can be as broad as this (Gostin, 2003). Yet this depends partly on how the principle and its core concept, harm, are understood.

Is it correct to assume that Sally, who does not know she is a hepatitis B carrier, and who has unprotected sex with Richard, is causing harm to Richard? Is Henry causing harm to his colleagues if he goes to work, unaware that he is a vector for a new and dangerous influenza virus? Paul got very ill and was admitted to a hospital, and now it appears that he has SARS and that he infected two nurses who cared for him. Did Paul harm the nurses?

Maybe Sally is causing harm if we assume that she and Richard should have taken precautions against sexually transmitted diseases anyway. If that is true, this may reveal that 'harming others' and even 'causing harm' are normative concepts, that only apply when certain moral norms are transgressed.[3] Joel Feinberg (1984: 36) indeed defines harm as a *wrongful* setback to the interests of another person, where 'wrongful' refers to transgression of a moral norm (Feinberg,[4]: 36). Certainly Henry can not be considered as harming his colleagues, if harm would involve the transgression of a moral norm: he just goes to work and is perfectly justified in doing so. Paul did not 'do' anything, and even though actually his admittance to the hospital did appear to be a threat, there is no sense in which *Paul* could have been responsible for it. This seems to imply that, if we emphasize the moral nature of causing harm, HP_1 only justifies compulsory measures towards persons who are in some sense responsible for the harm that they produce.[5] Compulsory policies towards persons who are unaware that they pose a threat to the health of others might not be justified on this interpretation of the harm principle.

---

[3] The example may provoke the reaction that Richard can not be said to have been harmed if he agreed to having unprotected sex (*volenti non fit injuria*), but this only affirms the claim that harm is a moral concept.

[4] However, Feinberg is specifically focusing on the role of the harm principle in the context of criminal law, and this may be a reason for thinking that the relevance of his concept of harm in the context of infectious disease control is limited.

[5] Note that this is not just a result of the definition of harm as such, but also in our understanding of *someone causing* harm. Did Henry cause harm to his colleagues, or was the harm caused by the virus? Statements of causal responsibility may seem purely empirical, but when they concern actions or omissions of persons, they will inevitably involve evaluative statements that presuppose some background of norms (Yoder, 2002).

Expanding the scope of the harm principle

However, the harm principle could also be interpreted in a less restricted way. In discussions of the harm principle it is unclear how broad its scope exactly is. Does the principle only justify compulsion or punishment of person A who is him/herself causing harm to person B? Mill suggests that the principle may also cover cases where A's omission to act (for example, to rescue) would result in harms for B. In other words, A's actions need not be the source of the harm. If we accept this, in fact we have adopted an alternative principle:

HP$_2$: It is justified to restrict the liberty of person A in order to prevent harm to others.

(Brink, 2007)

This principle neither requires causal responsibility nor moral responsibility of A for the harms that are to be prevented. Hence, on this principle also compulsory measures can be justified towards persons who are unaware that they pose a risk: for example, compulsory screening of travellers at airports or mandatory HIV tests for pregnant women. A policy by which all incoming travellers are screened for specific contagious diseases will lower the risk that outbreaks will occur within a country. Measures that temporarily prohibit the gathering of large groups of people will inhibit the spread of infection across a population. This principle could even support compulsory policies towards persons who are known to be not infected at all, for example vaccination policies of specific groups in order to prepare for a bioterrorist attack.

As attractive as this interpretation of the harm principle may seem for effective infectious disease control, it does raise a problem – at least for many libertarians. If it is irrelevant what or who caused the harm that is to be prevented, almost any compulsory policy that may promote or protect the health of others could be justified. For example, the state could openly force some persons into quarantine in order to convince the public that there is a serious threat to public health and that 'the state means business', thereby stimulating the public to comply all the better (Wilkinson, 2007). Parents could be required to have their children vaccinated against seasonal influenza, because that may reduce mortality among the elderly (Reichert et al., 2001). Citizens could be required to pay for vaccination and treatment of persons who cannot afford such forms of health care, etc. This is not to suggest that such policies would necessarily be wrong. However, these policies, and the revised version of the harm principle, may have little to do with the initial attractiveness of the harm principle in a liberal framework. The harm principle is often presented as a justification for compulsion and punishment that even the notorious libertarian could accept. This is because the principle (at least HP$_1$) is still consistent with allowing every person a maximum liberty.

The revised version of the harm principle, HP$_2$, however also justifies constraints on freedom of citizens if, for example, that would protect the health of persons who are relatively frail anyway. This would raise a discussion about whether such interventions 'really' aim to prevent harm to those persons, or 'just' confer benefits to them (Brink, 2007). Libertarians would complain that the revised version of the harm principle is not just aimed at the protection of liberty, but it is already trading off liberty against health and well-being. Such a trade-off however may well be acceptable – if not essential – in many other normative theories. Let us briefly focus on two such theories.

Consequentialist and egalitarian approaches to preventing harm

Contrary to what libertarians assume, it makes sense to hold liberty to be one value among others, and to reject the idea that freedom from intervention should always be given priority over other values, such as welfare or equality. Public health measures aim to protect people from diseases that are detrimental to their health and thereby undermine their opportunities to live a reasonably good life. Consequentialists will argue that it may be justified to constrain people's freedom if this would promote the general good. Infectious diseases may be detrimental to many different sources of well-being; consequently, effective prevention may promote well-being in various ways. Adequate protection against contagious diseases first of all promotes the good by preventing illness, suffering and premature death. Moreover, public health measures, such as surveillance, screening, testing and vaccination, and adequate structures to respond to disease outbreaks will also protect and facilitate people's societal life: to meet others, to go work, to receive education and to care for the elderly or the weak. If such measures require compulsion, this will be justified if the consequences are optimal. From a consequentialist perspective, the causal routes of the harms are rather irrelevant, and there are good reasons to prefer HP_2 over HP_1. Moreover, consequentialists may also acknowledge that compulsion can help to avoid a collective action problem. Suppose there is an actual threat of a smallpox outbreak, and it will be possible to contain the outbreak only if sufficient individuals will be vaccinated. The vaccine however is not completely safe. In such a case, individuals may forego vaccination and hope that they will benefit from the vaccination of other persons. However, if many people share this attitude, the public will not be protected at all, and hence all will be worse off. In order to avoid such problems, the state could compel the relevant groups to accept vaccination, for the sake of protection of all.

Liberal egalitarians, like consequentialists, may also support HP_2; though partly for different reasons. They see equality and fairness, next to autonomy, as fundamental values. Measures aimed at the prevention of infection can be considered as measures to reduce the risks of infection (hence the risk that harm will occur) within a population. Egalitarians will be concerned with a fair distribution of risks to health, but also with a fair distribution of the burdens of preventive measures. Health inequalities that are unjust, for example because they are caused by inequitable income distributions, need to be reduced. Infectious diseases may hit the rich as severely as the poor, but often there are clear correlations between social deprivation and increased prevalence of infectious diseases. Well-off groups will also have more possibilities to protect themselves against disease: they have better access to relevant information; they can afford special vaccinations, safe drinking water and hygienic living conditions; they may avoid places where infectious diseases are more common, decide to leave the city (or even their job) in case of an outbreak, and can afford therapeutic care when they get ill, etc. If it is left up to individual citizens to protect themselves, then arguably many people in socio-economically worse-off groups will be left unprotected. Egalitarians therefore support government interventions to protect the health of the public which go beyond the narrow version of the harm principle. Such interventions will at least aim at universal access to basic health care, paid from public resources, which includes basic preventive care and public health services (Daniels, 2001). Compulsory measures to reduce the risks of infectious diseases may also benefit the worse-off groups, and ensure that the burdens of protection are distributed equitably.

Although consequentialists and egalitarians may both support the expanded version of the harm principle (HP_2), there will also be differences. HP_2 fits within a general liberal framework which the consequentialist may not accept. HP_2 still focuses on *harm to others* and therefore does not cover paternalistic interventions that restrict someone's freedom in order to prevent harm to him or herself. For the consequentialist, all harms, including self-imposed risks, could be a reason for intervention. Moreover, consequentialists may argue that in the context of infection it will often be difficult to distinguish acts that are purely self-regarding. Most contagious diseases do not stick to persons who accepted the risk of being infected; they will spread from them to others as well.

Liberal egalitarians might respond that at least in some contexts, individuals have the possibility and responsibility to protect themselves against infection. Sexually transmitted diseases are a good example. Compulsory measures to prevent infection might be justified where individuals cannot be reasonably expected to protect themselves. If individuals can easily choose to have protected sex, public health authorities should be reluctant to intervene and compel them to take precautions. For that matter, compulsory measures would require interventions in people's private spheres – interventions which, if not impossible, would at least be highly impractical. Such pragmatic considerations will also be relevant to the consequentialist. Moreover, many consequentialists may aim at promoting well-being *and* freedom, and for them HP_2 will be a reasonable trade-off between both values.

Conditions for justified compulsion in public health

Let me briefly summarize the argument so far. The narrow version of the harm principle (HP_1) may offer justification for compulsory interventions that prevent people from deliberately or negligently infecting others, for example, infected persons who resist isolation or treatment. This justification is relatively uncontroversial as it can be based upon the value of freedom itself. For purposes of effective infectious disease control however, the scope of HP_1 is rather limited. Quarantining healthy persons in order to reduce the risk of contagion, or mandatory screening at borders, or compulsory tests for pregnant women, all involve situations where it is less clear whether the persons compelled are indeed *causing* harm to others – or even imposing risk on others. Such measures may fall within the scope of the expanded version of the harm principle (HP_2), because here the causal routes of harm and the moral connotations of our understanding of causing harm are irrelevant. The expanded principle can be coherent with several normative theories, notably consequentialism and egalitarianism. However, the scope of the principle may easily become too broad: the principle could support sacrificing innocent bystanders, if that would help in some way to reduce even minor risks within a population. Therefore, a solid justification for compulsory measures in terms of the prevention of harm should take into account several further constraints. Just the fact that a certain compulsory intervention may prevent harm is not enough to consider the intervention morally right.

Magnitude of harm

A first issue that will be relevant in any justification of compulsory measures is that the harm or risk to be averted should be significant and realistic. Chicken pox and the common cold are contagious, but, apart from special circumstances, do not create clear risks to individuals or the population. Symptoms of chicken pox may be very annoying for patients but it is questionable whether one should consider these as harms at all. Many other contagious diseases however have irreversible effects on the well-being of patients, or are otherwise mutilating or lethal. Therapeutic possibilities are limited which further decreases the prognosis for infected patients, as in the case of extremely resistant forms of tuberculosis. The magnitude of the harms that can be prevented does not only depend on how severe a disease is for a patient, but also on the mode and speed of transmission. Infections that lead to severe disease but that also spread rapidly within a population pose a serious threat to the public health at large. Such a disease, if not averted, will affect many individuals, and the ravages will not only be visible in each patient, but also on a population level.

Effectiveness and evidence

A necessary condition for any compulsory public health measure to be justified is that it should be effective in preventing infection and reducing the risks of disease. This condition may seem rather obvious: the rationale for controlling measures is indeed to control and prevent disease, and interventions that do not work make no sense. However, it is often difficult to evaluate and assess the effects of public health strategies. Evidence is often historical or anecdotal, supported by common sense. Randomized trials of policies like surveillance, isolation, or border control are rare if not impossible. Moreover, evaluation of effectiveness should not just focus on theoretical effects in ideal circumstances, but also on the feasibility of measures in times of crisis. Especially where measures are compulsory, people may try to find ways to avoid them. If persons who are tested positive for disease are isolated from their families, they may decide not to see a doctor if they have symptoms. Finally, judgments of effectiveness of planned interventions against future diseases, such as pandemic influenza, are complicated by many uncertainties about the characteristics of the virus and its effects (infection rate, transmissibility, mortality, risk groups, etc.).

These problems make clear that assessment of effectiveness is often not a simple matter of appealing to scientific evidence; it requires judgment on the basis of incomplete evidence.

Proportionality and the least restrictive alternative

A further requirement for controlling measures is that their impact on the liberties and well-being of individuals should be in the right proportion to the magnitude of harm that can be prevented. Major threats to public health – for example, a bioterrorist attack with smallpox – may require interventions like compulsory isolation and vaccination, yet such measures may be effective but not reasonable in order to contain an outbreak of less severe diseases, like rubella or measles.

Reasonable approaches to protect public health will also endorse the principle of the least restrictive alternative: measures may sometimes justifiably impose constraints on civil liberties, but such constraints should not be greater than strictly necessary. Mandatory HIV tests for all persons who visit a hospital may not be justified if routine (opting-out) tests are known to be equally effective. Detention and forced treatment of tuberculosis is wrong if directly observed treatment without detention is also possible and effective. In many cases however, it is less clear what the least restrictive alternative would be. Especially where there is much uncertainty about the risks of harm or about the effectiveness of various options, any intervention could be considered to be the least restrictive means necessary. One interpretation of the principle is that compulsory interventions should only be imposed where less restrictive measures have been tried, and have failed (Annas, 2002). This may be applicable to treatment of tuberculosis patients, where detention of a patient could be an option after more voluntary approaches to enhance compliance to therapy have been tried and failed. However, in emergency situations and public health crises there may be few possibilities to try voluntary approaches first. 'The least restrictive alternative' therefore makes sense as a general principle that urges public health authorities to compare options and reflect on which measures are really necessary, but it is not a criterion that can be simply applied.

Infectious disease control and public trust

Infectious disease control involves a range of measures that are necessary for the protection of public health, but which may interfere with the interests and rights of individual persons. Moreover, for most policies to be effective it is important that members of the public cooperate, even if that might not be in their best interests. But why would individuals voluntarily cooperate if they run the risk that their privacy is violated (case reporting; contact tracing), that they may not be allowed to enter or leave a country (airport screening); or that they will lose their job because they cannot go to work (isolation)? One answer could be that they have moral obligations to take precautions against infection and act in the interest of public health (Verweij, 2005). Yet even if citizens acknowledge that they have such a duty, they may not be motivated to act according to public health regulations if they do not fully trust that such regulations actually are for the common good, that policies are applied fairly and that adverse effects on well being are minimized. Hence, it is essential for effective infectious disease control that the public will trust public health authorities and have confidence in the interventions that those authorities impose. If there is a lack of trust in public health authorities, even compulsory policies will be futile. Conversely, if public health professionals and authorities can and do publicly justify regulations that are deemed necessary – especially those regulations that are compulsory in nature – they provide reasons for the public to trust such interventions.

Compulsory interventions should also be applied in a fair and non-discriminatory way; procedural due process for persons who are separated is then important. Public trust may be further strengthened if adverse effects of controlling public health measures are countervailed where possible (stigmatization, social isolation, health risks, economic losses, etc.), and if persons can expect reasonable compensation for economic losses they have as a result of such interventions.[6] Unfortunately, the possibilities for due process and full compensation schemes may be limited in large-scale public health emergencies, such as a bioterrorist attack or influenza pandemic. Emergency situations where many people are quarantined may not allow time for personal hearings and legal representation for each individual. And if a large part of the population faces economic losses due to public health measures, it may be impossible to compensate everyone. One might hope that citizens will accept the limitations of due process and compensation in a large-scale crisis if they have confidence in the public health measures.

---

[6] In fact, trust cannot be easily created or promoted. Meijboom *et al.* (2006: 432–4) argue that, ultimately, only trustworthiness strengthens trust. Yet if public health authorities publicly justify the measures they take, and if they are accountable for the implications for citizens (including fair compensation schemes, etc.), they do become more trustworthy.

Compulsory screening for dangerous infectious diseases, contact tracing, case reporting, isolation and quarantine, vaccination or treatment – all these measures can deeply interfere with people's well-being and freedom, and they require a strong moral justification. There should be sufficient evidence that a coercive measure is necessary to prevent significant harm to others. Paradoxically, the more this measure and its justification is endorsed by the public, the less force and compulsion may be required to protect public health.

Acknowledgement

I have had some very illuminating discussions with Franck Meijboom, Angus Dawson and Frans Brom that have helped me in developing the argument in this chapter.

References

Annas, G. J. (2002) Bioterrorism, public health, and civil liberties. *New England Journal of Medicine*, **346**(17): 1337–42.

Biraben, J. (1976) *Les hommes et la peste en France et dans les pays Européens et méditerranées. Tome II: Les hommes face à la peste*. Paris: Mouton.

Brink, D. (2007) Mill's moral and political philosophy. In *The Stanford Encyclopedia of Philosophy*. Available at: http://plato. stanford.edu/entries/mill-moral-political/ (accessed: 8/12/08).

Brody, S. N. (1974) *The Disease of the Soul: Leprosy in Medieval Literature*. Ithaca, NY: Cornell University Press.

Daniels, N. (2001) Justice, health, and health care. *American Journal of Bioethics*, **1**(2): 2–16.

Feinberg, J. (1984) *Harm to Others. The Moral Limits of the Criminal Law, Part I*. New York: Oxford University Press.

Gostin, L. O. (2000) *Public Health Law. Power, Duty, Restraint*. Berkeley, CA: University of California Press.

Gostin, L. O. (2003) When terrorism threatens health: how far are limitations on personal and economic liberties justified? *Florida Law Review*, **55**: 1105.

Gostin, L.O. (2006) Public health strategies for pandemic influenza: ethics and the law. *Journal of American Medical Association*, **295**: 1700–4.

Lerner, B. H. (1999) Catching patients: tuberculosis and detention in the 1990s. *Chest*, **115**: 236–41.

Meijboom, F. L. B., Visak, T. and Brom, F. W. A. (2006) Public health strategies for pandemic influenza: ethics and the law. *Journal of Agricultural and Environmental Ethics*, **19**(5): 427–42.

Mill, J. S. (1859) *On Liberty*. London: John Parker and Son.

Moote, A. L. and Moote, D. C. (2004) *The Great Plague: The Story of London's Most Deadly Year*. Baltimore, MD: The Johns Hopkins University Press.

Noordegraaf, L. and Valk, G. (1988) *De Gave Gods. De pest in Holland vanaf de late middeleeuwen*. Bergen: Octavo.

Porter, R. (1997) *The Greatest Benefit to Mankind. A Medical History of Humanity from Antiquity to Present*. London: Harper Collins.

Reichert, T. A., Sugaya, N., Fedson, D. S., Glezen, W. P., Simonsen, L. and Tashiro, M. (2001) The Japanese experience with vaccinating schoolchildren against influenza. *New England Journal of Medicine*, **344**, 12: 889–96.

Rennie, S. and Behets, F. (2006) Desperately seeking targets: the ethics of routine HIV testing in low-income countries. *Bulletin of the World Health Organization*, **84**(1): 52–7.

Rothstein, M. A. and Talbott, M. K. (2007) Encouraging compliance with quarantine: a proposal to provide job security and income replacement. *American Journal of Public Health*, **97**(Suppl 1): S49–56.

Roueché, B. (1953) *Eleven Blue Men and Other Narratives of Medical Detection*. Boston, MA: Little, Brown and Company.

Verma, G., Upshur, R., Rea, E. and Benatar, S. R. (2004) Critical reflections on evidence, ethics and effectiveness in the management of tuberculosis: public health and global perspectives. *BMC Medical Ethics*, **5**: 2.

Verweij, M. F. (2005) Obligatory precautions against infection, *Bioethics* **19**(4): 323–35.

Verweij, M. F. and Dawson, A. (2007) *The meaning of 'public' in 'public health'*. In *Ethics, Prevention, and Public Health*, ed. A. Dawson and M. F. Verweij. Oxford: Oxford University Press.

Wald, P. (1997) Cultures and carriers. 'Typhoid Mary' and the science of social control. *Social Text*, **15**: 181–214.

Wilkinson, T. M. (2007) Contagious disease and self-defence. *Res Publica*, **13**(4): 339–59.

Yoder, S. D. (2002) Individual responsibility for health: decision, not discovery. *Hastings Center Report*, **32**(2): 22–31.

Chapter

7

Population screening

Ainsley J. Newson

Introduction

At first glance, the idea of examining a group of asymptomatic individuals for signs of disease or illness would appear laudable, even essential. Who would not want to try to prevent or provide early treatment for serious conditions such as cancer or HIV/AIDS? The screening tests involved are often minor, can significantly reduce morbidity and can even be life-saving. The myriad population screening programmes now in existence are under-pinned by the rationale that screening can help optimize population health.

Yet issues such as impinging, however slightly, on people's liberty when offering a screening test mean that the introduction of this sort of health monitoring in populations should not be undertaken without careful factual and ethical analysis. Offering an unproven or ill-chosen test to an individual can have far-reaching implications for their future health care and well-being. Population screening may also conflict with valued ethical principles in health care, such as autonomy and consent. Ethical considerations arise with implications for health professionals, recipients and policy makers.

Conversely, the principles and frameworks for ethical analysis in a public health context (although methodologically uncertain) arguably differ from traditional analyses in medical ethics. It may be short-sighted to prioritize individual interests over those of society, as there are opportunities for rich ethical analysis in assessing the relative values of individual and collective interests in public health. Focusing on preventive medicine in asymptomatic populations raises the prospect of a collectivist ethic, in which communal life and the links that sustain it must be recognized (Jennings, 2007). Public health ethics also forces us to address difficult questions, such as the acceptability of reducing particular diseases in the community and the mechanisms by which this may be achieved.

This chapter reflects these broader tensions in public health ethics by highlighting and analysing some of the ethical considerations that should be borne in mind for population screening. It is divided into three sections. The first briefly describes what we mean by 'screening' and reviews the criteria for introducing screening programmes. In the second section, examples of screening programmes are presented and briefly described. The majority of the chapter is dedicated to the third section, in which the ethical issues arising from screening are presented and critiqued, with reference to the examples presented previously. It emerges that population screening is a complex field with many overlapping ethical tensions, with several key issues remaining unresolved.

Public Health Ethics, ed. Angus Dawson. Published by Cambridge University Press. © Cambridge University Press 2011.

What do we mean by 'screening'? When should a screening programme be introduced?

Definitions of 'screening'

Population screening is a diverse aspect of health care, offered in numerous formal (and sometimes informal) programmes. Broadly, the term 'screening' means the application of a straightforward but perhaps preliminary test for a designated health problem in an asymptomatic population, to find the few who are at increased risk. This population will often share a characteristic, but this may not be related to the condition being screened for. Individuals who return a 'screen positive' result will then be selected for further investigation (Riis, 1985; Shickle and Chadwick, 1994; Wilfond and Thomson, 2000; Press and Ariail, 2004).

Screening has two main purposes: primary and secondary prevention. Primary prevention is the detection of a risk of future disease in a completely asymptomatic individual, such as identifying a pregnant woman as a carrier of sickle cell anaemia. Secondary prevention involves detecting a disease in its very early stages in order to offer treatment to maximize prognosis, such as in mammography screening for breast cancer. Both purposes aim to reduce disease incidence in a population (Riis, 1985; Shickle and Chadwick, 1994).

The National Screening Committee (NSC) in the UK offers the following definition of screening:

> Screening is a process of identifying apparently healthy people who may be at increased risk of a disease or condition. They can then be offered information, further tests and appropriate treatment to reduce their risk and/or any complications arising from the disease or condition.
>
> (National Screening Committee, 2011)

This reveals some important ethical aspects of population screening programmes. First, screening usually involves a recommendation of testing to a previously unaware population. The suggestion to test comes proactively from a central organization and is not commissioned following an individual's request (Clarke, 2007).

Second, consequentialist/collectivist reasoning is predominant when assessing the ethics of population screening, in that a benefit–harm calculation is often used to justify screening programmes (Juth and Munthe, 2007). Screening aims to benefit the health *of the population*, as opposed to individuals. While individuals may benefit from screening, to keep costs down initial screens may not have the same degree of sensitivity and specificity that clinical tests may have. This is considered an acceptable trade-off as screening tests are generally low risk (Berlin, 1999; cited in Wilson, 2000), although they will not help every screened individual and may in fact cause harm. Such harm is a particularly significant issue if the term is interpreted broadly to include psycho-social factors such as anxiety and practical considerations such as time allocated to attending for screening.

Screening is distinct from clinical 'testing', although the boundaries are easily blurred and the terms are used interchangeably in the literature. Screening tests are generally fairly straightforward to administer and interpret and have a low unit cost. Testing is generally offered to individuals who are already at increased risk of a specific disease or condition. A diagnostic test may be more complicated, expensive or risky to administer than a screening test; but it will also be more accurate. The purpose of testing is diagnostic: 'Does this person *have this disease?*' and involves a definitive test. Screening instead asks: 'Is this person at higher identifiable risk for this disease?' and results may be probabilistic (Nuffield Council on Bioethics, 1993; Gostin, 2000; Wilfond and Thomson, 2000; Wilson, 2000; Press and Ariail, 2004).

This chapter is limited to discussions of 'population screening' – formal programmes implemented by an organization to promote public health objectives. Some forms of screening, for example whole body magnetic resonance imaging or prostate specific antigen screening, will not be addressed as they are not yet offered to the public via a formal screening programme.

Criteria for establishing screening programmes

Formal screening programmes are unlikely to obtain funding or other relevant support unless they are shown to uphold defined criteria. One of the earliest and best-known lists of criteria to be met before a screening programme can be established was published by Wilson and Jungner in 1968. These criteria are presented in Box 7.1.

Whether any hierarchy exists between these principles is unclear, as it will be very difficult for any one screening programme to meet all of them (Shickle and Chadwick, 1994). However, Wilson and Jungner did emphasize that the second principle (treatment) was particularly important.

The relevance of these principles remains today, although they have necessarily been adapted to meet changing health care contexts and priorities. For example the UK NSC has published its own criteria, all of which should be met before a screening programme is introduced (National Screening Committee, 2003). The 22 criteria incorporate Wilson and Jungner's first seven principles, while the eighth and ninth are re-worked to provide additional requirements for diagnostic testing and clinical management. Further NSC criteria require other primary prevention interventions and treatments to have been implemented, that no screening programme be introduced without quality randomized controlled trials, that the programme provides value for money and that the programme be managed and monitored. Yet whether these are adhered to in practice is sometimes questionable, as illustrated by the critique of then UK Prime

---

Box 7.1 Wilson and Jungner's principles for screening

1. The condition sought should be an important health problem
2. There should be an accepted treatment for patients with recognized disease
3. Facilities for diagnosis and treatment should be available
4. There should be a recognizable latent or early symptomatic stage
5. There should be a suitable test or examination
6. The test should be acceptable to the population
7. The natural history of the condition, including development from latent to declared disease, should be adequately understood
8. There should be an agreed policy on whom to treat as patients
9. The cost of case-finding (including diagnosis and treatment of patients diagnosed) should be economically balanced in relation to possible expenditure on medical care as a whole
10. Case-finding should be a continuing process and not a 'once and for all' project. (Wilson and Jungner, 1968: 26–7)

Minister Gordon Brown's proposals for screening programmes for diabetes, cardiovascular and renal disease (Tudor Hart, 2008; White, 2008).

The NSC criteria also explicitly account for ethical issues. Wilson and Jungner's sixth principle is supplemented by criteria requiring the complete screening programme to be clinically, socially and ethically acceptable to both health professionals and the public (NSC criterion 14). Criterion 15 requires benefits of screening programmes to outweigh physical and psychological harm. Informed choice (discussed further below) is included as the justification for providing good evidence-based information to participants.

The notion of a 'suitable test' for a screening programme (Wilson and Jungner's fifth principle) merits further discussion. Any screening test should provide an accurate basis for determining which participants require additional tests. The terms 'sensitivity' and 'specificity' are relevant here: sensitivity requires an acceptable percentage of affected individuals in the population to be positively identified by the test, while specificity denotes that a percentage of unaffected individuals need to be excluded from further testing by the initial screen. Sensitivity and specificity are necessarily offset in screening as optimizing both is impossible. Increasing sensitivity will raise false positives and increasing specificity leads to more false negatives (Shickle and Chadwick, 1994). Yet finding the right threshold is vital: a person incorrectly identified as potentially affected may suffer continuing anxiety, while parents of an ill child whose diagnosis was missed in an initial screening test may experience difficulty, delay and frustration in obtaining a diagnosis at a later stage.

Meeting screening criteria is often difficult. A condition being screened for may be an important health problem, yet it could be rare in the population. The rarer a disease is, the more specific a screening test needs to be, and therefore more expensive. The screening test will have to provide a trade-off between specificity and cost. Not all proposals for screening will receive funding, as a programme may not represent an appropriate allocation of financial and other resources comparable to other health interventions. Significant harm can also be caused if the threshold for sensitivity is set too low. In the early days of newborn screening for phenylketonuria (described below), some babies were misdiagnosed and erroneously treated. Tragically, this caused brain damage in some children who would have otherwise been of normal functioning and some children died (Fost, 1999).

Common screening programmes

Screening programmes are available to populations at virtually all stages of the lifespan. These include: the use of mammography in post-menopausal women to aid the detection of breast cancer, the use of cervical smear tests in women to detect the early stages of cervical cancer, faecal occult testing to screen for early signs of bowel cancer and genetic screening.

Genetic screening

From an ethical perspective, an interesting collection of screening programmes are those involving genetic conditions. The identification of more and more genes implicated in human disease, together with the decreasing cost and complexity of molecular methods of diagnosis, has led to a steadily increasing interest in using genetic testing on a population-wide basis to promote the public's health (President's Commission, 1983; Khoury et al., 2000; British Medical Association, 2005). Genetic screening programmes predict or diagnose genetic disease or determine genetic risk for future offspring. They can be used in the

Box 7.2 Genetic screening in practice – screening for β-thalassaemia in Cyprus

- β-thalassaemia causes abnormalities in haemoglobin structure. It requires lifelong blood transfusions, removal of excess iron from the blood and sometimes splenectomy. These treatments are expensive.
- If a couple each have a copy of the mutated gene, they have a 25% chance of having an affected child. In Cyprus, 1 in 7 people carried the mutated gene and 1 in 158 children were expected to be born with the disease, placing a demand on health resources.
- In the 1970s, a national policy was introduced to reduce new cases of thalassaemia, incorporating community involvement, public education, service improvement and initially a prevention campaign to discourage carriers from marrying (later replaced by a prenatal diagnosis campaign).
- The programme has led to a significant proportion of the population receiving screening and a 90% reduction in the number of children born with β-thalassaemia. (Angastiniotis et al., 1986)

general population or in recognized sub-groups known to be at risk for a designated condition (European Society of Human Genetics, 2003). For example, antenatal carrier screening in a couple can lead to a foetus being tested for thalassaemia (see Box 7.2) or adults may be screened for familial hypercholesterolaemia. As many genetic conditions are rare and the sensitivity of genetic tests varies, a genetic screening programme will usually only be developed when the disease has a significant prevalence and when the presence of a gene change (mutation) strongly predicts disease manifestation. Future genetic screening programmes may instead take advantage of whole genome sequencing technologies.

The purpose of genetic screening to prevent disease can be categorized slightly differently to the primary and secondary categories for screening discussed above. Genetic screening can also be said to focus on either phenotypic or genotypic prevention (Press and Ariail, 2004). Phenotypic prevention reflects primary and secondary prevention in that the purpose is to prevent the manifestation of a chosen genetic condition. Genotypic prevention is a form of primary prevention unique to genetic screening: the purpose is to prevent intergenerational transmission of a genetic disease in conjunction with promoting informed reproductive decision-making by couples. The outcome of genotypic prevention may prevent the existence of an individual and so gives rise to ethical issues such as making value judgements about the quality of life that those with genetic conditions must live with. The example of screening for thalassaemia in Cyprus, discussed in Box 7.2, also raises the issue of whether it is ever appropriate to explicitly set the reduction of a disease as the aim of a screening programme. These and other ethical issues in genetic screening are discussed below.

A consideration of any genetic screening programme will indicate that it may often be difficult, if not impossible, to meet those criteria set down by Wilson and Jungner or the NSC. This problem was recognized some time ago and alternate criteria have been suggested. Genetic screening should therefore:

1. Contribute to improving the health of persons who suffer from genetic disorders; and/or
2. Allow carriers for a given abnormal gene to make informed choices regarding reproduction; and/or
3. Move towards alleviating the anxieties of families and communities faced with the prospect of serious genetic disease. (Lappé et al., 1972, cited by Nuffield Council on Bioethics, 1993: 17)

Antenatal screening

Given the necessity of their contact with health care providers, pregnant women are principal recipients of offers of screening. In the past 30 years a large number of screening programmes have been introduced in this group, with the overall goal of optimizing the health of newborn babies. A secondary goal is to allow women to make informed choices about continuing a pregnancy when a foetus is at risk of developing a serious health problem. Tests related to this goal include ultrasound and maternal serum screening to measure biochemical markers in the pregnant woman's blood; both of which provide a risk profile for several diseases including Down's syndrome. Pregnant women may also be screened to determine their carrier status for conditions such as cystic fibrosis. Screening tests are offered at different stages of pregnancy and some women will receive more tests than others; relative to variables such as maternal age and ethnicity. Women obtaining higher-risk results from these screening tests will then be offered further invasive investigations.

Not all screening tests in pregnancy carry the implication of a potential termination of pregnancy. Since 1999, all pregnant women in the UK have been offered screening for the presence of HIV. The purpose of such testing is twofold: to provide affected women with appropriate treatment to optimize their long-term health; and to prevent maternal–foetal transmission of the virus. Other tests include anaemia, hepatitis B and Rhesus blood group status.

Newborn screening

Programmes to screen the health of newborn babies have been in existence for nearly 50 years (Guthrie, 1986; Fost, 1999; Kayton, 2007). Tests are performed on a small dried blood sample obtained during the first week of life. Screening aims to detect the presence of those congenital diseases where early intervention is beneficial, including phenylketonuria (PKU) and hearing.

Wilson and Jungner's criteria for screening are utilized in newborn screening, although more specific requirements have also been advocated. Clayton, for example, suggests the following factors:

- The disease has a devastating outcome;
- Treatment is highly effective in averting this outcome, but only if it is started early;
- Affected children cannot be detected on the basis of symptoms in time to start effective treatment; and
- Screening reliably detects most affected children. (Clayton, 2004: 1005)

Newborn screening is not without ethical concerns (Kerruish and Robertson, 2005). As programmes have developed and expanded, the degree to which the above criteria are still met is contentious (Wilford, 1995). While screening for PKU easily satisfies them, they are arguably less robustly adhered to in screening for conditions such as Duchenne muscular dystrophy – as little can be done to avert the onset of disease. Yet ancillary benefits can be identified, for example offering parents the chance to avoid subsequent diagnostic uncertainty, the opportunity for psychological adjustment and the ability to request prenatal diagnosis in future pregnancies.

Consent, or its absence, is also contentious – reflecting the broader tension in public health ethics. In most US states newborn screening for a large number of diseases, including mitochondrial disorders, is mandated. Parents in 46 states are technically able to refuse screening (Kayton, 2007), although whether this is actively communicated to parents is uncertain (Clarke, 1997). If they do refuse, the child may be removed for testing without their permission (Bratton, 2007) – a practice rejected elsewhere (Laurie, 2002). In the UK, parents are invited to make an informed choice about testing and refusals of testing are respected but not condoned.

As newborn screening expands, the criteria for testing will be stretched further. A current issue involves reporting carrier status results, for example after screening for cystic fibrosis. This approach may be criticized as inconsistent with policies for genetic testing in children, which generally stipulate that children should only be subjected to genetic testing when a direct health benefit can be shown. However, the finding of carrier status occurs as an artefact of the screening test and forms part of the health record, so is therefore legally accessible by parents. Empirical evidence suggests that parents are not adversely affected by receiving this information (Parsons *et al.*, 2003).

Further complexity in newborn screening is anticipated. As genes involved with multi-factorial diseases such as diabetes are identified, and as whole genome sequencing improves, the question of screening will arise. Will providing parents with information about their child's susceptibility to common diseases be a valuable tool for optimizing children's health? Or, will parents perceive their children as vulnerable? Early evidence suggests parents will not worry excessively (Gustafsson Stolt *et al.*, 2003; Kerruish *et al.*, 2007), yet ongoing monitoring will be important.

Screening in adults

Most of us can expect to be invited to participate in a series of screening programmes throughout our lives. These will include screening for transmissible viruses, such as HIV, and acquired conditions, such as cancer.

Modern screening programmes emphasize prevention and early detection. At various points in our lives – depending on our age, gender and ethnicity – we will be invited to undergo screening for HIV, bowel cancer, bone density, cervical cancer, breast cancer, diabetes, high blood pressure or coronary artery disease, among others (Muir-Gray and Pearce-Smith, 2007). All of these programmes are subject to cost–benefit calculations and give rise to ethical issues, discussed further below.

Although the diseases forming the focus for screening in the twenty-first century tend to be acquired or inherited instead of infectious, the SARS epidemic of 2003 illustrates that infectious disease can still have significant implications for public health. And in the developing world, the malaria pandemic is a significant cause of morbidity and mortality. The persistent threat of infectious disease gives rise to the question of whether and when the state can acceptably intervene to mandate screening of individuals for infectious disease, and if disease is detected what measures can be taken to restrict a person's liberty.

Ethical issues arising across screening programmes

The sometimes divergent approaches of public health ethics and the more traditional theories of health care ethics provide a key contention in ethical debates over population screening (Mann, 1997; Hodge, 2004). In traditionally conceived health care ethics (bioethics), significant emphasis is placed on individual rights and responsibilities. Principles such as autonomy, avoidance of harm and promotion of justice are emphasized. Although public health ethics has not abandoned individualism (indeed, the promotion of voluntariness in screening is increasingly prevalent, albeit not universally condoned), the focus for the promotion of health through population screening is more collective.

This juxtaposition of emphasis is reflected in some of the key ethical questions for population screening. When to introduce screening, whether it should be mandatory or voluntary and determining how to manage information gained are all important questions, reflecting some key themes in public health ethics (Hodge, 2004).

Defining 'success' in screening

Ultimately, for the state to support a screening programme and for that programme to be ethically justifiable, that programme needs to be successful. Gostin (2000: 397), for example, suggests that: 'Screening programs can be justified only if they effect a positive outcome that would not have occurred without the screening.'

In the context of genetic screening, Burris and Gostin (2004) have suggested that for a screening test to be ethical there must be a reasonable probability that it will reduce the incidence of a genetic condition or mortality from that condition in society or in a population facing a specific threat.

Preventing disease in the population cannot be all there is to 'success' in screening however, as prevention per se could come at a great cost to individuals within that population. One reason for ethical discomfort in screening is that much success is defined in terms of economics; specifically the chance to reallocate those costs that would otherwise have been spent on treating a case of disease. In an adult population this is not such a problem; most people would prefer not to develop a disease were it possible to avoid this outcome. But in antenatal screening, often the only way to prevent a case of disease is to terminate a pregnancy. The concern over defining success of screening in terms of cost savings is that it could lead to accusations of calculating the value of a life in purely economic terms or accusations of eugenic practice.

Labelling antenatal screening programmes as 'eugenic' could be used as an indefeasible rejection of this technology. However, the argumentation behind this critique is unclear (Chadwick et al., 1998). In this context, eugenics is taken to mean a deliberate use of screening to improve the quality of the human gene pool, leading to socially relevant changes. Chadwick et al. argue in response that maintaining a status quo can in itself be eugenic and that genetic screening is unlikely to cause suffering to future individuals (Chadwick et al., 1998). If we continue to respect the lessons learned from past eugenic mistakes (Wikler, 1999), screening is not per se problematic.

In the context of screening for Down's syndrome, published programme objectives are also notable for their absence of emphasis on economic considerations. Nor do they aim for a reduction in the incidence of the condition in the population. The main aim is to 'ensure access to a uniform screening programme', with a further aim to provide women with the necessary information to exercise an informed choice (National Screening Committee, 2011). This approach is laudable, but has been subject previously to criticism:

Programmes that claim to justify their existence by offering choice may find it difficult to put this into practice if the outcome measures they use are, in practice, those relating to uptake of screening, terminations of pregnancy and the birth incidence of affected infants. . . .

(Clarke, 2007: 429)

In defining 'success' in screening, the focus should be broad. Screening should not be seen as making a judgement about those with a disability. Outcomes should not only consider those identified as being at higher risk, but those who receive screen-negative results. But as more screening programmes are implemented, it will remain important to continue to reflect on the ethical assumptions behind the aims of a given screening programme, and to question whether it is appropriate to set the reduction of a disease as a goal. While uptake by a population may be taken as tacit acceptance of the goals of a screening programme, Clarke's above criticism suggests that participants in screening may not always base a decision to screen on complete information.

Informed consent and informed choice

Generally, for any diagnostic test in health care, no individual should be tested without full informed consent from that person or an appropriate surrogate. This upholds modern ethical and legal doctrines of bodily integrity and autonomy. But in population screening, where collectivist values are also relevant, should fully informed consent always be required?

To some, the need for informed consent to screening is equivalent to that for any diagnostic test. Though not endorsing this position, Gostin (2002) points out that screening can be intrusive; if imposed without consent it can invade personal autonomy and bodily integrity. For some, screening should therefore be preceded by provision of appropriate information, the recipient should be competent to make a decision and should decide voluntarily. The inherent power imbalance in professional–patient relationships could also undermine informed consent, as the mere offer of a screening test may be taken to imply that having the test is a 'good thing' and may lead to a 'compliance effect' on this ground alone (Shickle and Chadwick, 1994; European Society of Human Genetics, 2003).

But, encouraging fully informed consent may be resource-intensive to satisfy in practice. This begs the question that even if it is theoretically possible to obtain fully informed consent to screening, is it desirable? Informed consent will significantly raise the costs of screening programmes and so it may not always be justifiable, at least for some diseases where the value implications are less significant (for example, screening interventions that can be life-saving and are minimal risk). Also, if resource constraints are affecting information provision, participants may not be aware of the condition being screened for or may struggle to appreciate the (minimal) risks involved – raising the question of whether it is indeed wise to require informed consent at all times. Fostering autonomy could also manifest in a shifting of the burden of decision making to screening participants (Chadwick et al., 1998). It may be that the costs of obtaining fully informed consent can be traded off against other benefits to the population from screening.

These potentially competing concerns necessitate an assessment of priorities in screening in the developed world: high uptake or an informed decision (Raffle, 2001). Screening will not be effective in the absence of high uptake; if potential participants are put off by complex information, public health goals will not be achieved. Further, as screening targets a healthy population, the ethical assumptions of screening are different to those found in clinical practice. Effective screening will save lives or improve quality of life via early diagnosis.

Conversely, persuading people to receive screening tests (such as a cervical smear test or an antenatal screen for foetal abnormality) may be unethical without fully informed consent. Even if it harms a programme's success, open and frank communication about some screening programmes is vital to make participants equal partners in screening (Pfeffer, 2004). Making an informed decision should therefore be included as a measure of success in some screening programmes, in addition to measuring the numbers who take up an offer of screening (Raffle, 1997; Foster and Anderson, 1998; Marshall and Adab, 2003). Such an approach may not, however, be appropriate for all screening programmes – informed consent may on occasion be traded off in light of significant health benefits to the population.

HIV screening is one domain where concerns over informed consent have been raised. Testing for HIV is now offered on a routine 'opt out' basis in numerous domains, including at sexual health clinics and in antenatal screening. HIV is now a manageable condition and people's best interests are served by knowledge of infection status. Testing is strongly recommended and a high uptake is expected. In the antenatal context this has been criticized as undermining a pregnant woman's rights to bodily integrity and free choice (Bennett, 2004; Bennett, 2007) and empirical evidence suggests that only a minority of women have enough of an understanding of the screening test to meet standards of informed consent and that women are more likely to participate in screening if they spend less time discussing it (Sherr et al., 2006; de Zulueta and Boulton, 2007).

Bennett recognizes that pregnant women should know their HIV status, not least because mechanisms to prevent maternal-foetal transmission of the virus are so effective. Yet with this knowledge comes the expectation of compliance to a complex regime of treatments and interventions that can have serious side effects. To this end, she proposes that antenatal screening for HIV operate on a policy of 'informed choice,' to both promote screening and ensure women's trust (Bennett, 2004).

'Informed choice' for screening marks a recent departure from emphasizing screening as a public health activity designed to reduce the community burden of disease. The concept has been adopted in many domains of screening and is explicitly recognized in the NSC criteria (National Screening Committee, 2003) and can be defined as being '. . . based on relevant knowledge, consistent with the decision-maker's values and behaviorally implemented' (Marteau et al., 2001: 100). Applying this to screening:

> [A]n informed choice to undergo a screening test occurs when an individual has a positive attitude towards undergoing a test, has relevant knowledge about the test and undergoes it. An informed choice to decline a test occurs when an individual holds a negative attitude towards undergoing a test, has relevant knowledge about the test and does not undergo it.
>
> (Marteau et al., 2001: 100)

Compared with informed choice, consent involves a more active process of decision making and almost invariably involves contact with a health professional (Jepson et al., 2005: 193). It will be more time-consuming and resource intensive. Informed choice may offer a pragmatic and ethical alternative to fully informed consent. Yet informed choice is not a one-way exchange of information: any choice that is either based on poor quality information or is inconsistent with the decision maker's values will be uninformed and liable to ethical critique.

Care also needs to be taken regarding the nature of the information to be provided to facilitate informed choice, insofar as informed choice is appropriate to a particular screening programme. Unsurprisingly, the lay public process information differently to health professionals or policy makers and potential barriers must be identified. Pre-screen information should, in general, cover the purpose of screening, the likelihood of false positive or negative results, the implications of testing and plans for follow-up. But conveying these concepts is often difficult and may not assist in making an informed choice. Participants in screening may also want to receive information about the diseases being screened for and to hear narrative accounts from those who have already participated in the programme (Jepson et al., 2007).

Informed choice may offer an appropriate trade-off between high uptake and informed decisions, although a decrease in uptake of screening is possible. Appropriately implemented it can offer increased feelings of control, a reduction in anxiety and an improvement in behavioural change (Marteau and Kinmonth, 2002). How this is put into practice will vary with the participant population, the clinical significance of the condition being screened for, the risks associated with the test and resource or time constraints. Quality control and practitioner training are also important (Jepson et al., 2005).

When should consent be waived? Mandatory and routine screening

We have seen that informed choice can be an appropriate tool for the ethical delivery of screening programmes. Yet screening is not always voluntary: it can also be administered as mandatory or routine, with different or absent standards of informed choice. Although much routine screening is largely uncontroversial – as patients, we assume that contact with health services will at some point lead to screening (Wynia, 2006) – these departures from rigorous informed choice have been subject to criticism.

Newborn screening is effectively mandatory in most US states, as discussed above. This process is contested (Paul, 1999; Press and Clayton, 2000). Some have argued that if screening is important for a child's future health, then parents should not have the right to refuse (Faden et al., 1982a, 1982b). Spending valuable resources on seeking informed consent could also be inequitable. Further, as virtually all parents agree to the screening test, the extra anxiety they may suffer through being informed could outweigh any autonomy-based considerations around informing them.

The increasing involvement of patients in health care can be cited as reason to reject mandated screening, although whether this translates from a medical to a public health context is contentious. That said, the ability to make an informed choice about this practice helps promote trust in the health professions and allows parents to exercise their right to be accorded respect in making decisions for their child (Clarke, 1997). It also offers a valuable opportunity to educate families about the value of this screening (Friedman Ross, 2002) and will minimize harm and promote parental cooperation in the event that an abnormality is detected. Even if a parent refuses screening, the chances a child will be harmed are small but are nonetheless real. It may be that even if mandated screening is unacceptable, parents who refuse newborn screening may be legitimately encouraged to have the test by health professionals (Newson, 2006).

An emerging problem for informed choice and newborn screening is the rapid expansion of these programmes. Should information be provided about the myriad of conditions to be tested for, and how? A balance needs to be struck between empowering parents and ensuring viability of the screening programme. While mandatory screening seems unjustified in the absence of a significant risk to the child, a pragmatic approach may have to be adopted. Although this de-emphasizes fully informed consent, some degree of informed choice can still be used. Some interventions in medicine may indeed be collective in nature and as such are unsuitable for individual decision-making (Nijsingh, 2007).

Mandating screening of competent adults is more difficult to justify, as patients have a general right to refuse medical treatment even if it harms their interests. Despite this, in some countries mandatory screening for diseases such as tuberculosis is carried out at some sampling points, such as admission to hospital. But again, should a screening test being implemented to further public health goals be assessed using the same ethical principles as health care? Screening may also be more acceptably mandated if an infectious disease outbreak occurs, for example SARS. Grounds for justification of mandatory screening are that screening tests are unlikely to be invasive and the outcome can have significant impact on personal and public health. This demonstrates the Millian 'harm principle', in that individual autonomy can be restricted in order to prevent harm to others (Bayer et al., 1993). The right to privacy is usurped by the need to prevent the spread of disease. The mandating of any screening programme should, however, only be carried out once high standards of safety and efficacy are demonstrated. Reversal is also difficult post-implementation (Fost, 1999).

Pregnant women are an ideal group for screening from a public health perspective. They are necessarily in contact with health services and screening could improve health outcomes for the next generation. For these reasons a large number of antenatal screening programmes are now routinely offered. These programmes aim to protect the health of pregnant women and their foetuses.

One aspect of antenatal screening focuses on the foetus' future health. This is unique in public health in that if an abnormality is detected it could lead to the prevention of a being's existence by terminating a pregnancy. The active promotion of these screening tests in light of their potentially far-reaching implications has led some to criticize their routinization as an implicit yet strong recommendation in favour of testing by health professionals. This may lead to a downturn in informed choice and may be at odds with individually held values surrounding disability. Empirical studies have also suggested that not all women make an informed choice when having this screening, particularly those who accept the tests (Green, 2004; van den Berg et al., 2005, 2006).

While antenatal screening tests should be made available to women who desire them, it needs to be experienced by women as a considered choice and not something that merely happens to them while they are pregnant (Clarke, 2007). So-called 'institutional directiveness' towards abnormality screening in pregnancy can be avoided by providing sound and unbiased information to pregnant women, ensuring they understand the potentially significant results the test may provide.

Screening and the right to remain in ignorance

Just as we have a right to obtain knowledge to inform our health care, our right to make autonomous decisions also implies we should have the right to refuse at least some public health screening tests. In the genetics literature for example, the 'right not to know' one's genetic status has received significant attention (Raikka, 1998; Bennett, 2001; Andorno, 2004). Broadly, the right to genetic ignorance has two aspects: the right not to know one's mutation status, and the right not to know that one is at risk at all. The former of these is most relevant to the screening context given that screening by definition involves an at-risk population and so respecting the second sense of the right would be incompatible with education or recruitment policies. That said, individuals who are identified as being at risk of a condition that will have implications for their relatives should exercise due caution when considering an unsolicited disclosure of risk to other members of their family.

Broadening out the right not to know from the genetic context may not always be appropriate. Generally, the right not to know that one is at risk of disease is straightforward to respect, although some have argued it precludes full autonomy and may cause us to fail to fulfil our obligations to others (Rhodes, 1998; Harris and Keywood, 2001). It also undermines the collectivist values that underscore ethical analysis in public health. Physically restraining a person to obtain a sample for screening would be unacceptable in all but extreme cases, such as testing for a highly infectious disease when significant concerns arise about third-party harm.

Potential for stigma and discrimination

The term 'stigmatization' is used to describe the negative labelling a person can experience following an event, in this context screening. The Nuffield Council on Bioethics has defined stigma as 'the branding, marking or discrediting . . . of a particular characteristic' (1993: para 8.8; cited by Chadwick et al., 1998). Stigma can be experienced as a self-regarding trait, or something placed upon a person by others. Self-regarding stigma involves feelings of negative perception following a change in personal status, including the receipt of a test result. Discrimination is related to stigmatization, but is not the same. Simply, discrimination involves treating like people differently. It leads to differential treatment in light of a person's status. Any screening programme that led to stigma or discrimination would be problematic and steps would be needed to minimize this occurring.

Concerns over stigma can arise when a specific population is targeted for screening. Perhaps the most notorious example arose from the well-intentioned yet ill-fated sickle cell anaemia screening programmes in the USA in the 1970s. During this decade, many US states mandated screening in African-Americans to identify carriers of this recessively inherited genetic condition, with a view to providing health and reproductive advice and counselling. However, this was not the only effect. Due to misinformation about the nature of carrier status, those found to have one copy of the mutated gene (who were healthy) were discriminated against by employers and insurers who believed carriers would become unwell. Moreover, the African-American population themselves indicated little interest in testing and were not explicitly consulted during policy development. Additionally, sickle cell became widely known as a 'black disease' (Kenen and Schmidt, 1987; Fost, 1999; Wilfond and Thomson, 2000: 64; Bayer et al., 2006: 352).

In the 1980s, screening for HIV also carried concerns over stigma, with potential access to results by third parties causing significant concerns. In 1990, Almond and Ulanowsky observed that:

> [T]he social and financial implications of a positive diagnosis are serious. Health and life insurance, mortgages and house purchase may all be affected. There may be problems for some types of employment . . . .
>
> (1990: 16)

They also show that HIV illustrates how branding can occur:

> AIDS . . . has been particularly associated . . . with certain clearly defined groups – gay and bisexual males, IV drug users, and haemophiliacs . . . .
>
> (1990: 16)

While treatment for HIV has dramatically improved over the past two decades, with a consequent positive impact for morbidity and quality of life, people with HIV arguably do still suffer some degree of stigma. Wynia (2006) suggests this could actually be due to the exceptional treatment of HIV in screening, given the requirements for in-depth counselling and pre-test advice. Regardless of its mechanism, the potential for branding or otherwise derogatively marking people who have HIV remains a problem and must be taken into account by screening programmes.

A more recent, yet less widely discussed example of potential stigma arising from screening in target populations is the use of genetic screening for a panel of diseases known to have a higher prevalence in the Ashkenazi Jewish population (ACOG Committee on Genetics, 2004; Leib, *et al.*, 2005). This includes Tay–Sachs disease, Gaucher Disease, Canavan Disease and Fanconi anaemia. A significant difference between this programme and earlier genetic screening programmes is the degree of consultation with, and involvement of, the target population. Yet problems with stigma may still arise, in two ways. First, these conditions may be (and in some places, have been) labelled as 'Jewish' diseases, when they in fact arise across most populations. Second, members of the Jewish population may be labelled as particularly susceptible to disease. Despite this, the Jewish population's experiences with screening have been positive and this group exhibits a strong desire for screening.

Discrimination following testing has been discussed at length in the genetic screening literature. The main concern has been access to results by third parties; notably insurers or employers. This has been discussed at length elsewhere, but can be summarized as concerns that:

- Individuals will be denied life or other insurance, or charged a disproportionately high premium, after undergoing a screening test;
- Genetic screening will become a prerequisite to employment or obtaining insurance;
- Individuals or groups will be excluded from some workplaces due to a genetic risk they pose, whether or not that risk is related to the particular role; and
- Workplaces will decrease their safety standards; instead only hiring employees with low-risk screening results. (Nuffield Council on Bioethics, 1993: chs 6, 7)

Difficulty in accessing insurance can have devastating consequences, especially in those jurisdictions lacking a national health service. However, companies providing insurance products are commercial entities and cannot be expected to act as charities. Adverse selection, in which consumers disproportionately increase their insurance to counter a known (but undisclosed) genetic risk could have significant commercial implications and would raise premiums for all. Therefore, all contracts of insurance should be made on a level playing field, with full disclosure on both sides.

Potential discrimination in access to insurance has been taken seriously by policy-makers in several countries. The UK, for example, currently has an industry concordat and moratorium on the use of results of predictive genetic tests by insurers (Department of Health, 2005). This gives a high level of consumer protection and as such a legislative approach is not deemed to be required. In the USA, however, the Genetic Information Nondiscrimination Act 2008 does provide legal protections for individuals in relation to employment and health insurance.

In the employment context, it needs to be recognized that employers can already legitimately request medical information in some circumstances. Further, testing may not necessarily have to exclude employees – screening could be used to indicate whether any additional risk-avoidance strategies are required. Mass screening programmes of employees are not only introduced to exclude people and maximize profits; they may also lead to a reduction in occupational disease (Nuffield Council on Bioethics, 1993).

Despite this, employers should not act to provide screening without due cause. Indeed, one US employer has been sued for coercing employees to take non-indicated tests (Philipkoski, 2001). The Nuffield Council on Bioethics has recommended that screening is used only where a connection between a specific disease that seriously endangers health and a workplace has been shown; and for which nothing can be done (Nuffield Council on Bioethics, 1993: 64). Others have recommended, in addition to standard requirements for privacy and predictive value, that the genetic factor should be positively correlated with adequate job performance and that a plan is in place for the use of any data gained (Lappé, 1983; Murray, 1983; Schulte and DeBord, 2000).

Overall it appears that, with some minor exceptions, concerns about discrimination and stigma following screening remain unsubstantiated. Additionally, as Western populations become more mixed, some governments have opted to broaden out screening programmes initially targeted at specific populations; the recent change in practice in the National Health Service antenatal and newborn screening programmes for sickle cell anaemia and thalassaemia in the UK being one example (National Health Service, 2006). With an emphasis on policy monitoring and broad education, concerns over stigma and discrimination can be mitigated. Routinization of screening for other diseases such as HIV could also help reduce stigma.

Provision of pre-test counselling

For genetic screening in particular, until recently most screening programmes incorporated a counselling element, to try to ensure participants make an informed decision that reflected their values. Indeed, the provision of counselling (before or after screening) has been recommended by several authorities in the field (see, for example, Clarke, 1995; European Society for Human Genetics, 2003). More recently, the growing number of genetic tests that can detect conditions for which treatment is readily available and which have little reproductive implications has led some to question whether such tests are really exceptional when compared to standard screening tests in medicine. Thus the requirement for pre-test counselling could be relaxed and values more associated with public health (namely high uptake) could be emphasized. The inherited condition familial hypercholesterolaemia (FH), for example, can cause morbidly high cholesterol if untreated, can be effectively screened for (using either genetic or clinical means) and a diagnosis has no reproductive implications. Once a case is identified in an individual, the care team will 'cascade' out to that person's relatives, in an attempt to identify some of the thousands of undiagnosed individuals with this condition. Once diagnosed, cholesterol can be controlled via diet, exercise and statin drugs if needed. For conditions such as FH, counselling should arguably not be required. If an individual's best interests are served by knowledge of mutation status, a good intervention is available, the test has no reproductive implications and stigma is unlikely, then many of the reasons why pre-test counselling is offered are mitigated. A pre-test counselling process could instead cause potential participants to be more concerned about what is really a straightforward test, increasing refusal rates. Waiving the need for counselling will not be appropriate in all circumstances, but adopting a 'one size fits all' approach to counselling in population screening programmes is equally unwise.

Screening and the potential for psychological harm

A primary ethical principle underpinning screening is that the benefits of early diagnosis need to be counterbalanced against potential harms. A hallmark of all screening programmes is that they tend to be offered to otherwise healthy populations. This can have the effect of introducing concepts of illness and disease to groups which otherwise had no cause for concern regarding their health. This may cause harm, for example, problems caused by misleading results leading to unnecessary further testing.

The aspects of screening programmes most likely to give rise to concerns about psychological harm are the potential for false positive (identifying disease in a healthy person) or false negative (failing to identify the disease of interest) results, caused by the necessarily imperfect specificity and sensitivity of screening tests. These rates are not insignificant: screening tests for some cancers have a 10–20% false negative rate.

Both false negative and false positive results can give rise to harm. A false negative result can potentially mean that a screening recipient will go on to develop the condition or disease being screened for, although this risk can in some circumstances be mitigated if the person participates in regular screening and seeks health care when unusual symptoms develop. A false positive result can give rise to serious feelings of morbidity and anxiety, even some months after the initial test and despite continuous reassurance (Brett et al., 1998; cited in Wilson, 2000).

In the context of newborn screening, around 1% of parents will receive a false positive diagnosis, received at an important point of parent–baby bonding. The effect of this has been the subject of many empirical studies exploring possible harms such as parental anxiety or hyper-vigilance about the child's health. While early studies described the problem of 'PKU anxiety syndrome' (Rothenberg and Sills, 1968), more recent data suggests that parents display no adverse behavioural attitudes towards their children (Pollitt et al., 1997; Green et al., 2004). A minority do have lingering concerns about their children's health (Pollitt et al., 1997; Green et al., 2004), yet this harm from a false positive diagnosis can be minimized if good quality information is provided during follow-up (Green et al., 2004).

False negative results can also have repercussions for individuals, as the example of cervical screening illustrates. Litigation in response to false negative results for breast and cervical cancer has occurred in several countries, including the UK and Australia (Wilson, 2000). This has, in some cases, led to a drop in the number of people presenting for screening, an increase in referrals for invasive tests in patients who have slightly abnormal results and a demand for more accurate yet vastly more expensive screening tests (Stanley, 1996; Wilson, 2000). Wilson comments that the enthusiasm for screening promoted by health agencies has provided recipients and the legal fraternity with a false sense of security as to accuracy.

The possibility of facing further testing following screening can also cause harm. Combined nuchal and maternal serum screening, for example, is a minimally invasive way for some pregnant women to reduce their background risk of foetal abnormalities. However, the test is inherently uncertain and presents results probabilistically. This can cause anxiety or can establish women on a path to invasive testing that they may not have contemplated at the outset. As this test is only capable of obtaining meaningful results after 12 weeks' gestation women who do later discover their foetus carries an abnormality will face a decision about termination of pregnancy later than they may feel comfortable with. They may also experience their pregnancy as 'tentative' until these tests are conducted (Katz Rothman, 1993). Some argue that the test has also medicalized pregnancy for the many younger women who previously experienced pregnancy without screening interventions (Lippman, 1991).

In offering routine antenatal screening, careful counselling and information provision is required to ensure that women make informed decisions. Yet ensuring this is achieved within the myriad of other tests, interventions and information pregnant women receive is no easy task.

In light of these concerns, Shickle and Chadwick (1994) argue that a full risk–benefit calculation must always be performed before a screening programme commences and that health authorities must be prepared to accept the fact that this may mean that a screening programme should on occasion not be implemented.

Access to screening programmes – justice and distribution

Determining how to allocate scarce resources is inherent to any domain of health care; and public health is no exception. Appropriate use of funding in public health is imperative to its success, as this will satiate funders and help ensure public confidence in screening programmes. Thus any screening programme, and certainly those funded from public resources, will need to be targeted in some way, otherwise the benefits of screening will be undermined by the inefficiency that inevitably arises when too broad a population is screened. A consequence of such targeting in screening is that some who may benefit from screening will be excluded, or may not even be made aware of the programme's existence.

Screening programmes will almost always be competing for resources from a finite pool of funding. While equity in access to screening regardless of finances is ethically laudable, it ignores the reality of resource allocation. Distributing funds between groups is often difficult, as is comparing the value of different interventions. How can we justly compare the benefits of cervical screening with newborn hearing tests? Both of these appear to be 'important health problems', but prioritizing this importance may be difficult and could involve the use of potentially problematic factors such as ethnicity, socio-economic status or gender (Chadwick et al., 1998).

Any screening programme should aim to use funds primarily to increase the marginal health of the population – which will require a sound demonstration of the screening test's efficacy and efficiency. This involves a consideration of more than mere cost-effectiveness. Population screening for prostate cancer is not currently provided using public funds in the UK because evidence for benefits of screening is not strong enough to outweigh the potential harm of false diagnosis of this condition (National Health Service Executive, 1997).The psycho-social impact of any screening test is also relevant. Burris and Gostin (2004) point out that in the context of genetic screening a test result will be experienced by a person within a complex set of social links and relationships. Not only are test recipients at risk of stigma or other kinds of psychological harm, they may suffer economic burdens through increased health care costs or denial of access to other resources.

A further issue affecting the provision of screening programmes is access to relevant treatments and/or preventive measures should a person be deemed to be at high risk of disease following screening. A programme should not be instigated until other basic necessities are in place, such as availability and affordability of the relevant treatment or preventive tool, or control of the relevant environment (European Society for Human Genetics, 2003).

In establishing or extending any screening programme, its impact on other populations who may benefit from screening but whose needs are less 'visible' should also be assessed. Screening programmes will be problematic if the outcome deliberately or inadvertently excludes those who may benefit or if the screening process causes harm. For these reasons, the equity and effectiveness (broadly construed) of all programmes should also be monitored once they are established.

Involvement of the private sector

The risk of some individuals or groups being excluded from a screening programme will also depend on how the programme is provided – through the public sector, via a charity, in the course of a research project or on a fee-for-service basis. If publicly funded, cost constraints will inevitably determine the definition and boundaries of the target population. Under privately funded service provision, cost may instead become the primary barrier to access, while the programme itself may be provided to a wider cross-section of participants.

The potential for competing interests between the financial motivation of commercial providers and the avoidance of harm for participants in screening has not gone unnoticed, particularly in discussions of genetic screening (Chadwick *et al.*, 2001). Many companies now offer genetic testing direct to consumers, usually via the Internet. Although these services are subject to some concerns, most fall outside the scope of this chapter in that they are not explicitly screening programmes. Concerns may arise, however, if a screening programme is deemed important enough to be established, yet is then provided by a commercial entity.

Concerns underpinning private provision of screening echo those arising in other areas of health care. These include:

- Denying justice to those who are already disadvantaged.
  People who have less financial means may not be able to pay for commercial screening services. But members of lower socio-economic groups may also stand to gain huge benefits from screening.
- The value to public health will be lost.
  If screening becomes accessible only to those who can pay for it, then the potential for benefit from screening programmes may be reduced. This will then reduce the efficiency of the programme, which may undermine it being offered at all.
- The introduction of a screening test before validity is certain.
  Commercial entities will be keen to recoup their costs in developing a test and so may offer it in the private market before the recommended evaluations have been carried out. If a test proves not to be beneficial then people would have wasted their money investing in it.
- Screening will exploit the 'worried well'.
  Private entities offering screening are very likely to heavily market their tests in order to ensure maximum customer uptake. Those who do take the test may feel more in control of their health; yet they are also at risk of taking an ineffective or inappropriate test.

- Unbiased counselling may be compromised.
  Evidence suggests that people who receive a higher risk result after screening do suffer a degree of anxiety, albeit one that resolves in the longer term. However, this does not mean it should not be addressed when it occurs. How will private or commercial entities handle pre-test counselling? Will it be possible to offer independent counselling, or will this become confused with the need to 'sell' the test? Further, will distressed patients be pushed back into the public sector to have their problems addressed?
- Confounding factors if screening is offered by the charity or research sectors.
  If screening is offered by charities, it will be dependent upon funding and donations. These can at times become unstable, which could affect continuity of service provision. If screening is offered in the course of a research project, the nature and duration of that programme will be constrained by the aims and timeline of the particular project. (Clarke, 1995; R. E. Ashcroft, pers. comm., 2005)

In his thoughtful book, Jim Thornton (1999) argues in favour of a limited programme of private screening, discussing equity, health needs and free markets. Regarding screening in adult populations, he argues that consumers are the best persons to judge their own health. Some screening programmes are ineffective while others may cause actual harm. For these reasons, adult screening should be provided by the private sector. Some screening programmes may also cause harm. Children and those yet to be born, however, are not capable of advocating their best interests and so the State must protect them via quality programmes. And if public screening is being requested, the burden of proof for justification lies with those advocating for it.

If private commercial entities are to be involved in screening, then this should be entered into with caution and with transparent and rigorous regulation, including oversight of marketing and advertising. Steps need to be taken to ensure appropriate linking in with a participant's primary care provider and, in the case of genetic screening, to help the proband identify relatives who may also wish to be screened. Factors such as marketing and pre-screen information should be monitored and the need for an oversight authority should be considered (Chadwick et al., 2001).

Emerging issues

Population screening is not a static programme. As more and more screening is performed for a wider array of conditions or clauses, further ethical issues are sure to arise. For example, the vast number of biological samples collected during screening can pose problems around consent and control of future use. Many samples are used again, for example in research or public health monitoring. This necessitates a balancing of the right to control access to biological data with the practicality and cost of obtaining fully informed consent for these kinds of uses. Legislation and policy is also relevant here and in some jurisdictions is complex.

In the field of genetics, genes contributing to complex human diseases and conditions, such as coronary artery disease, diabetes and cancer, are frequently identified. DNA sequencing technology is also constantly improving; becoming faster and less expensive. 'Personalized genomics', whereby we will all be able to obtain a complete sequence of our genome with an indication of disease risk is already commercially available and is receiving attention from policy makers (Fink and Collins, 2000). The use of DNA chips (microarrays) also enables the detection of several hundred gene changes at once. The possible implications of such testing for geneticization of health, our self-understanding and discrimination and stigma requires more attention.

Screening programmes also tend to be offered by health systems in developed countries, leading to further discrepancies in global health worldwide. The equitable and ethical introduction of health screening worldwide is a significant challenge for the twenty-first century (Ballantyne, 2006).

Conclusion

Population screening for public health offers myriad complexities; drawing together considerations of ethics, economics, effectiveness and equity. Ethical issues in population screening tend to be assessed using a utilitarian framework applied consistently with ethical standards in clinical practice, although some have suggested that as screening programmes are essentially large-scale experiments a research ethics framework is more appropriate (Skrabanek, 1990; cited by Jepson et al., 2007). Appropriately analysing these overlapping considerations and frameworks requires knowledge of each of these domains, and the literature is illustrative of the collaborations and cross-considerations currently taking place between academics, health professionals and policy makers.

This chapter has offered an overview of the many debates ongoing in this fascinating area of health care. Ethical issues arise at all stages of screening programmes, from establishing a case for a new screening test, to recruitment, testing and monitoring. A balancing of individual and community values is required, with a key theme of prioritizing benefit over harm to benefit the population and promote and protect health. Screening is not, however, without risk and to some extent there remains a question mark over whether risks are always accurately safeguarded against, or what risks it is acceptable to trade-off to promote population health. Additionally, the issue of evidence to support screening can be contestable, particularly if screening is time consuming or invasive.

Acknowledgements

The author would like to thank Dr Angus Dawson, Professor Robyn Martin and Professor Richard Ashcroft for helpful discussions and assistance during the preparation of this chapter.

References

ACOG Committee on Genetics (2004) Prenatal and preconceptional carrier screening for genetic diseases in individuals of Eastern European Jewish descent. Obstetrician and Gynecologist, 104: 425–8.

Almond, B. and Ulanowsky, C. (1990) HIV and pregnancy. Hastings Center Report, 20(2): 16–21.

Andorno, R. (2004) The right not to know: an autonomy based approach. Journal of Medical Ethics, 30: 435–40.

Angastiniotis, M., Kyriakidou, S. and Hadjiminas, M. (1986) How thalassaemia was controlled in Cyprus. World Health Forum, 7: 291–7.

Ballantyne, A. (2006) Medical Genetic Services in Developing Countries: The Ethical, Legal and Social Implications of Genetic Testing and Screening. Geneva: World Health Organization.

Bayer, R., Gostin, L. O., Jennings, B. and Steinbock B. (eds) (2006) Public Health Ethics: Theory, Policy and Practice. New York: Oxford University Press.

Bayer, R., Dubler, N. N. and Landesman, S. (1993) The dual epidemics of tuberculosis and AIDS: ethical and policy issues in screening and treatment. *American Journal of Public Health*, 83: 649–54.

Bennett, R. (2001) Antenatal genetic testing and the right to remain in ignorance. *Theoretical Medicine and Bioethics*, 22: 461–71.

Bennett, R. (2004) Routine antenatal HIV testing and its implications for informed consent. In *Ethics and Midwifery*, ed. L. Frith and H. Draper, 2nd edn. Edinburgh: Books for Midwives, pp. 74–90.

Bennett, R. (2007) Routine antenatal HIV testing and informed consent: an unworkable marriage? *Journal of Medical Ethics*, 33: 446–8.

Berlin, L. (1999) Malpractice issues in radiology: screening versus diagnostic mammography. *American Journal of Roentgenology*, 173: 3–7.

Bratton, A. J. (2007) Deputies seize baby to test blood against parents' will. *Iowa State Daily*, 22 October.

Brett, J., Austoker, J. and Ong, G. (1998) Do women who undergo further investigation for breast screening suffer adverse psychological consequences? *Journal of Public Health Medicine*, 20: 396–403.

British Medical Association (2005) *Population Screening and Genetic Testing: A Briefing on Current Programmes and Technologies*. London: BMA. 'Available at: http://www.bma.org.uk/images/ ScreeningBriefing2_tcm41-20993.pdf (accessed: 04/04/11).

Burris, S. and Gostin, L. O. (2004) Genetic screening from a public health perspective: three 'ethical' principles. In *A Companion to Genethics*, ed. J. Burley and J. Harris. Oxford: Blackwell, pp. 455–64.

Chadwick, R., ten Have, H., Husted, J., *et al.* (1998) Genetic screening and ethics: European perspectives. *Journal of Medicine and Philosophy*, 23: 255–73.

Chadwick, R., ten Have, H., Hoedemaekers, R., *et al.* (2001) Euroscreen 2: towards community policy on insurance, commercialization and public awareness. *Journal of Medicine and Philosophy*, 26: 263–72.

Clarke, A. (1995) Population screening for genetic susceptibility to disease. *British Medical Journal*, 311: 35–8.

Clarke, A. J. (1997) Newborn screening. In *Genetics, Society and Clinical Practice*, ed. P. S. Harper and A. J. Clarke. Oxford: Bios Scientific Publishers, pp. 107–17.

Clarke, A. (2007) Genetic counselling. In *Principles of Health Care Ethics*, 2nd edn, ed. R. E. Ashcroft, A. Dawson, H. Draper and J. R. McMillan. Chichester: John Wiley, pp. 427–34.

Clayton, E. W. (2004) Genetic testing and screening: newborn genetic screening. In *Encyclopedia of Bioethics*, 3rd edn, ed. S. G. Post. New York: Macmillan Reference, pp. 1004–7.

Department of Health (2005) *Concordat and Moratorium on Genetics and Insurance*. London: Department of Health. Available at: http://www.dh.gov.uk/en/ Publicationsandstatistics/Publications/ PublicationsPolicyAndGuidance/ DH_4105905 (accessed: 27/11/07).

de Zulueta, P. and Boulton, M. (2007) Routine antenatal HIV testing: the responses and perceptions of pregnant women and the viability of informed consent. A qualitative study. *Journal of Medical Ethics*, 33: 329–36.

European Society of Human Genetics, Public and Professional Policy Committee (2003) Population genetic screening programmes: technical, social and ethical issues. *European Journal of Human Genetics*, 11(Suppl. 2): S5–S7.

Faden, R., Chwalow, A. J., Holtzman, N. A. and Horn, S. D. (1982a) A survey to evaluate parental consent as public policy for neonatal screening. *American Journal of Public Health*, 72: 1347–52.

Faden, R., Holtzman, N. A. and Chwalow, A. J. (1982b) Parental rights, child welfare and public health: the case of PKU screening. *American Journal of Public Health*, 72: 1396–400.

Fink, L. and Collins, F. S. (2000) The human genome project: evolving status and emerging opportunities for disease prevention. In *Genetics and Public Health in* the 21st Century, ed. M. J. Khoury, W. Burke and E. J. Thomson. New York: Oxford University Press, pp. 45–59.

Fost, N. (1999) Ethical implications of screening asymptomatic individuals. In New Ethics for the Public's Health, ed. B. Steinbock and D. E. Beauchamp. New York: Oxford University Press, pp. 344–52.

Foster, P. and Anderson, C. M. (1998) Reaching targets in the national cervical screening programme: are current practices unethical? Journal of Medical Ethics, 24: 151–7.

Friedman Ross, L. (2002) Genetic testing of children: who should consent? In A Companion to Genethics, ed. J. Harris and J. Burley. Oxford: Blackwell, pp. 114–26.

Gostin, L. O. (2000) Public Health Law: Power, Duty, Restraint. Berkeley, CA: University of California Press.

Gostin, L. O. (ed.) (2002) Public Health Law and Ethics: A Reader. Berkeley, CA: University of California Press.

Green, J. M., Hewison, J., Bekker, H. L., Bryant, L. D. and Cuckle, H. S. (2004) Psychosocial aspects of genetic screening of pregnant women and newborns: a systematic review. Health Technology Assessment, 8(33): 1–124.

Gustaffson Stolt, U., Ludvigsson, J., Liss, P.-E. and Svensson, T. (2003) Bioethical theory and practice in genetic screening for Type 1 diabetes. Medicine, Health Care and Philosophy, 6: 45–50.

Guthrie, R. (1986) Newborn screening: past, present and future. In Genetic Disease: Screening and Management, ed. P. Carter and A. M. Wiley. New York: Alan Liss, pp. 319–39.

Harris, J. and Keywood, K. (2001) Ignorance, information and autonomy. Theoretical Medicine and Bioethics, 22: 415–36.

Hodge, J. G. (2004) Genetic testing and screening: public health context. In Encyclopedia of Bioethics, 3rd edn, ed. S. G. Post. New York: Macmillan Reference, pp. 1016–20.

Jennings, B. (2007) Community in public health ethics. In Principles of Health Care Ethics, 2nd

edn, ed. R. E. Ashcroft, A. Dawson, H. Draper and J. R. McMillan. Chichester: John Wiley, pp. 543–8.

Jepson, R. G., Hewison, J., Thompson, A. G. and Weller D. (2005) How should we measure informed choice? The case of cancer screening. Journal of Medical Ethics, 31: 192–6.

Jepson, R. G., Hewsin, J., Thompson, A. and Weller D. (2007) Patient perspectives on information and choice in cancer screening: a qualitative study in the UK. Social Science and Medicine, 65: 890–9.

Juth, N. and Munthe, C. (2007) Screening: ethical aspects. In Principles of Health Care Ethics, 2nd edn, ed. R. E. Ashcroft, A. Dawson, H. Draper and J. R. McMillan. Chichester: John Wiley, pp. 607–15.

Katz Rothman, B. (1993) The Tentative Pregnancy: How Amniocentesis Changes the Experience of Motherhood. New York: W.W. Norton.

Kayton, A. (2007) Newborn screening: a literature review. Neonatal Network, 26: 85–95.

Kenen, R. and Schmidt, R. (1987) Social implications of screening programs for carrier status: genetic diseases in the 1970s and AIDS in the 1980s. In Dominant Issues in Medical Sociology, ed. H. D. Schwartz. New York: Random House, pp. 145–54.

Kerruish, N. J. and Robertson, S. P. (2005) Newborn screening: new developments, new dilemmas. Journal of Medical Ethics, 31: 393–8.

Kerruish, N. J., Campbell-Stokes, P. L., Gray, A., Merriman, T. R., Robertson, S. P. and Taylor, B. J. (2007) Maternal psychological reaction to newborn genetic screening for type 1 diabetes. Pediatrics, 120(2): 324.

Khoury, M. J., Burke, W. and Thomson, E. J. (2000) Genetics and public health: a framework for the integration of human genetics into public health practice. In Genetics and Public Health in the 21st Century, ed. M. J. Khoury, W. Burke and E. J. Thomson. New York: Oxford University Press, pp. 3–24.

Lappé, M., Gustafson, J. and Roblin, R. (1972) Ethical and social issues in screening for genetic disease. New England Journal of Medicine, 286: 1129–32.

Lappé, M. (1983) Ethical issues in testing for differential sensitivity to occupational hazards. *Journal of Occupational Medicine*, **25**: 797–808.

Laurie, G. (2002) Better to hesitate at the threshold of compulsion: PKU testing and the concept of family autonomy in Eire. *Journal of Medical Ethics*, **28**: 136–7.

Leib, J. R., Gollust, S. E., Hull, S. C. and Wilfond, B. S. (2005) Carrier screening panels for Ashkenazi Jews: is more better? *Genetics in Medicine*, **7**: 185–90.

Lippman, A. (1991) Prenatal genetic testing and screening: constructing needs and reinforcing inequities. *American Journal of Law and Medicine*, **17**: 15–50.

Mann, J. M. (1997) Medicine and public health, ethics and human rights. *Hastings Center Report*, **27**(3): 6–13.

Marshall, T. and Adab, P. (2003) Informed consent for breast screening: what should we tell women? *Journal of Medical Screening*, **10**: 22–6.

Marteau, T. M., Dormandy, E. and Michie, S. (2001) A measure of informed choice. *Health Expectations*, **4**: 99–108.

Marteau, T. M. and Kinmonth, A. L. (2002) Screening for cardiovascular risk: public health imperative or matter for individual informed choice? *British Medical Journal*, **325**: 78–80.

Muir-Gray, J. A. and Pearce-Smith, N. (2007) *Screening Specialist Library*. NHS National Electronic Library for Health. Available at: http://www.library.nhs.uk/screening/ (accessed: 22/11/07).

Murray, T. H. (1983) Genetic screening in the workplace: ethical issues. *Journal of Occupational Medicine*, **25**: 451–4.

National Health Service (2006) *NHS Sickle Cell and Thalassaemia Screening Programme*. London: NHS Antenatal and Newborn Screening Programmes. Available at: http://sctscreening.nhs.uk/ (accessed: 04/04/11).

National Health Service Executive (1997) *Population Screening for Prostate Cancer*. London: Department of Health. 'Prostate Cancer EL (97)12. Leeds: Department of Health'.

National Screening Committee (2003) *Criteria for Appraising the Viability, Effectiveness and Appropriateness of a Screening Programme*. London: Department of Health. Available at: http://www.screening.nhs/uk/criteria (accessed: 04/04/11).

National Screening Committee (2011) Aims and Objectives of the NHS Down's Syndrome Screening Programme. London: Department of Health. Available at: http://fetalanomaly. screening.nhs.uk/cms.php?folder=2452 (accessed: 04/04/11).

National Screening Committee (2011) *What Is Screening?* London: Department of Health. Available at: http://www.screening.nhs.uk/ screening (accessed: 5/04/11).

Newson, A. (2006) Should parental refusals of newborn screening be respected? *Cambridge Quarterly of Healthcare Ethics*, **15**: 135–46.

Nijsingh, N. (2007) informed consent and the expansion of newborn screening. In *Ethics, Prevention, and Public Health*, ed. A. Dawson and M. Verweij. Oxford: Oxford University Press, pp. 198–212.

Nuffield Council on Bioethics (1993) *Genetic Screening: Ethical Issues*. London: Nuffield Council on Bioethics.

Parsons, E. P., Clarke, A. J. and Bradley, D. M. (2003) Implications of carrier identification in newborn screening for cystic fibrosis. *Archives of Disease in Childhood: Fetal and Neonatal Edition*, **88**: F467–F471.

Paul, D. (1999) Contesting consent: the challenge to compulsory neonatal screening for PKU. *Perspectives in Biology and Medicine*, **42**: 207–19.

Philipkoski, N. (2001) Genetic testing case settled. *Wired Magazine*. Available at: http:// www.wired.com/science/discoveries/news/ 2001/04/42971 (accessed: 27/11/07).

Pfeffer, N. (2004) 'If you think you've got a lump, they'll screen you.' Informed consent, health promotion, and breast cancer. *Journal of Medical Ethics*, **30**: 227–30.

Pollitt, R. J., Green, A., McCabe, C. J., *et al.* (1997) Neonatal screening for inborn errors of metabolism: cost, yield and outcome. *Health Technology Assessment*, **1**(7).

President's Commission for the Study of Ethical Problems in Medicine and Biomedical and Behavioral Research (1983) *Screening and Counseling for Genetic Conditions: A Report on the Ethical, Social and Legal Implications of Genetic Screening, Counseling and Education Programs.* Washington, DC: US Government Printing Office. Available at: http://www.bioethics.gov/reports/past_commissions/geneticscreening.pdf (accessed: 04/04/11).

Press, N. and Clayton, E. W. (2000) Genetics and public health: Informed consent beyond the clinical encounter. In *Genetics and Public Health in the 21st Century: Using Genetic Information to Improve Health and Prevent Disease*, ed. M. J. Khoury, W. Burke and E. J. Thomson. New York: Oxford University Press, pp. 505–26.

Press, N. and Ariail, K. (2004) Genetic testing and screening: reproductive genetic testing. In *Encyclopedia of Bioethics*, 3rd edn, ed. S. G. Post. New York: Macmillan Reference, pp. 996–1004.

Raffle, A. E. (1997) Informed participation in screening is essential (letter) *British Medical Journal*, **315**: 1762.

Raffle, A. E. (2001) Information about screening: is it to achieve high uptake or to ensure informed choice? *Health Expectations*, **4**: 92–98.

Raikka, J. (1998) Freedom and a right (not) to know. *Bioethics*, **12**: 49–63.

Rhodes, R. (1998) Genetic links, family ties and social bonds: rights and responsibilities in the face of genetic knowledge. *Journal of Medicine and Philosophy*, **23**: 10–30.

Riis, P. (1985) Ethical issues in mass screening procedures. In *Ethical Issues in Preventive Medicine*, ed. S. Doxiadis. Dordrecht: Martinus Nijhoff Publishers, pp. 84–89.

Rothenberg, M. B. and Sills, E. M. (1968) Iatrogenesis: the PKU anxiety syndrome. *Journal of the American Academy for Child Psychiatry*, **7**: 689–92.

Schulte, P. A. and DeBord, D. G. (2000) Public health assessment of genetic information in the occupational setting. In *Genetics and Public Health in the 21st Century*, ed. M. J. Khoury, W. Burke and E. J.

Thomson. New York: Oxford University Press, pp. 203–19.

Sherr, L., Fox, Z., Lipton, M., Whyte, P., Jones, P., Harrison, U. and the Camden and Islington Steering Group (2006) Sustaining HIV testing in pregnancy: evaluation of routine offer of HIV testing in three London hospitals over 2 years. *AIDS Care*, **18**: 183–8.

Shickle, D. and Chadwick, R. (1994) The ethics of screening: is 'screeningitis' an incurable disease? *Journal of Medical Ethics*, **20**: 12–18.

Skrabanek, P. (1990) Why is preventive medicine exempted from ethics constraints? *Journal of Medical Ethics*, **16**: 187–90.

Stanley, F. (1996) Litigation or science: what's driving medical decision-making? Australian Law Reform Commission. Available at: http://www.austlii.edu.au/au/other/alrc/publications/reform/reform69/ALRCR69LITIGATIONORSCIENCE.html (accessed: 16/7/07).

Thornton, J. (1999) *Should Health Screening be Private?* London: Institute of Economic Affairs.

Tudor Hart, J. (2008) A few lessons in screening for Gordon Brown. *British Medical Journal*, **336**: 123.

van den Berg, M., Timmermans, D. R., ten Kate, L. P., van Vugt, J. M. and van der Wal, G. (2005) Are pregnant women making informed choices about prenatal screening? *Genetics in Medicine*, **7**: 332–8.

van den Berg, M., Timmermans, D. R., ten Kate, L. P., van Vugt, J. M. and van der Wal, G. (2006) Informed decision making in the context of prenatal screening. *Patient Education and Counseling*, **63**: 110–17.

White, C. (2008) Prime minister promises raft of screening tests. *British Medical Journal*, **336**: 62–3.

Wikler, D. (1999) Can we learn from eugenics? *Journal of Medical Ethics*, **25**: 183–94.

Wilfond, B. S. (1995) Screening policy for cystic fibrosis: the role of evidence. *Hastings Center Report*, **25**(3, Suppl.): S21–S23.

Wilfond, B. S. and Thompson, E. J. (2000) Models of public health genetic policy development. In *Genetics and Public Health in the 21st Century: Using Genetic Information to Improve Health and Prevent Disease*, ed. M. J. Khoury, W. Burke and E. J. Thomson. New York: Oxford, pp. 61–82.

Wilson, J. M. G. and Jungner, G. (1968) Principles and practice of screening for disease. In *Public Health Paper Number* **34**. Geneva: World Health Organization.

Wilson, R. M. (2000) Screening for breast and cervical cancer as a common cause for litigation. *British Medical Journal,* **320**: 1352–3.

Wynia, M. K. (2006) Routine screening: informed consent, stigma and the waning of HIV exceptionalism. *American Journal of Bioethics,* **6**: 5–8.

Vaccination ethics

Angus Dawson

Introduction

Ever since it began as an intervention designed to protect against smallpox, vaccination has been controversial. However, the passion that people bring to debates about vaccination is not always supported by a fair review of the evidence and issues. In this chapter I will outline and discuss a few of the key arguments about this important area of public health.

I begin with some clarifications about the limits of this chapter. First, vaccination at its broadest can be taken to involve some form of artificial stimulation of the immune system as a response to actual or potential bacterial or virological infection. Vaccination might be either preventive (given prior to potential infection) or therapeutic (given in response to infection). This chapter is deliberately termed 'vaccination ethics' as I will restrict my discussion to priming of the immune system *before* contact with any disease. This means we can exclude from this chapter discussion of other forms of immunization such as the giving of immunoglobulin after possible exposure to, or after infection with, a disease. This is not because such techniques are unimportant, but because both the use of immunoglobulin and therapeutic vaccination might be thought of as primarily *clinical* interventions rather than *public health* activities. This chapter will concentrate on preventive vaccination as this is the core controversial issue. Second, the classic image of vaccination consists of an injection (into the muscle or under the skin). However, in some cases the relevant material is given orally (and absorbed through the digestive tract) or through a nasal spray, or in the future it might be delivered in some other way (such as through the consumption of fortified foods). Lastly, most preventive vaccination is carried out in childhood. This is because this is the time when the immune system can be primed to the greatest advantage, but also it is a time of greatest threat to the individual from many diseases. However, it should not be forgotten that many other vaccinations are carried out with adolescents and adults. Such vaccination might be for a number of reasons: boosters for childhood vaccinations, because older individuals might be at threat of disease due to travel or because they are held to be at increased risk for some medical reason (for example, medical conditions related to immune suppression or general old age) or some expected lifestyle change (for example, human papilloma virus vaccination prior to sexual activity). I will focus on childhood preventive vaccination for the rest of this chapter unless I specify otherwise.

I outline three key arguments in the following sections: the nature of our obligation not to bring about harm to others; the idea of best interests; and a discussion of harms and benefits. I end with a short discussion of the possible grounds for compulsory vaccination.

Public Health Ethics, ed. Angus Dawson. Published by Cambridge University Press. © Cambridge University Press 2011.

Harm to others

Much contemporary bioethics assumes a broadly liberal set of background commitments. How might this approach be related to vaccination? Traditional liberals (such as John Stuart Mill [1859] and Joel Feinberg [1973]) commonly make a distinction between actions likely to cause harm only to self and those likely to result in harm-to-others. They hold that this makes a vital difference to the legitimacy of interfering in someone's freedom of action. On this approach third parties have fewer justifiable reasons to intervene on harm-to-self grounds. While health care professionals may have a duty to warn about a risk of harm or provide relevant information, any attempt to bring about a vaccination for someone's own good will be met with the charge of paternalism.

What is paternalism? Paternalism can be defined as acting (or not acting) with the intention of reducing harm or bringing about greater good for the particular individual affected by the action (or omission). On this definition it is left open whether a paternalistic action is morally justifiable: there are two separate judgments. Is it paternalism? If it is, is it morally justified? However, many liberals believe that we can use a distinction between hard/strong or soft/weak paternalism to settle the issue of justifiability. On this view it is argued that strong paternalism is where an action will overrule the action or decision of a competent individual. (In the liberal's view this is usually held to be unjustifiable.) In contrast, weak paternalism is where an action is performed on behalf of an incompetent individual (for example, young child; adult with serious learning difficulties; adult with dementia, etc.). (In the liberal's view this is usually held to be justifiable.)

Routine childhood vaccinations are usually carried out on very young children, so, if we are talking about paternalism at all, we are talking about weak paternalism. The issue under discussion will not be whether someone should make decisions on behalf of children just a few months old, but who should do so. As we are talking about incompetent individuals here, we can set aside the harm-to-self argument and concentrate upon harm-to-others considerations. With young children, 'harm-to-self' considerations end up being, at best, only a component of a judgment of best interests (as we will see below). In the case of young children, any argument about harm-to-others considerations related to vaccination will focus on the potential harm (to third parties) as a result of the parent's decision not to vaccinate their child.

However, note that harm-to-others considerations are likely to be an important consideration in relation to decisions about the vaccination of competent adults as well as children. For example, an adult traveller might knowingly put others at risk of harm if they refuse to be vaccinated for a contagious disease. A related issue is whether certain individuals or groups have special obligations to protect others from harm. For example, in many parts of the world, health care workers are required to be vaccinated for conditions such as hepatitis B as a means of reducing the risk of being infected themselves but also of passing on infections to others. There has been a recent lively discussion about whether there is an obligation upon workers in care homes to be vaccinated against influenza (van Delden et al., 2008).

As suggested above, while liberal political philosophy generally leaves it to the individual to make decisions about their own lives, there is an important exception: where your actions might result in harm-to-others. (Such compulsory powers of detention can be seen in most jurisdictions and in the International Health Regulations as a means to ensure that individuals are protected from a potential source of infectious disease, particularly if treatment is refused.) We can construct a harm-to-others argument related to vaccinations as follows:

1. Contagious diseases that might result in (more than trivial) harm can be passed on to others through non-intentional action.
2. This could be prevented through vaccination of any potential source individual in advance (where a relevant vaccine exists).
3. We have a general moral obligation not to cause harm to others through our own actions and inactions.
4. Given 1 and 2, an individual can reduce the risk of causing (non-trivial) harm to others through vaccination for (serious) contagious disease.

Conclusion: given 3 and 4, we are morally obligated to have vaccinations for (serious) contagious diseases (where available).

Of course there are many issues to discuss in exploring such an argument (Dawson, 2007). However, support for this view comes from the fact that, as mentioned earlier, a decision not to vaccinate (against contagious diseases) does not just put the non-vaccinated individual's health at risk. A failure to vaccinate is not like a failure to consent to a blood transfusion. In the latter case it is only the individual themselves that is harmed, whereas in the vaccination case others may be harmed as a result of an individual's choice or a parent's decision not to vaccinate their child. In other words, where there are serious public health issues at stake it is possible to argue that we are under a moral obligation to be vaccinated or ensure our children are vaccinated on the grounds of potential harm to third parties (Dawson, 2007).

It should be noted that harm-to-others arguments are not paternalistic, because the reason for intervention is nothing to do with the good or potential harm relating to the particular individual we are concerned about. The justification for action is the potential harm to third parties flowing from the parent's decision about their child. This argument is potentially powerful in the vaccination case, because of the highly contagious nature of many vaccine-preventable childhood diseases. However, some will object to such an argument, because they will say that the presumption in favour of parental autonomy should not be overturned on these grounds in relation to vaccination, perhaps because the risk of harm resulting from a particular instance of non-vaccination will be too remote. However, even if this is true, the harm-to-others argument will become stronger the more imminent and the greater the threat of harm resulting from the decision.

The 'best interests' argument

Liberal democracies, rightly, value individual liberty. As a result competent adults are usually considered to be the appropriate persons to make decisions about their own health care treatment. This freedom is usually extended to parents in relation to decisions about their children's health. Such a position could be supported on a number of different theoretical and practical grounds. For example, it is sometimes argued that a parent might be considered to know better than anyone else what is in an individual child's best interests, because they can reasonably be expected to know that particular child better than anyone else. They are also likely to know what will benefit their child, and be aware of the societal and cultural context within which the child will be raised (and so, what is likely to make that child's life go well). Parents might also argue that such decisional authority is part of what it is to be a parent. While this latter claim may consist of an assertion of ownership or control, it need not do so; for example, parents might, alternatively, link the idea to the responsibilities they have as a parent. Ultimately, however such a view is justified, there seems a reasonable claim at its root, as it will be the parents that have to deal with any negative or positive consequences that result from any decision made. Another possible argument in support of parental authority might be based on the idea that the family is a private institution, and that it is inappropriate for the state to intervene in decision making relevant to the family, except in exceptional circumstances. Each of these claims has different merits and problems. Luckily, we do not need to debate them here. We can just accept that liberal philosophy, however supported, will normally give parents decisional authority in relation to their children.

How does this relate to vaccinations? Parents generally make decisions about childhood vaccinations. Is it appropriate for parents to refuse vaccination on behalf of their child? The child has no say in the matter, and by the time they are competent, damage might have been caused to the child as a result of the parents' decision. While most will agree that the presumption in favour of parental authority can be overturned in cases where it is a matter of potential life or death, or serious and significant harm, is there a role for the state to step in to protect the child from parental decisions and provide vaccinations? Certainly such a power is used in other health and social contexts. Let us focus on pre-school vaccinations. If an older child is held to be competent, then we can treat them as we do adults. An argument can be constructed in favour of vaccinations on the grounds of best interests as follows:

1. Medical decisions about incompetent patients should be made on the basis of what is in their best interests (where prior wishes are unknown or non-existent).
2. Pre-school infants are incompetent (and have no prior wishes).
3. Therefore, decisions about the medical care of infants should be made on the basis of what is in their best interests.
4. Best interests in relation to infants should be determined by seeking to balance the potential harms and benefits of possible actions and inactions.
5. Where the parents make a decision about an infant's care which is likely to result in substantial risk of significant harm to that infant then third parties (such as the state) have an obligation to intervene to protect the infant from the consequences of that decision.
6. Given 4, what is in the best interests of infants in relation to vaccinations is to be decided by seeking to balance the harms and benefits associated with vaccination versus non-vaccination.
7. Given 3, 5 and 6, where it is in an infant's best interests to be vaccinated (or not vaccinated) and the parents decide the other way then the state (or other legitimate third parties) have an obligation to ensure that the infant is protected from the consequences of such a decision.

Conclusion: parental decision making about childhood vaccinations can be overruled legitimately in at least some cases.

This argument requires a lot of explanation and discussion over issues such as what constitutes 'best interests'. All I suggest here is that it might be possible to construct such an argument assuming that parents do not *by definition* decide what is in their child's best interests: that is, parents can *in fact* be error about what is in their child's best interests (Dawson, 2005). On this view best interests are decided on the basis of an overall welfare judgment, and on at least some occasions other parties may step in to ensure that children are protected from the consequences of their parents' decision making.

A possible objection is that a judgment about best interests is always made in relation to an individual child. In circumstances where herd protection exists in a population, it looks as though a judgment about best interests may favour non-vaccination (assuming there is *any* possibility of harm resulting from that vaccination). Some might argue that there is a potential issue of justice here and that such parental decision making is essentially free riding upon the actions of others (Cullity, 1995). There is a sense in which this is true, but it is not clear that objections based on free-riding are sufficient to impose an obligation to vaccinate in such circumstances (Dawson, 2007). In addition, it should not be forgotten that there will be individual benefits from vaccination as well (for example, the child might travel to another population where herd protection does not exist) and there will always be strong pragmatic reasons in favour of vaccination even where herd protection exists (Dawson, 2005, 2007).

Harms and benefits

Arguments related to the balancing of harms and benefits are important to vaccination policies. You don't need to be committed to consequentialism to accept this, and it is important to see that this is not the only possible moral argument about vaccination. The vital and difficult issue to decide is: what are the relevant harms and benefits? In this section I will begin by suggesting some relevant considerations, and then argue that in vaccination policy (like in many preventive programmes) the focus cannot just be on harms and benefits in relation to particular individuals but that any such judgment needs to take into account the consequences for populations not just individuals. This complicates the ethical discussion.

Vaccination brings potential benefit to the individual receiving the vaccination because they are less likely to develop that particular disease if they come into contact with it. However, there is also an important benefit to society if sufficient members of that population are vaccinated to create herd protection (Paul, 2004). Herd protection means that all members of the community are at reduced risk of attack by infectious disease. This is because if such a disease enters the population it is far less likely to become an epidemic or pandemic as any diseased individual is unlikely to pass on the infection if the surrounding individuals have been vaccinated prior to contact. In addition, any unvaccinated individuals in the population are better protected, as they are less likely to come into contact with an infected individual. (At least some unvaccinated individuals are not at risk due to their own decisions. For example, neonates might not be old enough to be vaccinated; the ill and those with compromised immunity might be unvaccinated for sound medical reasons; vaccination might fail or be insufficient to give immunity; scheduled vaccinations might have been missed due to population movement, etc.) Herd protection offers all these groups their *only* vaccine-related protection against the risk of disease.

The supporters of vaccination will argue that few other medical interventions have had such a positive impact upon the world's health (CDC, 2006). Smallpox could not have been eradicated without vaccination and poliomyelitis (despite some problems) is close to eradication as a result of global efforts and a sustained vaccination programme. Much effort has gone into the preparation of a vaccine in response to the latest influenza pandemic as a direct means of preventing the spread of such a disease. If routine vaccination for all recommended diseases were available to everyone across the world the impact on global health would be hugely significant (WHO, 2002). Despite this, some authors have expressed scepticism about the scale of the contribution of vaccination to the dramatic reduction in childhood mortality from infectious disease since the mid-nineteenth century (Keown, 1976). They suggest that improvements in nutrition, water quality and sanitation have had more impact upon the disease-related mortality figures. I would argue that these factors have certainly contributed to this fall, as a healthy child is better able to fight infection. However, Keown's thesis almost certainly underestimates the impact of vaccination in preventing or reducing the force of waves of disease. The (additional) impact of vaccination can be seen by looking at infection rates for such diseases as diphtheria in the UK where the number of infections (and deaths) plummeted after routine vaccination was introduced in the 1940s and 1950s (Salisbury and Begg, 1996: 68).

Ironically, in the developed world it is the very success of vaccination in maintaining unprecedented low rates of many infectious diseases that has proved to be part of the reason why vaccination has become such a controversial issue at times. Few adults in the developed world have any experience of previously very common infectious diseases (for example, diphtheria, measles, pertussis), and so it is easier to downplay or ignore the risks of such diseases and overemphasize any potential risks from a vaccine. Of course, vaccinations can cause harm. Such harms range from inflammation and pain at the site of injection through to anaphylaxis and death. However, any adverse events are rare, and serious adverse events are very rare indeed for most vaccines. Occasionally, the public can lose confidence in a particular vaccine as happened in the UK during the 1970s with pertussis and MMR since 1998. In some cases, with particular vaccines, the risks of vaccination can be higher than would be acceptable for a routine vaccination programme and this can lead to poor uptake in target populations (for example, recent smallpox vaccination among 'first responders' in the USA was held to be disappointing. See Yih et al. [2003]). Media reports, rumours and misunderstandings can feed these concerns. However, vaccines are subject to at least the same rigorous development standards as any other medicinal products. In practice, though, risks tend to be much lower because of the need to administer vaccines to very large asymptomatic populations. We can distinguish between the perception of risks and the statistical reality of risks but the former matter as vaccination programmes need to be acceptable to the target population (Verweij and Dawson, 2004).

Different vaccines have different adverse event profiles depending upon how they are made. Vaccines can be manufactured using live but weakened (attenuated) pathogens, dead pathogens, part pathogens, inactivated toxins, or recombinant techniques (a kind of genetic engineering). In some cases there is a choice of vaccines for the same disease (as with polio) and they will have different modes of operation and side-effects (Paul and Dawson, 2005). In other cases, the choice of a particular strain might make a difference to the likelihood of side-effect as some strains will be more virulent than others (see Kretzschmar et al., 2006, on smallpox vaccines). In addition, the vaccine will not just contain an active ingredient designed to induce immunity but also other things including adjuvants (ingredients to stimulate an immune reaction) as well as preservatives. Sometimes these elements can be the reason for concern, such as in the recent discussion in the USA about the role of mercury as a preservative in vaccines (Institute of Medicine, 2004). Vaccine development involves a constant process of refinement and improvement with the aim of trying to reduce any potential risks to a minimum.

There are some other possible 'harm-related' objections to vaccination that I will leave to one side. For example, it might be claimed that there is no risk of harm involved in common childhood diseases, or that the risk of harm from vaccines is disproportionate to the threat from such diseases. Such arguments tend to be over-generalized or involve dubious empirical claims. Much of the popular anti-vaccination material available in the public domain is based on no or poor evidence, with little attempt to consider the issues fairly (Sorell, 2007). Objections to vaccinations *as such* will not be considered here (although I do not think they make any sense, as any harm–benefit judgment can only be focused on a consideration of an individual vaccine and disease).

As mentioned earlier, it is important that in considering harms and benefits in relation to vaccination we do not merely focus on how these issues affect individuals but also how they affect the whole population. This is vital in relation to vaccination because of the issue of herd protection. Herd protection is a good example of a benefit that exists at the population level. However, this population benefit is not an instance of a mere aggregation of individual benefits. Where herd protection exists, the benefit extends much further than the sub-group of the total population that have been vaccinated. One way of conceptualizing this population-benefit is in terms of seeing it as a public good. A public good is a good that cannot be created by any individual alone: it takes collective efforts. It cannot be broken down into individual goods and distributed among the members of a population. All benefit in a population, if it exists. None can enjoy it, unless all benefit. There are various problems associated with the creation and maintenance of public goods, but the importance for this section is that such a benefit as herd protection cannot be easily entered into any simple harm/benefits calculation in relation to individuals: the population level is relevant to such deliberations (Dawson, 2007).

It is important to see that this appeal to population benefits does not mean that individuals need to be sacrificed for the good of the population, just that the relevant benefits to the population as a whole are a relevant consideration in any deliberations about harms and benefits. While it can be argued in relation to at least some preventive public health policies that risks are run by individuals, while benefits accrue to the population, this is not true of vaccination policies (Dawson, 2004). Vaccinated individuals do benefit from their participation in the programme; it is just that they will gain an *extra* benefit if herd protection exists. Where herd protection is an explicit aim of a vaccination programme and vaccination is strongly encouraged, it is very important to consider the question of compensation for any possible vaccine-related harm: even the perception of injustice, of unnecessarily sacrificing individuals for the good of the population, should be avoided if possible (Paul and Dawson, 2005).

In addition to seeing herd protection as a public good, we might also see it as a common good. Common goods are those goods that are created and maintained through social interaction in a joint or common project: they are about what 'we' do together. They often include the kinds of things that are related to the background conditions for a flourishing life. Common goods are the product of shared social norms and meanings, and they are not maintained through potential enforcement (unlike at least some public goods, that may involve state pressure to ensure participation).

Common goods in relation to vaccination can perhaps be best seen at certain historical periods. For example, the pursuit of a vaccination for polio in the USA during the 1940s and 1950s was largely driven by a collective sense of threat and widespread support through small charitable donations to groups such as March of Dimes. The discourse of common goods is not often used these days, for a number of reasons. Talk of common goods does not fit well with the general focus in today's society upon individual choices and rights, but this does not mean that such a common or joint sense of activity does not continue to exist in relation to vaccination. We can see the collective reduction of risk to a society as a whole, through the creation and promotion of herd protection, as being a clear example of this (despite the fact that this is not the way it is talked about). Vaccination, where herd protection is a plausible aim, provides a way for us to think about responding to common threats to our society and our way of life, and how 'we' as a group can respond and protect. When I choose to vaccinate my children, I do more than protect them in an individual sense, as I am also contributing to a collective project. If I choose not to vaccinate them, I am not only putting them at increased risk of harm as individuals, but also failing to contribute to the maintenance of a common good. Of course, it may be objected that parents will make the decision based upon what is in their child's interests. This is fair enough, but it is worth drawing people's attention to the fact that, once again, we can see that choices about vaccination do not merely have consequences for the direct individuals involved, but for the whole of society (a society that all such individuals belong to). Our connectedness to others becomes more and more invisible, and we are starting to lose the language of such social connections. However, invoking the idea of common goods, and promoting a sense of public health ethics that contains such a notion, will, arguably, result in a richer and more socially based view of ethics in general. Such a view would allow us to invoke other positive, non-individual values such as solidarity, reciprocity and social justice. The idea of common goods can also be used, in turn, to offer further support for other moral arguments in favour of vaccination, such as those based on both harm-to-others and best interests. A society with a declining sense of the values we share is contributing to an increased possibility of harm, and one with a commitment to common goods is clearly in the best interests of a child. In conclusion, this suggests that such values ought to at least be on the table, and we should not just assume that the only relevant values are those related to individuals, or are those that have come to the fore in medical ethics over the last forty years (see Dawson, Chapter 1).

Compulsion?

Such arguments based on shared or common values are not going to be acceptable to everyone. However, one of the interesting things about vaccination is that we can produce many different arguments about it. Even if someone wants to remain within the framework of values derived from medical ethics and its dominant liberal discourse, certain arguments in favour of vaccination remain powerful. For example, on the latter approach, appealing to both the idea of harm-to-others and best interests might provide some justification for a moral obligation to vaccinate a child in at least some circumstances. Let us assume this is the case – does it follow that compulsion is therefore justified? It always seems slightly odd to me that many people consider this to be the most important ethical issue in relation to vaccination. It is, of course, possible to have legally compulsory vaccination, but in many cases this is not necessary. Compulsion may be tempting for legislators for a number of reasons, such as where public health structures are weak; there is a lack of trust or little feeling of social solidarity; or where there is a social or political culture committed to individual freedom as the primary value of public policy. However, in many parts of the world, such measures are not necessary, and vaccination rates remain sufficient for herd protection to exist. Rather than seeing the justifiability (or not) of compulsion as *the* central issue in vaccination ethics, we can almost take the fact that this is an issue for public policy as a sign that something has gone wrong with the sense of values in such a population. A society without what we might call *active* social values (that is, social values that have purchase within discourse about public policy) is a failing society. A society that agrees upon the state's central role as being one of coercing free citizens into acting in various ways (including accepting their moral obligations) is to accept an impoverished model of social relations: one where making sense of public health becomes very difficult, if not impossible. There is an odd paradox here. A society that privileges the value of individual liberty above all others ends up needing compulsion to ensure reasonable consideration for other valuable considerations, such as freedom from potential harm, whereas a society that actively embraces a range of values may have little need for compulsion at all. As a result, to frame the debate in terms of being in favour or against compulsion is already to miss the point.

Whatever a reader thinks of this last point, it is important to see that the issue of legal compulsion is different from that of the existence of a moral obligation. An argument for compulsion requires a further step to move from our moral condemnation of a parent, to an act of interference in the family to ensure a certain end. However, in certain circumstances the latter might be justified, for example where the risk of harm was great enough, or perhaps where a court orders vaccinations after a parental dispute (Dawson, 2005). Of course, 'compulsion' in the everyday sense implies the use of force or legal sanctions such as fines. However, related activities might count as 'indirect' compulsion and these can cover a range of cases from the requirement to have vaccinations before enrolment in school, to a presumption in favour of vaccination with little possibility to opt out and little attempt to offer the relevant information for an informed consent. Of course, direct compulsion will generally be an action of last resort. In many cases there will be strong arguments against, because if it is not proportionate it might actually result in a decline in vaccination uptake. However, some people will be opposed to compulsion on principle, so in the rest of this section I will consider some categorical objections to compulsory childhood vaccination.

First, it might be argued that it can never be appropriate to overrule parents' decisions about vaccinations, because vaccination is a preventive rather than a therapeutic measure, and in most cases the diseases are trivial and low risk. Invoking the powers of the state to interfere in the family in such a case, it could be argued, is just inappropriate. However, it is not clear that this argument will succeed as any attempt to draw a morally significant difference between an action based upon the fact it is either preventive or therapeutic is potentially problematic. It can be argued that it should be a balance between all relevant harms and benefits that matters (Dawson, 2004). In addition, any risk of disease must be balanced against the risk of vaccination. As previously suggested, any risks of vaccination related to common diseases are low. While the risk of contracting such a disease in the developed world is also usually low, if contracted, the potential impact of many of these diseases should not be underestimated. (Neither should it be forgotten that the calculations of such risks and benefits might vary widely depending upon the background societal conditions. In many parts of the developing world childhood diseases are endemic and millions of children die each year from vaccine-preventable diseases.)

Second, it might be argued that parents can invoke a right to refuse this medical intervention. Presumably such a claim would have to involve some kind of justification for seeing this particular right as taking precedence over other rights, including a right of the child to be protected from potential harm. I do not have space to consider rights discourse in any detail here, but it is worth pointing out that the parents' refusal in this case is not governing their own care, but that of their child. This may make a significant difference to the case. Even if such a right to refuse treatment is held to be central to the debate about vaccinations, it is only likely to block any best interests argument, leaving the harm-to-others argument untouched.

Third, parents might use another form of appeal to rights. In this case, they may argue that the child has a right to bodily integrity, and that this will be transgressed in the case of compulsory vaccination. Once again, the important thing about rights is that there are many such rights and, when they are invoked, it is a requirement of their defender to produce an argument not just to say why we have such a right, but explain why that particular right is supposed to take precedence in our moral deliberations. While such an argument can, no doubt, be produced, it can surely be contested. Once again, while such a right might, at most, have some claim in relation to arguments about best interests, it is not clear how it might deflect any harm-to-others argument.

While all of these objections may be important, as the risk of harm-to-others from the relevant disease grows, it becomes more and more difficult to hold that any such rights take precedence. Even in relation to best interests, we might doubt whether these arguments are decisive. This is because any deliberations about best interests mean that no parent has an absolute right to do as they want with a child. Parents have a great deal of leeway about how they choose to bring up their children, but there are serious constraints upon what will count as being legitimately in the best interests of any child.

Conclusion

These different arguments will work in different ways depending on the nature of the particular disease, vaccine and potential recipient(s). Determining the most relevant and effective vaccination policy is not easy. However, it will certainly involve a consideration of the risks of harm and benefits from vaccination and non-vaccination, as well as more theoretical arguments about harm-to-others and best interests. Considering the ethical issues related to vaccination requires new thinking because the focus of traditional bioethics has been on the individual. This is unhelpful as it misses the fact that vaccination is not just about individuals and their choices but population health as well.

Acknowledgement

This chapter is a revised version of a chapter, used with permission, that first appeared as: Dawson, A. (2007) Vaccination ethics. In *Principles of Health Care Ethics*, 2nd edn, ed. R. Ashcroft, A. Dawson, H. Draper and J. McMillan. Chichester: Wiley.

References

CDC (2006) Vaccine preventable deaths and the global immunization vision and strategy, 2006–2015. *MMWR*, 12 May, **55**(18): 511–15. Available at: http://www.cdc.gov/mmwr/preview/mmwrhtml/mm5518a4.htm (accessed: 1/9/06).

Cullity, G. (1995) Moral free riding. *Philosophy and Public Affairs*, **24**(1): 3–34.

Dare, T. (1998) Mass immunizations programmes: some philosophical issues. *Bioethics*, **12**(2): 125–49.

Dawson, A. (2004) Vaccination and the prevention problem. *Bioethics*, **18**(6): 515–30.

Dawson, A. (2005) The 'best interests' argument and childhood vaccinations. *Bioethics*, **19**(2): 188–205.

Dawson, A. (2007) Herd protection as a public good: vaccination and our obligations to others. In *Ethics, Prevention and Public Health*, ed. A. Dawson and M. Verweij. Oxford: Oxford University Press.

Feinberg, J. (1973) *Social Philosophy*. Engelwood Cliffs, NJ: Prentice-Hall.

Institute of Medicine (2004) *Immunization Safety Review: Vaccines and Autism*. Washington, DC: National Academies Press.

Kretzschmar, M., Wallinga, J., Teunis, P., Xing, S. and Mikolajczyk, R. (2006) Frequency of adverse events after vaccination with different Vaccinia strains. *PLoS Medicine*, **3**(8).

McKeown, T. (1976) *The Role of Medicine: Dream, Mirage, or Nemesis*. London: The Nuffield Provincial Hospitals Trust.

Mill, J. S. (1859) *On Liberty*. Reprinted 1974. Harmondsworth: Penguin.

Paul, Y. (2004) Letter: Herd immunity and herd protection. *Vaccine*, **22**: 301–2.

Paul, Y. and Dawson, A. (2005) Some ethical issues arising from polio eradication programmes in India. *Bioethics*, **19**(4): 393–406.

Salisbury, D. and Begg, N. (eds) (1996) *Immunisation Against Infectious Diseases*. London: HMSO.

Selgelid, M., Battin, M. and Smith, C. B. (2006) *Ethics and Infectious Disease*. Oxford: Blackwell.

Sorell, T. (2007) Parental choice and expert knowledge in the debate about MMR and autism. In *Ethics, Prevention and Public Health*, ed. A. Dawson and M. Verweij. Oxford: Oxford University Press.

van Delden J. J. M., Ashcroft R., Dawson A., Marckmann, G., Upshur R. and Verweij, M. F. (2008) The ethics of mandatory vaccination against influenza for health care workers. *Vaccine*, **26**(44): 5562–6.

Verweij, M. and Dawson, A. (2004) Ethical principles for collective immunisation programmes. *Vaccine*, **22**: 3122–6.

World Health Organization (2002) *State of the World's Vaccines and Immunization*. Geneva: WHO.

Yih, W. K., Lieu, T. A., Rêgo, V. H., *et al.* (2003) Attitudes of healthcare workers in U.S. hospitals regarding smallpox vaccination. *BMC Public Health*, **3**: 20.

Chapter

9

Environment, ethics and public health

The climate change dilemma

Anthony Kessel and Carolyn Stephens

In this chapter we explore the relationship between the environment, ethics and public health (Kessel, 2006). To do this we take the theme of climate change and public health (with climate representing the natural environment), and we examine the relationship between our climatic environment and public health ethics. We illustrate the changing relationship between public health and the environment, and examine the place of ethics in the relationship between the environment and public health. In particular, we critique the status of utilitarianism as a moral foundation for public health. The importance of environmental justice, environmental philosophy and development ethics to the future of public health are discussed.

Background: definitions and methods

As an introduction to this chapter it is important to refer to some difficulties around definitions, and also to briefly describe the methods used. To philosophers definitions are often key to their debates. For one philosopher in particular, Ludwig Wittgenstein, issues to do with definitions are at the root of all philosophical problems (Elliott, 2001). A look at the words used in the title of this chapter readily illustrates the challenges of writing on this topic. To Socrates, ethics was about how we ought to live, and why. More contemporarily, however, ethics has been divided into normative ethics (systematic examination of organized theories) and speculative (or reflective) ethics (Honer *et al.*, 2006). In this chapter we look at moral theories as well as adopting a more speculative approach.

The environment, likewise, has different meanings to different people in different contexts, all of which are relevant to health debates. There is the physical (sometimes called the built) environment, for instance buildings and urban infrastructure. The social environment, in contrast, tends to refer to demographic factors in populations (age structures, ethnic groups, inequalities), and the natural environment usually relates to aspects such as air, water, green spaces (for example, parks, forests), and biodiversity. In this chapter we are largely discussing the natural environment. Within the public health literature the term 'environmental health' has tellingly been used – as will be returned to later in this chapter – largely to capture the impacts of man-made contamination of the environment on human health (for example, chemical hazards, toxins), rather than to describe the intrinsic health of the natural environment per se (Environmental Health Commission, 1997; Jukes, 1999).

Public Health Ethics, ed. Angus Dawson. Published by Cambridge University Press. © Cambridge University Press 2011.

What is meant by public health is also open to debate. In 1988, Donald Acheson led an inquiry into the future of public health in the UK and – drawing on Winslow's 1920 definition – described public health as 'the art and science of preventing disease, promoting health, and prolonging life through organized efforts of society' (Department of Health, 1988: 1); the Institute of Medicine in the USA had similarly drawn on Winslow in a report of the same year (Institute of Medicine, 1988). The health historian Dorothy Porter has, in a related vein, labelled public health as 'collective action in relation to the health of populations' (Porter, 1999: 4).

In 2002, the Faculty of Public Health Medicine (UK) was still using Acheson's definition, and added that public health is '. . . concerned primarily with health and disease in populations, complementing, for example, medical and nursing concerns for the health of individual patients' and its 'chief responsibilities are monitoring the health of a population, the identification of its health needs, the fostering of policies which promote health, and the evaluation of health services' (FPHM, n.d.). What this definition illustrates is the perceived difference between professional public health (practitioners trained in the speciality) and non-professional public health (anyone working to improve population health). There are other qualitative distinctions that characterize the various interpretations of public health, some of which relate to the different histories of public health in different countries, but in this chapter we predominantly use Porter's definition, except when referring specifically to the professional component.

This is an inter-disciplinary chapter. The over-arching academic framework is ethical theory and philosophy, but discussions about history, public health science and policy are integrated within the analysis (Baum, 1995; Green and Thorogood, 2004).

Climate change and public health

In the approach taken to dealing with climate change, the debate about our environment has provided the opportunity to rethink the relationship between mankind and nature, and the moral dimensions of public health theory and practice. Often referred to synonymously as greenhouse warming, climate change presents an instance of the health effects of western lifestyles being borne by those at a distance in time and place. Unlike those affected by, say, passive smoking, those affected by climate change have little or no connection with the perpetrators, yet are left with the consequences. And this raises fundamental questions about the geographical, temporal and moral boundaries of public (health) responsibilities, as well as the place of utilitarianism in public health theory.

The scientific background to the process of climate change is well described in the literature, and will not be repeated here (McMichael, 1995; IPCC, 1996, 2001; Hamilton, 1999). The consequences of climate change to human health are similarly well articulated and most conveniently grouped into direct and indirect effects (McMichael, 1996). The direct effects result from increased exposure to thermal extremes (heat waves and severe cold) and associated climatic changes (deaths in vulnerable groups, domestic violence, civil disturbances and riots, floods, storms, cyclones, hurricanes and bushfires, injuries, psychological disorders and infectious diseases). Indirect effects stem from disturbances to complex ecological systems (changes in the ranges and activity of vectors and infective parasites such as those responsible for malaria, dengue fever, trypanosomiasis and the viral encephalitides), and changed food productivity will result in malnutrition, hunger, impaired child development and growth, with increased morbidity and mortality (Epstein, 1995; McMichael and Haines, 1997).

Climate change and public health philosophy

From the perspective of public health philosophy, what is fascinating about climate change is that it throws open three new aetiological dimensions to population health and disease. First, the causes of greenhouse warming and the resultant climate change and its health effects are anthropogenic. Excluding 'lifestyle' diseases – which an individual predisposes him- or herself to through personal activity[1] – there are plenty of examples of illnesses created by human activity, such as occupational cancers or the passive smoking example mentioned earlier. But in these situations only the populations that create the environmental hazard experience the consequences.

What is different about climate change is that certain communities (and the individuals within them), through their adopted activities, will affect the health of other communities that may well not have taken up such activities. And this opens up interesting, hitherto unexplored questions about personal responsibility, and also about the relationship between public responsibility and how this is expressed through policies such as those concerning public health. In other words, how do such responsibilities fit into the public health philosophy and practice of the perpetrating communities?

Second, the health effects of climate change are, to a substantial degree, likely to impact at a large geographical distance from their source. Aside from the equity issues relating to the *differential* impact and ability to mitigate or adapt accordingly – which are looked at later in this chapter – it is difficult to think of any other example[2] in which the activities of one community could so connectedly affect the health of a population afar. War is perhaps the closest parallel. Related to this point, the third new aetiological dimension that climate change throws up is that the health impacts of current (and past) activities will likely be the burden of generations to come. Once again, it is difficult to recall any similar example in the history of public health. So the question arises again of how do these spatial and chronological dimensions fit into the public health philosophy and practice of the perpetrating communities?

Like much public policy, public health is informed heavily by one moral theory: utilitarianism. Yet utilitarianism is problematic and seems out of touch with the world's current problems. As a guide for both personal and public morality, traditional utilitarianism appears anachronistic. Indeed, the roots of all the new dimensions of health effects of climate change outlined above, can be tracked against the deficiencies of utilitarian theory.

So the next section looks specifically at utilitarianism, its moral limitations and the relevance of these to climate change and public health philosophy. After that, the first major challenging moral framework for public health is considered, one based on John Rawls's vision of social justice.

---

[1] Personal choice, however, such as the ability to stop smoking, may be affected by factors such as employment status and social support, both of which are linked to deprivation.
[2] Apart from other economic activities related to human lifestyles.

Utilitarianism, climate change and public health

Utilitarianism falls into the consequentialist class of moral theories, in which the rightness or wrongness of an action, or rule, is determined by the consequences of that action or rule. Despite relentless ongoing criticism utilitarianism has proved a remarkably tenacious moral theory, the corner-stone to liberal democracy, and both its persistence in and significance to western political philosophy inevitably tie utilitarianism to ethical issues in public health.

Utilitarianism became applied politically in the eighteenth century, and is most famously associated with Jeremy Bentham (1748–1832) and, a little later, John Stuart Mill (1806–73). But utilitarianism had antecedents, and the main tenets of the theory were laid down earlier by philosophers such as John Locke (1632–1704) and David Hume (1711–76).

Bentham was a lawyer and was most interested in the relevance of his ideas to legislation. This element connected him strongly to one of his followers, Edwin Chadwick, because of a shared belief in improving the lot of those worst off through reform. However, Bentham's concept of equality was strikingly at odds with that of certain successors, such as Marx and Engels, who provided a very different explanation for the historical processes determining how inequalities arose and what should be done to redress them. To Bentham, equality formed the basis of a calculus[3] in which each individual was of equal value (Russell, 1991).

Bentham's theory was founded on two linked principles, the principle of association and the principle of utility. The principle of association was a deterministic account of linked mental occurrences, akin to the modern 'conditioned reflex' but without the physiology. The principle of utility, or the greatest-happiness principle is, however, what Bentham is best known for, and rests on the premise that what is good is pleasure, and what is bad is pain. Bentham came to this position through the belief, articulated in his 1789 *Introduction to the Principles of Morals and Legislation*, that human beings are subject to, and slaves to, two poles of sensation (Scruton, 1996). Bentham took the leap of designating happiness as the moral goal, and his principle of utility '. . . approves or disapproves of every action whatsoever, according to the tendency which it appears to . . . augment or diminish the happiness of the party whose interest is in question; or what is the same thing in other words, to promote or to oppose that happiness' (Bentham, quoted in Rachels, 1993: 91).

Extrapolated from the individual to the larger, social domain, the principle of utility states that '. . . the greatest happiness of all those whose interest is in question . . . [is] . . . the only right and proper and universally desirable end of human conduct' (Bentham, quoted in Scruton, 1996: 224). So, one set of affairs is better than another if there is a greater balance of pleasure over pain, or a smaller balance of pain over pleasure. Empiricism was thus brought firmly into the foreground, as the right action could – in theory at least – be determined by summing up individual experiences of these two sensations. This process of quantification was Bentham's 'felicific' calculus,[4] in which the 'audience' to be considered was all those affected by the action, each counting equally.

In his 1863 book *Utilitarianism*, John Stuart Mill, like Bentham, extended moral consideration to the whole of sentient creation but, differently, made qualitative

---

[3] The calculus referred to a calculation, rather than the modern understanding as a particular method in mathematics.
[4] Also known as the optimific, or hedonic, calculus.

distinctions between pleasures (Harris, 1997: 128). Although critiques of modern utilitarianism, and their relevance to public health, will be looked at a little later, it is necessary to point out here a serious problem with the theory's early forms. That is, utilitarianism as depicted by both Bentham and Mill, makes a conceptual leap of inferring from what 'is' in the world to what 'ought' to be. Bertrand Russell (1991: 744) is straightforwardly damning:

> John Stuart Mill, in his Utilitarianism, offers an argument which is so fallacious that it is hard to understand how he can have thought it valid. He says: Pleasure is the only thing desired; therefore pleasure is the only thing desirable. He argues that the only things visible are things seen . . . and similarly the only things desirable are things desired. He does not notice that a thing is 'visible' if it can be seen, but 'desirable' if it ought to be desired. Thus desirable is a word presupposing an ethical theory; we cannot infer what is desirable from what is desired.

With this seemingly mistaken leap in mind, it is perhaps surprising that utilitarianism has endured. Yet few would demur that utilitarianism strongly underpins much of contemporary moral and political thinking and action. Good national policies are judged to be those that increase overall wealth, the modern euphemism for the greatest happiness, and good public health policies are judged to be those that demonstrably improve population health.

However, the pursuit of happiness has become something closer to a 'taken-for-granted', a lifelong endeavour shaped by society, unquestionably accepted and followed. And the inevitably elusive chase finds happiness disguised as, inter alia, healthism, obsession with risk aversion and consumerism (Forde, 1998; Porter, 1999). Not surprisingly therefore, faced with the significant lifestyle changes that would be required to offset climate change and its global health effects, most individuals do not really want to sacrifice or undermine pursuit of their own happiness-oriented goals, despite superficial environmental soundings to the contrary.

Picking up on this, the philosopher Alasdair MacIntyre has put the blame for today's moral ambivalence squarely on the shoulders of utilitarianism, and the selfishness it has engendered. He (1989: 243) argues that '. . . the individualism of modern society and the increasingly rapid and disruptive rate of social change brings about a situation in which for increasing numbers there is no overall shape to the moral life but only a set of apparently arbitrary principles inherited from a variety of sources'. Further, MacIntyre (1989: 237–8) holds the early utilitarians directly responsible for today's woes, and emphatically questions the price to be paid:

> The concept of happiness is, however, morally dangerous in another way; for we are by now well aware of the malleability of human beings, of the fact that they can be conditioned in a variety of ways into the acceptance of, and satisfaction with, almost anything. That men are happy with their lot never entails that their lot is what it ought to be. For the question can always be raised of how great the price is that is being paid for the happiness.

Critiques of utilitarianism, and relevance to climate change

The first criticism is that utilitarianism, in its classical or present economic form, necessitates the enumeration and summation of utilities in some shape or form. And utilitarianism then uses the results of this process as the moral basis to guide actions or policies. In its early form an obvious difficulty was how to quantify happiness, along with the problem outlined earlier of whether happiness is an appropriate moral goal in the first place. Preference- and welfare-based utilitarianism circumvent the latter issue, but do not get around the issue of quantification.

In fact, modern versions of utilitarianism do precisely the opposite. They are reliant, perhaps more than ever, on empirically obtained information as the basis for acting. They place, metaphorically, all the moral eggs in the basket of a positivist conception of science. In a classic book containing essays for and against utilitarianism, the philosopher Bernard Williams describes contemptibly the appeal of utilitarianism in that it picks up 'little of the world's moral luggage', preferring instead to place huge demands on information because 'even insuperable technical difficulty is preferable to moral unclarity, no doubt because it is less alarming' (Williams, 1991: 137).

This moral side-step may be economically and politically advantageous, in the short term at least, but it raises almost insuperable problems for climate change. There may be a general consensus now on the scientific proof that climate change is actually happening, but there is no agreement about what should be done about it (Menne and Bertollini, 2005; DEFRA, 2006).

More subtly, however, centralizing utilitarianism in the climate change debate raises the important point that some elements are more amenable to scientific enquiry and analysis than others. The environment, for example, is excluded from investigation. After all, how do you place a utility function on the value individuals may, or may not, place on retaining a beautiful area of wilderness, or an unpolluted atmosphere? It is clearly easier to calculate the economic costs of climate change and the mitigation strategies to prevent it, than to reliably quantify the health impacts or environmental utilities, so creating a bias in areas of consideration; and this does not even touch the question of how to compare different utilities. This is a fundamental issue recognized by Williams (1991: 148):

> For to exercise utilitarian methods on things which at least seem to respond to them is not merely to provide a benefit in some areas which one cannot provide in all. It is, at least very often, to provide those things with prestige, to give them an unjustifiably large role in the decision, and to dismiss to a greater distance those things which do not respond to the same methods. Just as in the natural sciences, scientific questions get asked in those areas where experimental techniques exist for answering them, so in the very different matter of political and social decision weight will be put on those considerations which respected intellectual techniques can seem, or at least promise, to handle.

The second criticism of utilitarianism, and its framing of climate change policies, relates to proximity. As has been described, classical and modern versions of utilitarianism involve quantification and summation of individual utilities, whether happiness, preferences or interests. But who should be included in the arithmetic? Bentham and Mill predicated that the pleasures and pain of all affected by the action, the audience, should be considered, including – to a lesser degree – non-human animals.

Although circumstances in the nineteenth and twentieth centuries were more contained than today by the technological allowances of the time, the focus on individuals (the audience members) close in space and time applies to both eras. This is because, as before, the utilitarian calculus favours consideration of issues around which there is greater certainty. The philosopher Robert Goodin (1997: 247) highlights that utilitarians may want to include the utilities of all those affected by an action in any given calculation, but in practice it is unlikely:

. . . utilitarians can go on to say, perfectly properly, that as a purely pragmatic matter their calculations will often lead us to show some apparent favouritism toward those near and dear to us. It is easier to know what people nearby need, and how best we can help; . . . Those are purely contingent, pragmatic considerations, to be sure. In the ideal world, they may be absent. But in the real world, they are powerfully present.

This creates special problems for policies relating to climate change. At the national level, and at the local level within countries, policy makers usually take into account the effects of their policies on individuals within their immediate boundaries. Climate change would appear to open up the borders by demanding that those from afar are considered too. But it is hard at present to know how to incorporate such requirements, and it remains difficult to believe that such tough decisions will be made by politicians with national, party, and their own interests at heart. The limited concessions to date in the high profile international climate change meetings affirm the somewhat bleak outlook.

So far, the focus of this second criticism has related to geographical proximity. But utilitarianism also has a temporal bias. The utilitarian philosopher J. J. C. Smart (1991) argues that it is impossible to envisage the total future situation because it stretches to infinity. According to Smart it is unnecessary in practice to consider very distant consequences, as these in the end approximate rapidly to zero like the furthermost ripples on a pond after a stone has been dropped into it. He (1991: 33–4) defends this presentism:

The necessity for the 'ripples in the pond' postulate comes from the fact that usually we do not know whether remote consequences will be good or bad. Therefore we cannot know what to do unless we can assume that remote consequences can be left out of the account.

This issue is particularly acute for climate change, and policies related to it, as the environmental, financial and health effects will not only occur in the future, but in the distant future. Economists have a general way of dealing with this phenomenon called 'discounting', an analytical tool to compare economic effects that occur at different points in time.[5] But there are different discount rates available and 'the choice of discount rate is of crucial technical importance for analyses of climate change policy, because the time horizon is extremely long, and mitigation costs tend to come much earlier than the benefits of avoiding damages' (IPPC, 1996: 8).

There has been extensive, unresolved debate about discounting in assessment of climate change policies, a debate which reminds us that facts alone cannot provide moral judgements. The recent IPCC publication (2001: 97) emphasizes that uncertainty regarding the discount rate 'relates not to calculation of its effects, which is mathematically precise, but to a value judgement about the appropriateness of the present generation valuing services for future generations'. Environmental philosophers have pointed out that any form of discounting devalues the environment, and the benefits that the environment holds for future generations.

The final criticism of utilitarianism relates to equity. The summation and averaging of utilitarian calculations insufficiently recognizes the importance of how utilities are distributed within the population under consideration. Whether the utility is health or wealth, there is scant difference between a population in which a small number have a lot of (good)

---

[5] The basic premise behind discounting is that a million pounds to me now is of more value than a million pounds in a year's time.

health and the remainder have poor health, and a population in which everyone is reasonably healthy. And this does not sit comfortably with our common-sense morality, as Williams (1991: 142–3) states:

> In this light, utilitarianism does emerge as absurdly primitive, and it is much too late in the day to be told that questions of equitable or inequitable distribution do not matter because utilitarianism has no satisfactory way of making them matter. On the criterion of maximising average utility, there is nothing to choose between any two states of society which involve the same number of people sharing in the same aggregate amount of utility, even if one of them is relatively evenly distributed, while in the other a very small number have a very good deal of it; and it is just silly to say that in fact there is nothing to choose here.

So, if climate change illustrates that utilitarianism is a limited moral determinant of public health policies, an alternative is needed. And here, recent developments in the climate change debate suggest an alternative might be emerging.

Social justice and climate change

There is a huge literature on justice stretching back as far as the Greeks. Aristotle, for instance, in the *Nicomachean Ethics* considers just actions, and likens the characteristic of being just to the other 'excellences' – or virtues of character. For Aristotle justice is a mean, injustice represents the extremes and the just man[6] recognizes how to determine an individual's appropriate share (Urmson, 1998).

In contemporary times, however, social justice has come to embody aspects of the last part of Aristotle's definition, fairness and proportionality. In contrast with legal and retributive justice, social justice is about the distribution of society's benefits and burdens and the socio-political mechanisms that enable such distribution to occur (Daniels, 2000).

This climate change dilemma has certainly extended the boundaries of moral debate in areas of public, and public health, policy making. Because the causes and effects of climate change are differentially distributed, the reasonableness of basing decisions purely on utilitarian economic thinking has been questioned.

As a result, there has been a flurry of academic work looking at equity considerations in the climate change debate. One way of determining how to distribute the costs of climate change mitigation and adaptation policies would be *not* to try to 'falsely' distribute such costs at all, but to allow the market to decide. But libertarian, or market utilitarian, approaches would likely lead to rich countries not valuing or wanting to pay for such policies and poor countries being unable to afford them. Unless there was some kind of catastrophic threat from climate change, poor countries might well be left to simply deal with the consequences.

An alternative framework would be contractarian, also sometimes called administrative utilitarian. In this approach, the limits of using total sum or average utility as a sufficient determinant of policy are acknowledged, and efforts are made to incorporate

---

[6] We are using man here, rather than person, to represent Aristotle's depiction, which focused predominantly on men.

additional dimensions to economic calculations to allow for more informed and, apparently fairer, distribution.

This framework has been argued is more egalitarian and has drawn strongly on the concept of social justice. In fact, one person's theory has been stressed within this dimension of the debate, John Rawls, whose name can be found scattered among the articles, discussion papers, and policy-related documents on equity issues in climate change. Rawls's (1999) *A Theory of Justice* was first published in 1971 and 40 years later the impact remains remarkable. There has been much discussion of Rawls's theory, and a number of expositions, and it is not appropriate to detail these here. However, a very brief recap is necessary as a prelude to the following sections.

Rawls thinks of justice as fairness. He starts from the premise that utilitarianism is an inadequate, inappropriate, and ultimately unjust moral or politico-economic tool for making distributive decisions in society. For Rawls (1999: 3), justice *denies* that '. . . the loss of freedom for some is made right by a greater good shared by others.' And justice does *not* allow '. . . that the sacrifices imposed on a few are outweighed by the larger sum of advantages enjoyed by many'. Instead Rawls (1999: 5) defines justice as '. . . a characteristic set of principles for assigning basic rights and duties and for determining what they take to be the proper distribution of the benefits and burdens of social cooperation'.

Rawls makes two other key assertions. First, he argues that people's perceptions of entitlement – and so too of justice or fairness – are inevitably shaped by their own backgrounds, interests and social organizations. While Rawls accepts that human beings naturally have certain interests – for instance striving for basic primary goals – most interests are not of this nature and any agreed notion of justice needs to be reached before the undue influence of unnatural interests. Second, he predicates that any social advantages obtained through chance – by birthright or natural endowment – are essentially unfair.

Putting these together Rawls sets out to establish the principles of justice for the basic structure of society that would be agreed by individuals in an 'original' (or abstract pre-existence) state. Taking the form of a social contract these principles are those that '. . . free and rational persons concerned to further their own interests would accept in an initial position of equality as defining the fundamental terms of their association' (1999: 10). This initial, or 'original', position corresponds to the state of nature in the traditional theory of the social contract. Rawls purports that the 'original position is . . . the appropriate initial status quo, and the fundamental agreements reached in it are fair.' This, he (1999: 11) continues, '. . . explains the propriety of the name "justice as fairness": it conveys the idea that the principles of justice are agreed to in an initial situation that is fair'.

Fairness issues in the climate change debate

Armed with the basics of Rawls's theory of justice, it is possible now to return to the climate change debate. The starting-point for the distributive concerns in climate change are three related questions: who is responsible for the problem; who will suffer (most) from the problem, and how; and who will bear the costs of abatement? The four fairness issues in climate change policy that correspond to these questions have been expressed as follows (Reichart, 1998; Rayner *et al.*, 1999):

1. What is a fair allocation of the costs of preventing the global warming that is still avoidable?
2. What is a fair allocation of the costs of coping with the social consequences of the global warming that will not, in fact, be avoided?
3. What background allocation of wealth would allow international bargaining (about the first two points) to be a fair process?
4. What is a fair allocation of greenhouse gases over the long-term and during transition to the long-term allocation?

In trying to address the fairness issues in climate change, debate has actually focused on an administrative utilitarian (or contractarian) approach, drawing in, to a degree, some Rawlsian ideas of social justice. The IPCC, for example, distinguishes two categories of equity as significant to climate change analyses: procedural equity and consequentialist equity. The former is largely about making policy, focusing on the criteria and methods for implementing fair procedures for design of, and participation in, the decision-making processes, as well as respect for legal rights. It is about inclusion, fairness and openness at all stages in the policy making processes and corresponds to item four on the list above.

Consequentialist equity, in contrast, and is about the outcomes of climate change (and policies addressing climate change): justice and fairness in respect of the *impacts* of climate change, and justice and fairness in respect of *abatement*, in other words the distribution of burdens and allocation of benefits associated with reducing greenhouse gas emissions and managing climate change. Consequentialist equity has been further divided into *intragenerational* equity (although actions by individuals in contributing to greenhouse gas emissions may affect anyone, impacts reflect vulnerability and are borne differentially by social groups or countries depending on their geography, economic development and so forth) and *inter*generational equity (costs of abatement may be borne now but benefits may not be realized well into the future). Consequentialist equity takes on board the widely heralded 'precautionary principle', which dictates that when there is serious doubt about likely environmental impacts and consequences, decisions should be made that err on the side of safety (Hayry, 2003).

Climate change and climate justice

The intellectual and theoretical developments described in the previous section have been mirrored in two parallel, connected sets of processes in the climate change debate: developments in international policy around managing climate change; and growth in the campaigning efforts of pressure groups. There is not scope here to look at how international policy developments have captured Rawls's ideas, although these are described elsewhere (Kessel, 2006). Instead, climate justice will be explored here.

In parallel to policy developments and negotiations (and sometimes providing evidence for them) there has been a groundswell in 'independent' think tanks, non-profit making organizations, and other new bodies established to press for fair and generally more aggressive policy targets relating to climate change. A number of these have expressed their opinions and activities in terms of global justice, and their mix of conscience-driven academics and pressure-group campaigners has provided both the intellectual base and the energy needed to drive activities forward. There is the feel of a throwback to the lobbying efforts of the first half of the twentieth century to clean the skies of air pollution.

The Global Commons Institute (GCI), for instance, was set up in 1990 in London, and has been encouraging awareness of its solution to climate change called *Contraction and Convergence*. Put forward as the suggested international framework for the arrest of greenhouse gas emissions *Contraction and Convergence* has argued that economic growth can continue at current ('business as usual') rates only provided large efficiency gains are made and nearly all energy comes from renewable sources (Global Commons Institute, n.d.; Meyer, 2000).

Another group, the cleverly named US-based EcoEquity, is committed to advancing equal rights to global commons resources, in particular the principle of equal per capita rights to the atmosphere. Lamenting both US rejection of the Kyoto Protocol and also the Byrd-Hagel resolution,[7] EcoEquity (n.d.) has argued that fairness '. . . cannot and will not mean that the rich go on as before', and that a climate treaty will have to embody a '. . . fairness that is acceptable in China as well as the United States'. EcoEquity has intended to deepen and clarify the meaning of climate justice through drawing together academics and non-government organizations into the global justice movement: 'What will we be doing?' has been asked or the EcoEquity (n.d.) website 'Working to bring the many threads now being spun around climate justice together into a stronger web, one that can support a broader political strategy.'

There are other individual groups or organizations, but a powerful coalition of groups – including CorpWatch, Friends of the Earth International, OilWatch Africa and the World Rainforest Movement – gathered as the 'International Climate Justice Network' at the final preparatory negotiations for the Earth Summit in Bali in June 2002. The coalition developed a set of principles aimed at 'putting a human face' on climate change. The 'Bali Principles of Climate Justice' first outline the nature of the problem (caused primarily by the rich, and felt disproportionately by small island states, coastal peoples, women, the poor and others; violating human rights), then state 27 core principles of the international movement for Climate Justice (CorpWatch, n.d.).

Within the context of this chapter – climate change dilemmas as a theme to explore the relationships between the environment, ethics and public health – these principles illustrate that Rawls's social justice has provided an alternative moral framework to utilitarianism for public health. The climate change debate has spawned a range of academic, policy and pressure group writings reflecting ideas articulated by John Rawls. Connected to this, the climate change debate has also become an arena for expression and discussion of the perceived reasons for many of the world's ills: the impact of industrialization and of modern western lifestyles, global poverty, and the conceptual imperialism of economics (Victor, 1999; Anthanasiou and Baer, 2002; Brown, 2002).

Discussion: environmental ethics, environmental justice and public health

Professional public health in the UK emerged at a time of great social and philosophical change and its conceptual framework was immediately linked to the utilitarian thinking of the period. Around the turn of the twentieth century, as the bacteriological model of disease pathology became widely accepted, medical and public health theory became increasingly

---

[7] A campaign prior to the Kyoto negotiations of 1997 led to 95 US senators demanding developing countries also take on firm reduction commitments, so challenging the UNFCC principle that developed countries take the lead in reducing emissions.

underpinned by science and epidemiology. Huge strides have since been made in western medico-science but, in parallel, both medicine and public health have become more distanced from the environment.

The climate change dilemma illustrates the limitations of public health theory, founded on utilitarianism, to cope with modern challenges such as climate change. And at a less global level, public health practitioners, through the twentieth century, have found it increasingly hard to engage in real issues about the health of the environment. Such developments have not occurred in isolation.

Separation of public health and the environment

The origins of today's environmental problems, and the relevance of this to public health, can be traced through the inter-connected paths of progress in scientific medicine, public health and political philosophy over the past few hundred years.

Before the era of Descartes, the relationship between mankind and nature was more integrated. In the centuries of Hobbes and Locke, however, this outlook changed dramatically. The development of mechanistic philosophy and the progression of science somewhat removed humans from the natural environment, which itself was mechanistically objectified. The era of individualism had begun, with justification of self-interested behaviour and an emphasis on individual and private rights. Personal morality no longer had a special relationship to the state, whose role became that of partner in a dispassionate arrangement that primarily provided an environment suitable for promotion of the individual (Cohen, 2001). Mary Midgley (2001: 159) captures this well:

> Since the Renaissance, this kind of contraction has in any case been happening in political philosophy in the West. Political thinkers of the Enlightenment systematically shrank morality by making it essentially a civic affair – a matter of mutual bargaining between prudent citizens within a limited society. Contract thinking sought to abolish the idea of duties towards anyone or anything outside that society . . . But this move had unintended side-effects. It now makes it quite hard for us to make sense of our responsibility towards humans outside our own society, and almost impossible to explain our responsibilities towards non-human nature.

The seventeenth-century philosopher John Locke's emphasis on individual rights and property rights illustrate how the era also proclaimed mankind's dominion over nature. The natural environment was articulated in inert, demarcated terms, largely devoid of value, and humans would be morally justified in manipulating it any way necessary to further legitimate personal interests. This tied in with ownership, rather than stewardship, of nature and began to set in stone an image of the natural environment – detached and there for human needs – which has only relatively recently been challenged by environmentalists (Passmore, 1974).

In fact, despite some romantic inclinations, this image of nature was reinforced during the eighteenth and nineteenth centuries as utilitarian political philosophy took hold (Rousseau, 1762). As discussed earlier, utilitarianism has (indirectly) reinforced moral justification for individual pursuit of that which gives pleasure, with maximizing human happiness as the overall goal. Manipulating nature to meet these ends has ethical validation and modern welfare economics – the corner-stone of liberal democracies – is grounded in these ideals. Yet utilitarianism focuses proximally, both in terms of the 'audience' within its calculation (failure to include impacts on those at a distance) and with regard to time – the difficulty of incorporating the needs and desires of future generations. And there is little or no accounting for the intrinsic worth of nature.

Utilitarianism emerged politically at a time of corresponding changes in science, medicine and biology. The connection of human health with nature through miasmatic theories of disease was gradually replaced at the end of the nineteenth century by bacteriological explanations, which catalysed the reductionism of medical science. And at that time Darwin and his colleagues were providing a vision of nature that placed self-interested behaviour at its very core, the driver for change, integrally related to adaptation to, and manipulation of, the environment (Dawkins, 1976).

Through the twentieth century individuals have often been seen as disconnected from other individuals and the natural world, with purpose, values and goals narrowly defined. Midgley (2001: 69) again captures this well:

> It is the *social atomism that lies at the heart of individualism* – the idea that human beings are essentially separate items who only come together for contingent reasons of convenience [original emphasis]. This is the idea expressed by saying that the state is a logical construction out of its members, or that really there is no such thing as society. A social contract based on calculations of self-interest is then supposed to account for the strange fact that such things as human societies do actually exist.

These developments have clearly impacted on how public health has progressed. Public health theory and practice has become distanced from the environment. Within contemporary public health the term 'environmental health' has come to signify how degraded aspects of the environment affect human health, rather than reflect the true health of the environment *per se*.

There has, however, been a recent counter-vision, in the form of environmental ethics, which has provided a different way of understanding the world. A look at environmental ethics, and the related areas of development ethics and environmental justice, will enable a synthesis of the implications for public health.

Environmental ethics

Although environmental ethics has blossomed as an academic activity over the last two decades, its main tenets can be traced back to earlier this century. And, though these fundamentals have been subject to considerable theoretical and philosophical debate, they have also become inescapably linked to socio-political ideologies and movements (Light and Holmes, 2003).

It is difficult to place the various philosophical perspectives on the environment into a bag labelled 'environmental ethics', as they differ in many important aspects, but what they share is a fundamental questioning of the value, or values, ascribed to nature. Yet even here there are different approaches, or ways in, to examining this core. One such approach, a sort of starting point in environmental ethics, is to distinguish between anthropocentric (human-centred) and non-anthropocentric ethics. This is seen as a good place to begin because an oft shared belief in environmental ethics is that the roots of today's environmental problems lie in the moral favouritism given to human interests; this is in itself linked to developments in science and political philosophy discussed in the previous section. The moral favouritism, the anthropocentric ethical framework, is then disapproved of in different ways and for different reasons.

In trying to summarily address what an environmental ethic is, Robert Elliot captures this overview and presents five sub-divisions. The first, 'human-centred ethics', has modern utilitarianism as an exemplar, in which facts are needed to calculate the happiness yielded by options, but only humans are treated as morally considerable, that is, are included in the calculus. An 'animal-centred ethic' treats individual animals as morally considerable, but may allow ranking to account for different interests and capacities. Treating equal interests equally and unequal ones unequally, for example, would accommodate human ranking above animals based on a different capacity for rational autonomous action. A 'life-centred ethic', on the other hand, counts *all* living things as morally considerable, not just humans or non-human animals. However, while some would ascribe equal moral considerability to all life, such as the 'biotic egalitarianism' of Norwegian philosopher Arne Naess, others allow differentiation, for instance by complexity. This may favour, for example, the biosphere over humans and leads to a special kind of life-centred ethic termed 'ecological holism', which grants moral considerability to wholes, such as large ecosystems or the biosphere: individuals or species are only important in relation to these wholes. The final environmental ethic, called 'rights for rocks' by Elliot (1997), extends moral considerability to all as an 'everything ethic'.

Underlying these divisions, or different perspectives, is the question of what makes something worthy of moral considerability – worthy of consideration when judging the morality of action (Goodpaster, 1978). Humans are morally considerable because they have interests that can be promoted or harmed, based on their human capacities – for rational thought and action, and sentience. However, not only is sentience shared by some animals (which could extend moral consideration to them), but moral considerability could lie elsewhere, in some other intrinsically valuable property, for instance complexity or even beauty. This in turn would shift moral considerability to non-sentient animals, plants,[8] ecosystems or the wilderness, and could include non-living[9] entities.

The different perspectives within environmental ethics lie along a spectrum, which stretches from humans to animals, plants, all living and non-living things, incorporating different concepts of what matters morally. Des Jardins, for example divides the spectrum up a little differently, but it still incorporates the same elements. His grouping are: biocentric ethics, which is centred around (all) life and has correlative duties[10]; ecological ethics, which focuses on ecological communities and embraces ethical holism; the 'land ethic', articulated first by Aldo Leopold in 1949, which embraces living things, ecosystems and the land (Callicott, 1979); 'deep ecology', especially that of Naess, which emphasizes the deep roots of environmental crises, the radical cure needed (personal and cultural trans-formation) and forcibly expresses its distinction from shallow anthropocentric environ-mentalism; and social ecology and ecofeminism, which explore how social structures serve the interests and power of certain groups, reflected in (and reinforced by) domination over nature (Des Jardins, 1997).

However the continuum within environmental ethics is separated out, academically or theoretically, a common thread is the difficulty, or failure, to ascribe 'inherent' value

---

[8] The difference between having interests and goals has been stressed by philosophers. A plant may grow towards light or a tree may wither and die, but neither the plant nor the tree, arguably, has attitudes towards these happenings.

[9] The distinction between living and non-living is often neither biologically nor philosophically clear. For instance, a rock may be considered non-living or inert, but what about soil?

[10] These are non-maleficence (to any organism), non-interference, fidelity (to not betray or deceive wild animals) and restitutive justice (to restore balance if harm done).

to non-human nature, whether that is other animals, vegetation or alternative concepts of what might exist. The anthropocentric nature of western ethics gives, at best, 'instrumental' value to anything non-human; in other words wombats, wild flowers and the wilderness are of value only by way of serving human interests – as pets, for rambling or as potential new medicines. This has arisen because of entwined developments in science, medicine, and moral and political philosophy over several hundred years. It may be fair to reflect that dominion over beasts was heralded back in Aristotelian times, but the contemporary situation is rather different in terms of the success and value placed on liberal individualism, materialism and the socio-political structures enshrining these ideologies. The present situation is also vastly different in terms of the depth of environmental crises affecting the planet, of which greenhouse warming is just one example. The Australian philosopher Peter Singer (1999: 285), despite holding sentience alone as morally considerable, is sure of the seriousness of the problem, and the extent of change needed:

> Now we face a new threat to our survival. The proliferation of human beings, coupled with the by-products of economic growth, is just as capable as the old threats of wiping out our society – and every other society as well. No ethic has yet developed to cope with this threat. Some ethical principles we do have are exactly the opposite of what we need. The problem is that . . . ethical principles change slowly and the time we have left to develop a new environmental ethic is short. Such an ethic would regard every action that is harmful to the environment as ethically dubious, and those that are unnecessarily harmful as plainly wrong.

Singer then outlines his environmental ethic as including consideration of all sentient creatures now and well into the future, aesthetic appreciation of wild places and nature, rejection of materialistic ideals, promotion of frugality and reassessment of extravagance. He (1997) has espoused these views elsewhere in further detail. For Singer, and many others, the connection between environmental ethics and environmental activism (or environmentalism) is strong.

Environmental justice and development ethics

Environmental ethics, as a field within ethical theory, has not developed in a vacuum. Two complementary concepts have emerged in the same recent period: environmental justice and development ethics. We do not have time to explore these concepts fully but will outline them briefly in the context of discussion of climate change and environmental ethics because of their relevance to the theme.

Environmental justice originated in protests in the 1980s by community groups in the USA against the repeated siting of polluting factories and waste sites in predominantly black neighbourhoods and indigenous peoples' reservations. Civil rights protestors highlighted the disproportionate burden of negative environmental impacts these caused for the most vulnerable sectors of society (Stephens and Bullock, 2000).

In 1994, the issue reached the White House when then President Clinton issued Executive Order 128298: Federal Actions to Address Environmental Justice in Minority Populations and Low-Income Populations. This order reinforced the Civil Rights Act 1964 by requiring federal regulatory agencies to 'make environmental justice a part of all they do' (EPA, n.d.).

Environmental justice is generally defined in normative terms, specifying a set of conditions or expectations which should be aspired to, sought after or demanded. Two definitions provide examples. The US Environmental Protection Agency (n.d.) defines environmental justice as:

> . . . the fair treatment and meaningful involvement of all people regardless of race, color, national origin, or income with respect to the development, implementation, and enforcement of environmental laws, regulations, and policies. Fair treatment means that no group of people, including a racial, ethnic, or a socioeconomic group, should bear a disproportionate share of the negative environmental consequences resulting from industrial, municipal, and commercial operations or the execution of federal, state, local, and tribal programs and policies. Meaningful involvement means that: (1) potentially affected community residents have an appropriate opportunity to participate in decisions about a proposed activity that will affect their environment and/or health; (2) the public's contribution can influence the regulatory agency's decision; (3) the concerns of all participants involved will be considered in the decision making process; and (4) the decision makers seek out and facilitate the involvement of those potentially affected.

Environmental justice has also been conceived in terms of rights and responsibilities. For example, Stephens and Bullock (2000) assert that environmental justice means:

> . . . that everyone should have the right and be able to live in a healthy environment, with access to enough environmental resources for a healthy life

and

> . . . that responsibilities are on this current generation to ensure a healthy environment exists for future generations, and on countries, organizations and individuals in this generation to ensure that development does not create environmental problems or distribute environmental resources in ways which damage other peoples health.

This idea of rights and responsibilities has a strong modern resonance with climate justice discourse, and indeed the two movements have begun to come together. The notion of responsibility also resonates with Singer's concepts of ethics in the age of individualism. And to an extent, this notion has become part of modern consciousness in wealthy countries and is articulated through the growing trend towards organic and locally sourced foods, recycling of waste and more sustainable building design. None of these actions may have a direct benefit on the individuals doing them, but the notion of responsibility – towards the planet, other species and the future – seems to motivate people nonetheless.

A final stream of complementarity is with the emerging field of development ethics. The central concept of development ethics is a reflection on where we are going as a species: the clearest articulation of this is from the International Development Ethics Association (IDEA) formed in 1984. They argue that: '. . . international development ethics is ethical reflection on the ends and means of local, national and global development' (IDEA, n.d.). We do not have the space to expand their ideas fully, but their initial declaration outlines the framework (IDEA, 1989):

- the absolute respect for the dignity of the human person, regardless of gender, ethnic group, social class, religion, age or nationality;
- the necessity of peace based on a practice of justice that gives to the great majorities access to goods and eliminates the conditions of their misery;
- the affirmation of freedom, understood as self-determination, self-management, and participation of peoples in local, national and international decision processes;

- the recognition of a new relation of human beings with nature, facilitating responsible use, respectful of biological cycles and the equilibrium of ecosystems – especially those of tropical forests – and in solidarity with future generations; and
- the stimulus to construct a rationality suited to exploited peoples, one that accords with their cultural traditions, their thought, their interests, and their needs and that involves a new valuing of self-esteem based on their being subjects rather than objects of development.

There are strong themes of justice and respect in this statement. It also articulates a form of procedural justice in its emphasis on freedom and participation.

Both environmental justice and development ethics bring the field of environmental ethics into the more activist realm of human rights, and overall development policy. Linked to climate change, development ethics would argue that our whole development trajectory is flawed – built on wasteful materialism and pursuit of human happiness articulated through ever increasing material wealth. Utilitarianism would see no problem with this – but both environment justice activists and development ethicists would argue that, with the changes in our environment brought about by human material development, the entire human development trajectory needs to be reviewed.

Conclusion

To have purchase, attempts to seriously tackle problems such as climate change need simultaneously to address the roots that have bred liberal individualism, dominant utilitarian-based political philosophy, materialism and social atomism.

Environmental ethics reminds us that the roots of current environmental ideas lie deep. Several hundred years of separation in western thought of mind from matter, subject from object, values from facts, has resulted in the dominance of scientific reductionism over holism, and the devaluing of nature. Connected developments in moral and political philosophy have ingrained utilitarianism and liberal individualism, justifying self-interested behaviour and leading to social atomism. The depth of the problem means meaningful solutions need to be radical.

Within public health, the environment has predominantly been viewed rather than inherent value of instrumental, as concerned with the human health consequences of environmental damage. The climate change dilemma is illustrative of connections between environmental ethics and human welfare, and reflective of the limitations of utilitarianism as the underpinning moral theory of public health. The alternative of Social and environmental justice is presented.

Over the last two centuries the means to health have been thought to be through improved material well-being – initially clean water, sanitation, safe housing. While even these conditions are still lacking for a shocking majority of the world's population, for a minority the definition of material well-being is not only a selfish level of material consumption, but deeply damaging to the planet and its future. While environmental matters such as chemical hazards and even outdoor air pollution are undeniably important, they really only attend to the superficial end of the spectrum, representing shallow environmentalism.

For the future of the public's health a more substantial change in attitudes is required: the discipline of public health needs to embrace the ideals of environmental ethics and social justice, and incorporate the idea of development ethics with its emphasis on critical reflection on our very development model.

References

Athanasiou, T. and Baer, P. (2002) *Dead Heat: Global Justice and Global Warming*. New York: Seven Stories Press.

Baum, F. (1995) Researching public health: behind the qualitative-quantitative methodological debate. *Social Science and Medicine*, **40**: 459–68.

Brown, D. (2002) *Ethical Problems with the United States' Response to Global Warming*. Blue Ridge Summit: Rowman and Littlefield.

Callicott, J. B. (1979) Elements of an environmental ethic: moral considerability and the biotic community. *Environmental Ethics*, **1**: 71–81.

Cohen, M. (2001) *Political Philosophy: From Plato to Mao*. London: Pluto.

CorpWatch. (n.d.) *Bali Principles of Climate Change*. Available at: http://www.corpwatch.org/article.php?id=378 (accessed: 17/5/05).

Daniels, N. (2000) Accountability for reasonableness. *British Medical Journal*, **321**: 1300–1.

Dawkins, R. (1976) *The Selfish Gene*. Oxford: Oxford University Press.

Department for Environment, Food and Rural Affairs (DEFRA) (2006) *Tomorrow's Climate: Today's Challenge (Climate Change UK Programme 2006)*. London: HMSO.

Department of Health (1988) *Public Health in England: Committee of Inquiry into the Future Development of the Public Health Function ('Acheson Report')*. London: HMSO.

Des Jardins, J. R. (1997) *Environmental Ethics: An Introduction to Environmental Philosophy*. Belmont, CA: Wadsworth.

EcoEquity. (n.d.) About EcoEquity. Available at: http://www.ecoequity.org/about.html (accessed: 22/5/05).

Elliott, C. (ed.) (2001) *Slow Cures and Bad Philosophers: Essays on Wittgenstein, Medicine and Bioethics*. London: Duke University Press.

Elliot, R. (1997) Environmental ethics. In *A Companion to Ethics*, ed. P. Singer. Oxford: Blackwell, pp. 284–93.

Environmental Health Commission (1997) *Agendas for Change*. London: Chadwick House Groups.

Environmental Protection Agency (EPA) (n.d.) Environmental justice. Available at: http://www.epa.gov/compliance/environmentaljustice (accessed: 17/5/07).

Epstein, P. (1995) Emerging diseases and ecosystem health: new threats to public health. *American Journal of Public Health*, **85**: 168–72.

Faculty of Public Health Medicine (FPHM) (n.d.) A career in public health. Available at: http://www.fphm.org.uk/CAREERS/Careers.htm (accessed: 9/8/02).

Forde, O. H. (1998) Is imposing risk awareness cultural imperialism? *Social Science and Medicine*, **47**(9): 1155–9.

Global Commons Institute (n.d.) Basic climate scenarios. Available at: http://www.gci.org.uk/scenarios.html (accessed: 17/5/05).

Goodin, R. E. (1997) Utility and the good. In *A Companion to Ethics*, ed. P. Singer. Oxford: Blackwell.

Goodpaster, K. (1978) On being morally considerable. *Journal of Philosophy*, **75**: 308–25.

Green, J. and Thorogood, N. (2004) *Qualitative Methods for Health Research*. London: SAGE.

Hamilton, C. (1999) Justice, the market and climate change. In *Global Ethics and Environment*, ed. N. Low. London: Routledge. pp. 90–105.

Harris, C. E., Jr (1997) *Applying Moral Theories*. Belmont, CA: Wadsworth.

Hayry, M. (2003) European values in bioethics; why, what and how to be used? *Theoretical Medicine and Bioethics*, **24**(3): 199–214.

Honer, S. M., Hunt, T. C., Okholm, D. L. and Safford, J. L. (2006) *Invitation to Philosophy: Issues and Options*, 10th edn. Belmont, CA: Wadsworth.

Institute of Medicine (1988) *The Future of Public Health*. Washington, DC: National Academy Press.

Intergovernmental Committee on Climate Change (IPCC) (1996) *Climate Change 1995: Economic and Social Dimensions of Climate Change. Contributions of Working Group III to the Second Intergovernmental Panel on Climate Change*. Cambridge: Cambridge University Press.

Intergovernmental Committee on Climate Change (IPCC) (2001) *Climate Change 2001: Impacts, Adaptation, and Vulnerability*. Cambridge: Cambridge University Press (for IPCC).

International Development Ethics Association (IDEA) (n.d.) What is development ethics? Available at: http://www.development-ethics.org/default.asp?cid=5010 (accessed: 17/5/07).

International Development Ethics Association (IDEA) (1989) Mérida Declaration July 7, 1989, Mérida, Yucatan, Mexico. Available at: http://www.development-ethics.org/default.asp?cid=5011 (accessed: 18/5/07).

Jukes, G. (1999) Environmental health perspectives. In *Perspectives in Public Health*, ed. S. Griffiths and D. J. Hunter. Oxford: Radcliffe Medical Press.

Kessel, A. (2006) *Air, the Environment and Public Health*. Cambridge: Cambridge University Press.

Light, A. and Holmes, R., III (eds) (2003) *Environmental Ethics: An Anthology*. Oxford: Blackwell.

MacIntyre, A. (1989) *A Short History of Ethics*. London: Routledge.

McMichael, A. J. (1995) *Planetary Overload: Global Environmental Change and the Health of the Human Species*. Cambridge: Cambridge University Press.

McMichael, A. J. (1996) Global environmental change and human health. *Paper presented at seminar on Global Changes and Human Health*. Royal Swedish Academy of Sciences, Stockholm, 29 May.

McMichael, A. J. and Haines, A. (1997) Global climate change: the potential effects on health. *British Medical Journal*, **315**: 805–9.

Menne, B. and Bertollini, R. (2005) Health and climate change: a call for action. *British Medical Journal*, **331**: 1283–4.

Meyer, A. (2000) *Contraction and Convergence: the Global Solution to Climate Change*. Dartington: Green Books.

Midgley, M. (2001) *Science and Poetry*. London: Routledge.

Passmore, J. (1974) *Man's Responsibility for Nature*. London: Duckworth.

Porter, D. (1999) *Health, Civilization and the State: A History of Public Health from Ancient to Modern Times*. London: Routledge.

Rachels, J. (1993) *The Elements of Moral Philosophy*. New York: McGraw-Hill.

Rawls, J. (1999) *A Theory of Justice*, rev. edn. Oxford: Oxford University Press.

Rayner, S., Malone, E. L. and Thompson, M. (1999) Equity issues and integrated assessment. In *Fair Weather: Equity Concerns in Climate Change*, ed. F. L. Toth. London: Earthscan, pp. 11–43.

Reichart, J. E. (1998) 'The tragedy of the commons' revisited: a game theoretic analysis of consumption. In *The Business of Consumption: Environmental Ethics and the Global Economy*, ed. L. Westra and P. H. Werhane. Oxford: Rowman and Littlefield, pp. 47–66.

Rousseau, J. J. (1762/1959) *The Social Contract and Discourses*, Trans. G. D. H. Cole. New York: Dutton.

Russell, B. (1991) *History of Western Philosophy*. London: Routledge.

Scruton, R. (1996) *A Short History of Modern Philosophy*. London: Routledge.

Singer, P. (1997) *How Are We to Live? Ethics in an Age of Self-interest*. Oxford: Oxford University Press.

Singer, P. (1999) *Practical Ethics*. Cambridge: Cambridge University Press.

Smart, J. J. C. (1991) An outline of a system of utilitarian ethics. In *Utilitarianism: For and Against*. Cambridge: Cambridge University Press, pp. 3–74.

Stephens, C. and Bullock, S. (2000) Environmental justice: an issue for the health of the children of Europe and the World. In *The Environment and Children's Health in Europe*, ed. G. Tamburlini. Rome: World Health Organization.

Urmson, J. O. (1998) *Aristotle's Ethics*. Oxford: Blackwell.

Victor, D. G. (1999) The regulation of greenhouse gases: does fairness matter? In *Fair Weather: Equity Concerns in Climate Change*, ed. F. L. Toth. London: Earthscan, pp. 193–206.

Williams, B. (1991) A critique of utilitarianism. In *Utilitarianism: For and Against*. Cambridge: Cambridge University Press.

Issues

Public health research ethics

Is non-exploitation the new principle for population-based research ethics?

John McMillan

Introduction

The ethical principles that should govern public health research must accommodate public health's focus upon the health of populations, as well as the different research methodologies that it tends to use. Whereas biomedical research ethics has tended to emphasize the centrality of consent, research upon populations often raises additional ethical issues and consent may often be insufficient or inappropriate. The Belmont principles of respect for persons, justice and beneficence are intended to cover all biomedical and behavioural research involving human subjects, so should be applicable to public health research. However, because of the population-based focus of public health research work, the scope and application of these principles need to be reconsidered. An additional consideration is whether once their scope and application has been reconfigured, the three Belmont principles are suited to the ethics of public health research. Non-exploitation is a moral concept that has been mooted as an additional principle for biomedical research. Given that a principle of non-exploitation can be readily applied to populations and some unethical public research can be described as exploitative, this would appear at first to be a promising principle for public health research. This chapter will consider the merit of these claims and conclude that the Belmont principles can be interpreted so that they imply that exploitative public health research is wrong.

What is public health research?

Before considering the appropriate normative framework for public health research it is important to characterize this kind of research as clearly as is possible. In 'The meaning of "public" in "public health"' Verweij and Dawson (2007) note that 'Public Health' is a contested concept and that there are many competing definitions of this concept. While this is likely to be the case a working definition is useful for characterizing the domain under discussion.

The Institute of Medicine gave the following influential definition in 1988: 'Public Health is what we, as a society, do collectively to assure the conditions in which people can be healthy.' While this definition is influential and inclusive it gives little guidance to the methodology of public health and given that this is important for characterizing public health research, a sharper definition is helpful for my purposes.

Public Health Ethics, ed. Angus Dawson. Published by Cambridge University Press. © Cambridge University Press 2011.

Childress *et al.* (2002: 170) say:

> Public health is primarily concerned with the health of the entire population, rather than the health of individuals. Its features include an emphasis on the promotion of health and the prevention of disease and disability; the collection and use of epidemiological data, population surveillance, and other forms of empirical quantitative assessment; a recognition of the multidimensional nature of the determinants of health; and a focus on the complex interactions of many factors – biological, behavioral, social, and environmental – in developing effective interventions.

Like the Institute of Medicine these authors emphasize the importance of a population level view about the aetiology and prevention of disease, but they also point to the core activities and methodology that characterize public health. Given that health promotion and the prevention of disease and disability are some of the central activities of public health, this helps to characterize the domain of public health research. The last part of their definition emphasizes the complicated explanatory level that public health often operates at. Clearly, the explanatory complexity of public health influences the study methodologies adopted and in turn will have implications for the moral framework that is best suited to public health research ethics. While there is a broad array of research methodologies that can be considered public health research, epidemiology, population surveillance and other kinds of empirical quantitative assessment are the uncontroversial core of public health research.

While there are clear examples of public health research there are some interesting cases where it is less obvious whether the systematic collection of information counts as public health research.

As is the case in the social sciences there is still a significant debate within public health about the relative merits of qualitative and quantitative methodologies. It has been claimed that 'Methodological problems remain at the forefront of public health research because the ideology underpinning public health is often in flux' (Research in Health and Behavioral Change, 1989).

This is significant for thinking through the ethics of public health research. Those who advocate qualitative methods also insist that the ethical issues that need to be thought through for this kind of research are very different from those for quantitative methodologies. This is partly because qualitative research has a radically different account of what constitutes validity and the implications that this has for what is considered good study design. There are also some interesting differences in that some qualitative researchers see themselves as engaged in what is essentially, an empowering experience for the people taking part in the research (Punch, 1994). Certainly, it does seem the case that for many qualitative studies, the likelihood of physical harm is radically different from clinical trials and often a participant can exercise their right not to participate by clamming up and refusing to speak to the researcher. While there are *some* reasons for thinking that ethical scrutiny is less important for qualitative studies the very permissive situation does seems to be changing somewhat at least in the UK: an important change is the introduction of a requirement for all research funded by the Economic and Social Research Council (the major social science funding body in the UK) to be ethically reviewed (ESRC, 2006). The ethical principles that provide an adequate framework for public health research also provide an adequate framework for qualitative research. However to argue this thesis out fully would require another chapter because it would require a full exploration of qualitative methods.[1]

---

[1] For an introduction to the ethical considerations that are relevant to qualitative research see Gauld and McMillan (1999).

The scope of this chapter is limited to the issue of whether the conventional principles of research ethics can accommodate cases of exploitative public health research.

Another important ambiguity is whether we can determine whether collecting public health information in a systematic way is research or audit (collecting health information for the purposes of measuring care against already existing standards). This distinction matters because in many places there is an obligation upon researchers to gain approval from a research ethics committee if they are conducting research, which usually entails a significant amount of extra work and time. Audit can be considered an essential component of checking the quality of services that are provided and therefore is usually not reviewed by a research ethics committee. Wade (2005) has discussed some of the difficult boundary cases that are reasonably common in biomedical research. One common way in which this boundary can become blurred is when data is collected in a systematic way for the purposes of audit, which when analysed unexpectedly generates findings that are generalizable and likely to be of interest to a broader audience. In this kind of case what started out as audit and was not scrutinized has morphed into research that probably should have been subjected to ethical scrutiny. While these tricky boundary cases are reasonably common in biomedical research they are likely to be even more prevalent for public health, given the research methodologies commonly used. Because public health tends to function at a population level it can be hard to distinguish data collection that is part of routine public health from public health research, because they use common methods.

MacQueen and Buehler (2004) describe a number of possible public health scenarios where it would be unclear whether what's being done is research or a public health intervention. Their suggestion is that we should focus upon the 'primary intent' of the researcher/physician to distinguish whether this is a public health intervention or research (as we might to distinguish audit from research). In cases where the methods used for a public health intervention are very similar to those used for public health research then there seems little choice but to make this determination on the basis of what it is that is intended, although this will not avoid the problem of unexpected generalizable findings.

Codes and principles

Up until the 1980s there were relatively few codes of research ethics. The Declaration of Helsinki (2008), the Nuremberg Code (Annas and Grodin, 1995) and the CIOMS (2002) guidelines were and still are important moral touchstones for human subject researchers. While these codes lay down rules that have been very significant in shaping the conduct of human subject research, they are limited in a number of important respects. All codes of ethics contain a set of moral rules that are thought to be important guides to conducting research in an ethical way. Inevitably codes of ethics have to strike a difficult, and perhaps impossible, balance between being too restrictive and setting conditions that are unlikely to be met and being overly permissive or vague with the result that the code has little normative force. For example, the Nuremberg Code says that all research should have the voluntary consent of the research participant which has the virtue of being a clear and prescriptive rule but seems to make it impossible to do research upon those who are unable to give consent, even when this research would clearly be in their interests or could not have any impact upon the interests of that person (para. 1). The Declaration of Helsinki requires researchers to ensure that research participants have access post trial to study medication if trial medication is shown to be effective for participants (para. 30). This rule is likely to have the consequence that some important research in the developing world cannot be conducted because of the difficulty that researchers would face in ensuring that the infrastructure for the continuation of the same kind of care is in place.

While the moral rules of research ethics play an important role they need to be supplemented by moral principles or other foundational values that can:

- justify exceptions to moral rules;
- justify the refinement of moral rules;
- determine the scope and applicability of a moral rule;
- provide guidance in cases which are not covered by an appropriate rule.

Even though rule based codes of ethics are important we often need to move to a deeper level of moral analysis which can provide better justified moral reasons, instead of just relying upon the more precise prescriptions that tend to be expressed by rules.

In addition to the difficulties inherent in applying moral rules to the complex and novel moral scenarios that are common in research ethics, the large number of codes of research ethics makes it difficult to know whose rules should be followed. Since the 1980s, when Nuremberg, Helsinki and CIOMS were the most prominent codes, the amount of guidance on research ethics has increased hugely. Codes of research ethics have proliferated to the extent that it would be unusual for any professional body whose members conduct research to be without its own code of ethics. To a significant extent, codes are parasitic so there is a degree of consistency between them. However, there are also many examples where different professional bodies express rules about the same thing in significantly different ways. For example the Royal College of Physicians (1996: SS 7.3) *Guidelines* claim that the level of risk that is appropriate for healthy volunteer research should not exceed that which would be presented to people travelling by car but less than that which would be presented by travelling by pedal or motorcycle. While this rule has the virtue of clarity this degree of precision means that it is likely to contradict the rules of other professional bodies who also specify the level of risk that is appropriate. Making a judgement about which rule is applicable in a particular case can be made by moving to a level of analysis where the fundamental values underpinning these rules can be weighed and applied to the rule and case.

As I will argue in the following sections, the Belmont principles can be interpreted so as to specify the fundamental values that underpin public health research. If they are carefully applied and interpreted in exploitative cases they can explain the wrongness of these cases.

The Belmont principles

The Belmont Report (National Commission for the Protection of Human Subjects of Biomedical and Behavioural Research, 1979) attempts to articulate the core moral values that should be implicit in all ethical research involving human subjects. The Report's authors hoped to provide an analytic framework for considering the ethics of all human subject research. The idea is that by laying out the fundamental moral principles of research, argument about the appropriate rules and specific cases can proceed with a common basis in a set of shared moral commitments. The Belmont principles are:

- Respect for persons
- Beneficence
- Justice

The Report gives an account of what these principles mean and examples of some of the moral rules and practices that can be justified by reference to them.

The Report (1979: B1) interprets respect for persons as implying:

> . . . at least two ethical convictions: first, that individuals should be treated as autonomous agents, and second, that persons with diminished autonomy are entitled to protection. The principle of respect for persons thus divides into two separate moral requirements: the requirement to acknowledge autonomy and the requirement to protect those with diminished autonomy.

This way of explicating respect for persons emphasizes the centrality of autonomous individuals and their right to self determination. This account leads naturally to requirements such as informed consent and the right to have one's sensitive medical information protected which are fundamental practices and rules for public health research ethics. Belmont's authors are clear that these obligations are not the only obligations that follow from respect for persons which is consistent with their intention to provide a framework for moral analysis rather than a set of moral rules that will cover all cases. Nonetheless, their brief account of respect for persons does not mention some other aspects of this principle and this has led some to suggest that other principles need to be added to the Belmont three. In the following sections I will show that concerns about the relevance of non-exploitation to public health research are implied by a more developed account of respect for persons.

While Beauchamp and Childress (1994; Beauchamp, 2007) think that it is necessary to have four principles of biomedical ethics, the Belmont Report (rightly in my view) includes non-maleficence under its principle of beneficence.

> Persons are treated in an ethical manner not only by respecting their decisions and protecting them from harm, but also by making efforts to secure their well-being. Such treatment falls under the principle of beneficence. The term 'beneficence' is often understood to cover acts of kindness or charity that go beyond strict obligation. In this document, beneficence is understood in a stronger sense, as an obligation. Two general rules have been formulated as complementary expressions of beneficent actions in this sense: (1) do not harm and (2) maximize possible benefits and minimize possible harms.
>
> (1979: B2)

As I will show, the obligation to benefit research participants is the subject of a significant debate and some have argued that the principle of beneficence is not a core foundational value for research ethics. The Report's authors could have done more to show why beneficence is a core value, particularly research that is combined with professional care.

The Belmont Report (1979: B3) describes the question of justice as being primarily about

> Who ought to receive the benefits of research and bear its burdens? This is a question of justice, in the sense of 'fairness in distribution' or 'what is deserved'. An injustice occurs when some benefit to which a person is entitled is denied without good reason or when some burden is imposed unduly. Another way of conceiving the principle of justice is that equals ought to be treated equally.

The Report conceives of justice as being primarily a matter of justice in distribution. In the context of public health research ethics this will imply a number of things, including that the benefits and burdens of research should be distributed equally and account should be taken of any particular vulnerabilities that may lead to inequity. This might mean that public health research that is conducted upon those who have very poor access to care, puts a group at significant risk or cannot benefit members of that research group, distributes the benefits and risks of research in an unfair way. Applying the principle of justice to public health research might imply that care needs to be taken over the recruitment of groups with a particular vulnerability.

While the Report's authors are right to emphasize this as a core element of justice there are other ways in which the concept of justice can be relevant to public health research ethics. In *A Theory of Justice*, Rawls (1972) defends the idea of 'justice as fairness', which includes not only a principle of distributive justice but also a liberty principle which requires us to maximize the liberties of agents within a political community. This is significant because (as I will show) focusing upon this aspect of justice provides a way to value non-exploitation without adding another principle to the Belmont three.[2] A broader conception of justice is important for the ethics of public health more generally and a great deal more could be said about this. For my present purposes it will be sufficient to show interpreting the principle of justice in a fuller sense can accommodate worries such as exploitation.

All of the Belmont principles can be explicated by reference to different and often divergent moral theories. As is the case for justice, there are theoretical accounts of what respect for persons amounts to,[3] many of which emphasize different things and some of which might imply contradictory things. Defenders of principlist approaches can insist that this is one of the strengths of focusing upon principles rather than particular moral theories. The theoretical debates about, for instance, justice, are contested and complicated. When we need analytic tools for arguing about the ethics of applied topics such as public health research ethics we should aim at reaching a sound answer to an applied question rather than settling a theoretical debate about moral theory. Nonetheless, fleshing out moral principles in the way that I think we should, is consistent with the spirit of the Belmont Report and other authors who defend a principles based approach to research ethics. Moving towards consistency between moral judgements or rules and the principles of research ethics by a careful process of minor revision and elaboration can be considered an instance of Rawlsian reflective equilibrium.[4] The coherence of principles, rules and judgements is important for providing a consistent account of the morality relevant to public health research ethics. Inevitably this will require elaboration upon the scope and meaning of principles as well as the clarification, reformulation and possible rejection of the rules and judgements about research ethics.

Before considering how the Belmont principles can apply to public health research it is important to see the reasons why principles are useful moral tools for research ethics but perhaps are less obviously so in clinical medicine. Beauchamp and Childress (1994) defend the use of four principles of biomedical ethics for all areas of biomedicine. There are some good reasons for supposing that principles are more appropriately applied to the ethics of research than they are to clinical medicine more generally. Research very often has an international dimension that raises important ethical issues. Some of the most significant recent debates about the ethical standards of research have focused on whether

---

[2] Others have applied Rawls to health care. In *Just Health Care* (1985) Norman Daniels argues that Rawls's principle of justice should be applied when considering the just distribution of health care within a nation state.

[3] For a useful introduction to the ways in which autonomy (which is one reading of what respect for persons amounts to) can be a value in a health care setting, see Stoljar (1997) and Dworkin (1988).

[4] See Rawls (1972: 51) and Van Willigenburg (2007).

research in different countries should follow exactly the same moral rules or whether there are principled reasons for permitting different rules in different parts of the world. The most prominent recent example of this is the standard of care debate that followed the publication of Lurie and Wolfe's (1997) article on AZT trials conducted in the developing world and was continued in articles published in the *American Journal of Public Health* (Annas and Grodin, 1998; Bayer, 1998; Karim, 1998). One of the major arguments in support of a principles-based approach is that it provides a 'common morality' that can be interpreted and applied so as to take account of the particulars relevant to different contexts. In the debate over the AZT trials the extent and way in which our obligations under the principle of beneficence should be discharged in the developing world was one of the principal bones of contention. Principles are particularly useful for debates of this kind because they provide moral standards that are both universal and have the flexibility necessary to accommodate the particulars of different contexts. The Nuremburg Code was adopted during the trial of Nazi physicians so that the Nuremberg judges had a universal code which could be used for assessing the wrongs committed in the name of research.

Clinical medicine is different, at least to some extent. The prominence given to autonomy by Beauchamp and Childress is not emphasized to the same extent in all other parts of the world. Clinical medicine in some countries still operates on a predominantly paternalist model. Of course, it might be that these countries should move towards a model that embraces patient autonomy. However, this seems unjustifiably imperialistic in a way that it does not in the case of research ethics. It might be that there are a number of different reasons for this intuition, but one that is particularly important is the different ends of clinical medicine and research. The fundamental objective of clinical medicine is patient welfare. While it is right that research should also have the welfare of research participants as a core moral commitment, the fundamental objective of research is the production of knowledge. When clinical medicine fails to promote a patient's welfare, clinical medicine has, in this case, failed. When research fails to promote a research participant's welfare, it might still produce useful knowledge. A physician who wants to be a successful physician fails to succeed when she does not promote a patient's welfare. In his classic article 'Ethics and clinical research' (1966) Beecher described the incentives for young researchers to take ethical short cuts because of the importance for their careers of generating research funding and publications. Given that the incentives, as well as the success conditions for research, can differ significantly from what promotes the patient's welfare or autonomy this means that there is a greater need for articulating the core values that are relevant to research So long as clinical medicine succeeds by promoting the patient's welfare (and by this I mean welfare in an extensive sense comprising more than just the patient's medical interests) then failing to emphasize autonomy to the same extent seems more defensible, if not less bad.

The Belmont principles and population-level research

While the Belmont principles should be applied to public health research, they need to be reconfigured so as to accommodate the population-level emphasis of public health. In 'Ethical principles for the conduct of human subject research', Larry Gostin (1991: 191) shows how the Belmont principles can be applied to public health research:

> Ethical principles help support autonomy and self determination, protect the vulnerable, and promote the welfare and equality of human beings. But traditional ethics focuses primarily upon

individual rights and duties and does not always see individuals as part of wider social orders and communities. A person dominated medical ethic is insufficient for the task of setting moral and human rights boundaries around the conduct of research on populations.

Given that public health research interventions usually operate at a population level, principles that emphasize only the interests of individual actors are unlikely to capture what's ethically salient about public health research. The Belmont discussion of respect for persons emphasizes the centrality of consent without mentioning the other ways in which persons can fail to be respected. The Belmont discussion of beneficence emphasizes the importance of not causing harm to research participants and working towards an appropriate risk/benefit ratio. Given that public health research is more concerned with the health of populations, how can respect for persons and beneficence be made relevant to public health research?

Gostin describes a number of the problems that can result when respect for persons is taken to imply only informed consent. These include the problems that can result when there is a significant degree of mistrust between researchers and participants as well as the problems that can occur in countries where decision making is made on a communal basis. Gostin suggests that when applying respect for persons to public health research in addition to inferring informed consent we should also consider:

> ... the interrelated concepts of individual consent, consensus should be regarded as additional ethical obligations that are to be examined within the context both of international human rights norms and local cultural and ethical beliefs.
>
> (Gostin, 1991: 194)

Belmont emphasizes the importance of adopting appropriate measures when autonomy is compromised. In public health research this way of cashing out respect for persons implies that groups that might be considered vulnerable (for example, prisoners or sex workers) should also be considered more carefully so that individuals are respected as persons.

Gostin describes a number of ways in which the Belmont principles can be interpreted so as to provide rules that are relevant to public health research. Rather than evaluating all of these it is more relevant to examine the cases which are hard for the Belmont principles to accommodate that have led some to propose that Belmont needs to be revised.

Exploitation and unethical public health research

Many instances where the ethics of public health research has gone awry can be reasonably described as instances where researchers have exploited their research subjects. Researchers involved in the Tuskegee syphilis study failed to provide research participants with penicillin when it was clear that this would be an effective treatment for their condition (Caplan, 1992; Northington Gamble, 1997). Instead they were given 'heavy metals' therapy and other treatments that were unlikely to provide them with any benefit. While it would be hard to defend what was done, the Tuskegee study did produce useful results on the natural progression of syphilis in African American males. This seems a case where the wrong that has been committed is one that is naturally described as 'exploitation' and the actions of the researchers as 'exploitative'.

A more recent and perhaps more arguable example is a Baltimore public health study on lead abatement therapy that was considered in the judgement *Grimes* v. *Kennedy Krieger Institute Inc* 2001. The study ran from 1993 until 1995 and was part of a broader public health initiative to improve the quality of housing for those in lower socio-economic groups. The research aimed to identify the least expensive, effective level of lead abatement therapy.

> Identifying the minimal effective level of lead abatement was considered important because of the need to preserve availability of low-rent urban housing that might be abandoned by landlords if they had to pay for the expensive repairs needed to eliminate lead using standard abatement methods . . . 1068 Baltimore rental properties were classified into 5 groups. Three groups of housing received less than full lead abatement (a different level for each group); housing in the 2 control groups either had previously undergone full lead abatement or had been constructed without lead paint. Over a 2-year period, the researchers were to measure and compare lead dust levels collected in the housing with lead levels in blood samples drawn from children living in those homes. Informed consent was to be obtained, and parents were to be notified of their children's blood levels and the results of lead dust collection in their homes. Blood levels would provide evidence regarding the effectiveness of a particular level of abatement.
>
> (Mastroianni and Kahn, 2002: 1074)

The researchers might argue that the children benefited by being in the trial because for any of the arms they might be randomized to they would be likely to be better off than they otherwise would have been. If they were randomized to one of the two arms that had full abatement therapy they would be better off because there was no lead in those houses. If they were randomized to one of the houses with the partial lead abatement therapy they would be likely to be better off because they would have avoided the risk of being in a house with no lead abatement therapy. Even though the children in these three groups might have been better off if they had been in one of the two groups that provided full abatement therapy, the fact that they were in the study has made them better off than they otherwise would have been. Given that parental consent had been obtained, the researchers might argue that they had benefited the children as well as respecting them as persons via the process of gaining parental consent.

This moral argument not withstanding there is something wrong about allowing poor children to live in houses that have higher levels of lead contamination than is thought healthy to find out whether in fact living with that level of contamination is unhealthy. The court in *Grimes* v. *Kennedy* agreed and made comparisons with the Tuskegee syphilis study while describing the research as exploitative (Mastroianni and Kahn, 2002: 1075).

More needs to be said about what exploitation is before reaching a conclusion about its viability as a principle but on the face of it, it does seem to be a specific kind of wrong that can occur even when there is consent and research participants have not been made worse off over all.

Non-exploitation as a new principle for research ethics

In an influential article, Miller and Brody (2003) raise important critical questions about the normative basis of research ethics; questions that they think have important implications for the ethical conduct of research. They think that the authors of the Belmont Report made a mistake when they included beneficence as a principle of research ethics. According to Miller and Brody the obligation to benefit is not an obligation that should befall researchers and conflates the ethics of clinical care with the ethics that should be relevant to research. They (2003: 20) claim that: 'An ethical framework that provides normative guidance about a practice should accurately characterize the practice'.

In other words, research involving human subjects does not ordinarily involve a commitment to benefit research participants so it is inappropriate to impose this ethical norm when it is not part of the practice. There are a number of reasons why this is not a particularly good argument. First, it does not follow from the fact that a practice exists that normative guidance must accurately characterize it – there are plenty of immoral practices that need to be reformed. Second, bioethics has been criticized in the past for being merely a legitimating exercise, that is, whatever new technology or research practice emerges ethicists will end up providing a rationale for that activity. Insisting that ethical principles must be derived from practice runs the risk of bioethics uncritically accepting the practice when the appropriate question is whether the norms are right. A third problem is that the rules that the Belmont authors derive from beneficence are generally accepted as norms for research: minimizing harm and maximizing benefit are hardly controversial rules.

While Miller and Brody think that this is an important argument against an obligation to benefit research participants, it is not their main objection. They (2003: 20) think that applying the principle of beneficence to research involves a misguided attempt to bridge the ethics of research and therapy:

> In view of the nature and purpose of clinical research, the principles of beneficence and non-maleficence applicable to clinical research lack the therapeutic meaning that guides their application to medical care . . . and as treatment conducted by physicians who retain fidelity to the principles of beneficence and therapeutic non-maleficence that govern the ethics of clinical medicine. The doctrine of clinical equipoise has emerged as the bridge between medical care and scientific experimentation.

Miller and Brody seek to completely overhaul the rules and principles of research ethics. Instead of beneficence and the requirements such as clinical equipoise they think that we should adopt a set of rules derived from a principle of non-exploitation. They endorse some of the rules proposed by Emanuel *et al.* (2000) and suggest that at least some of these rules derive from a principle of non-exploitation. While many instances of unethical research do intuitively seem to be instances of exploitation it is important to consider whether non-exploitation is a viable principle for research ethics in general and public health research ethics in particular.

There is something intuitively right about the idea that exploitation plays an important role in identifying unethical research. The wrongs of the Tuskegee syphilis study, Willowbrook (Pappworth, 1968) and other instances of unethical public health research in the twentieth century were intuitively instances where research subjects were exploited. The therapeutic misconception is notoriously difficult to avoid in clinical research (Appelbaum *et al.*, 1987). While it is more likely that public health physicians/researchers can do more to avoid this, it still seems to be at the root of the problem for the examples of unethical public research discussed thus far. A useful initial way of characterizing exploitative research is that it uses an inequality so that persons can be used as research subjects. Beauchamp and Childress (1994: 441) note:

> . . . because investigators and subjects are unequal in knowledge and vulnerability – especially if sick patients are involved – public policy and review committees must act to prevent potentially exploitative contracts. . . .

While the power and knowledge differential between researchers and subjects provide good reasons for supposing that exploitation is a key problem for research it is also important to be able to give a coherent account of what it is that exploitation amounts to.

Wertheimer and exploitation

Arguably the most important recent theory of exploitation is that produced by the political philosopher, Wertheimer (1996). He sets himself the task of giving an account of what the wrong making features of an exploitative transaction are. Rather than merely giving an analysis of what the concept means he is concerned with producing an account that brings out the distinctive normative features of exploitative arrangements. This kind of account is what is required in order for exploitation to play a useful role in public health research ethics. Unless a reasonably coherent account can be given of what exploitation is and why it is bad then it will tend to function merely as a rhetorical device or term of art. While there are a number of theoretical explications of each of the Belmont principles all of them can be characterized in a way that makes their normative force clear and this seems like a reasonable prerequisite for any moral principle.

Wertheimer's account is the most plausible non-Marxist account of this kind and this reason alone is sufficient for using his account in this context. A second, perhaps more important, reason for using Wertheimer's analysis is that those who have suggested a principle of non-exploitation for research ethics have referred to his account and Wertheimer (2007) has recently spelled out some of the implications of his theory for research ethics. As I will show, Wertheimer's account is not as obviously useful for research ethics as many think. Wertheimer distinguishes a number of meanings of exploitation: 'harmful exploitation', 'wrongful use exploitation' and 'non-consensual exploitation'. He argues that a fourth sense: 'mutually advantageous, consensual, exploitation' is a moral concept that is distinct from other moral considerations such as respect for persons.

Harmful exploitation

The Tuskegee syphilis study resulted in large numbers of African Americans not being provided treatment for syphilis so that the natural progression of the disease could be observed (Caplan, 1992). It seems reasonable to describe the African Americans who suffered from untreated syphilis at a time when penicillin was available as being exploited in the most appalling way.

The problem is that for Wertheimer this kind of wrong is not unambiguously identified as being an instance of exploitation. His project is to discover the distinctive wrongness of exploitation. While the Tuskegee study is an appalling wrong, its wrongness can just as readily be explained in terms of the harm caused to these people and the failure to provide treatment when it was available. In other words this wrong making aspect of the situation is well covered by the principle of beneficence.

Wrongful use exploitation

Many commentators including Miller and Weijer (2009) take exploitation to mean what can be called 'wrongful use' exploitation. The idea here is that transaction X between agents A and B is exploitative if and only if X involves A and/or B being treated as a mere means. In other words, wrongful use exploitation violates the Kantian injunction against the instrumental use of persons. Clearly exploiting research subjects in this way is a very serious wrong and would provide a *prima facie* reason for criticizing any trial that did this. Most instances of wrongful use will be instances of harmful exploitation but there will be some cases where it might be plausible to describe a person as being used inappropriately even though they have not been made worse off or harmed, so it is worth treating this as a distinct kind of case.

However, if exploitation is to play a distinctive role as a key principle of research it should do moral work that is not already provided by extant moral principles. Wrongful useful exploitation is a paradigmatic violation of the importance of respect for persons. While the Belmont report mentions consent as one of the implications of respect for persons there is no reason why the principle does not also imply the wrongfulness of using human beings instrumentally and neglecting their humanity. Wrongful use exploitation is clearly morally significant and a serious wrong but it is a paradigmatic implication of respect for persons.

Non-consensual exploitation

One common objection to allowing payment for research participation is that it will 'induce' participants to take part in research. More needs to be said on the nature of what constitutes an inducement, but a number of important commentators, Faden and Beauchamp (1986) being two notable examples, think that inducements are problematic because they compromise the validity of consent. They give the example of a woman who agrees to take part in risky and unpleasant research because of her desperate need and the large amount of money that she will receive for participation. Faden and Beauchamp are overly paternalistic in claiming that this will compromise her ability to consent and make this arrangement 'non-consensual'. It might be that she makes a cool assessment of what is in her interests on the basis of good information about the study and the usefulness of the money that it will provide. (For more on this see Wilkinson and Moore, 1997.) Nonetheless let us assume for argument's sake that this offer is what Wertheimer would call 'seductive' and results in her making a serious error in judgment about what is in her interests. We might be tempted to say that the researchers have exploited this woman's vulnerability with the result that she takes part in research that she would otherwise have refused. This would be an instance of what Wertheimer calls 'non-consensual exploitation' and while this clearly is morally problematic it's not unambiguously an instance of exploitation. This is because this kind of case is well covered by respect for persons and the importance of informed consent. While 'exploitation' might be a convenient label for this kind of case it is not of novel normative significance.

Mutually advantageous, consensual, exploitation

Having put non-consensual, harmful and wrongful use cases to one side Wertheimer gives a series of examples that he thinks bring out the distinctive wrongness of exploitation. The specific instances that he thinks are revealing are what he calls instances of mutually advantageous, consensual, exploitation (MACE). In other words these are unfair transactions or arrangements where an individual has given valid consent and will not be harmed by the arrangement, yet is exploited nonetheless.

It is an open question whether there is anything wrong with this kind of exploitation. As Feinberg (1990) suggests, if a person gives valid consent to an arrangement that will do them no harm then there is a serious question about whether or not they have any grounds for complaint. Nonetheless Wertheimer (1996: 22) does generate a number of plausible instances of this kind of exploitation that show that there is at least something wrong with transactions of this kind.

> An unexpected blizzard hits an area and people rush to the hardware store to buy a shovel. The
> hardware store owner sees the opportunity to make an abnormal profit and raises the price of the

shovel from $15 to $30. If B agrees to pay $30 for the shovel, because the shovel is worth more than $30 to B under the circumstances, then the transaction is clearly Pareto superior. Both parties gain. But B feels exploited because B gains less (or pays more) than B thinks reasonable. A similar structure applies to some of the other cases of alleged exploitation . . . profits from the AIDS drug AZT, surrogate motherhood contracts, organ sales. We need not deny that B benefits from these transactions, all things considered.

This idea of one party contributing more than they should or perhaps benefiting less than they should is very close to the heart of what was thought by many to be wrong about the AZT trials conducted in the developing world. Those who argued for the acceptability of these trials often pointed to the fact that no treatment was available for HIV/AIDS in many of these countries and that research subjects were therefore not made worse off and in many cases benefited from these trials. Nonetheless it is hard to dispute that it is unfair that subjects in these trials did not receive therapy that they would have if they lived in North America or Europe. Of course it is another argument to say that these trials should not have been conducted on the basis of this unfairness or that those who designed or conducted the trials had an obligation to provide this benefit.

The Baltimore lead abatement study also had this kind of moral problem. While questions were raised about whether parents were informed about all of the risks, the primary moral objection appears to have been the fact that although taking part in this research can be argued to have benefited them, their participation was obtained because a vulnerability was exploited. In other words the participation of the Baltimore subjects was mutually advantageous and possibly consensual but exploitative because of the lack of options for these subjects.

So far so good. These examples do suggest that MACE is relevant to at least some important examples in public health research ethics. Although Wertheimer aims to give an account of MACE he does not think that it always necessitates interference. So while in the snow shovel example B might have grounds for feeling exploited by A it does not follow that anything should be done to stop A exploiting B in this way. This is not in and of itself a reason to dismiss exploitation as a moral principle because all principles should be considered *prima facie*. However in more recent work Wertheimer has suggested that MACE as a concept won't help us determine whether or not an exploitative arrangement is wrong (2007: 253).

Problems for MACE

While Wertheimer's account is very influential he now concedes that his ideal market account of exploitation fails. Arneson has demonstrated that Wertheimer does not succeed in identifying the appropriate moral comparator for unfair transactions.

> Wertheimer argues that at least for an important range of cases, the baseline that fixes fair terms of interaction deviation from which qualifies as substantially unfair is the competitive market price for a good or service. If a perfectly competitive market actually exists, transactions under these conditions are not exploitative. If a perfectly competitive market does not exist, but we can envisage these conditions obtaining, then this hypothetical perfectly competitive price sets an appropriate baseline for determining whether actual terms of trade are substantially unfair.
>
> (2001: 890)

Arneson is referring to Wertheimer's (1996: 232) substantive account of what would make a MACE transaction fair and this says:

When a market is perfectly competitive, no one is able to take special advantage of particular defects in the other party's decision-making capacity or special vulnerabilities in the other party's situation.

In a public health research context this might imply that research participation is not exploitation when neither researcher nor participant has any vulnerability that either part could take advantage of. It's worth thinking of exploitation as being possible from both directions: while it does not seem very likely it is possible that a participant could exploit a researcher if the researcher were particularly desperate for their participation. Participants in the Baltimore lead abatement study might have been in a fairly competitive research participation market place if they had not been disadvantaged by their lack of a reasonable alternative for housing.

Arneson (2001: 890) points out that there are problems with this account because:

... suppose there is a perfectly competitive market for child care and house cleaning services in the city where I live and I am hiring John to care for my children. Nothing constrains me from offering him an above market wage. The market wage may be abysmally low.

A second counter example:

A perfectly competitive market for doctors' services may obtain, but this situation does not prevent Dr Ann from reflecting on what she ought to do and deciding to work at a medical clinic that serves poor people and pays her a below-market price for her services.

(Arneson, 2001: 891)

The point of these counter examples is that perfect competition does not have the normative significance that Wertheimer thinks and that perfect competition does not provide a standard for a just price. Wertheimer's account of MACE and the problems with it might appear to have drifted a little way away from the present concerns about public health research ethics. Nonetheless the important point here is that the most viable theoretical account of exploitation has problems that its author thinks decisive. Wertheimer does not think that this means that he has misidentified MACE but instead he has not succeeded in giving us an account of to what extent these cases are wrong. In other words consensual, mutually advantageous exploitation is a wrong without a viable theoretical underpinning.

This matters because it is reasonable to expect that a moral consideration that is to play the role of a principle should have at least one plausible theory that underpins it. One of the motivations behind Beauchamp and Childress's insistence that there should be four principles is that there are a number of plausible theoretical accounts of autonomy, beneficence and justice. A principle of non-exploitation is either redundant or applies only awkwardly in a limited number of cases.

MACE, justice and public health research ethics

A precondition for a principle being a plausible moral principle is that it has grounding in at least one reasonable theory and this does not appear to be the case for Wertheimer's analysis of exploitation. The other senses of exploitation, harmful, wrongful use and non-consensual are important values for public health research ethics but they are all implied by the Belmont principles.

Nonetheless MACE does seem to pick out the wrongness of the Baltimore lead abatement study and the AZT trials (on the assumption that they were wrong). Wertheimer's account of

MACE might be cashed out by coming up with a normative baseline that is more appropriate for public health research ethics. Even if Arneson had not shown the competitive market place to be a mistake it's a comparator that is tricky to apply to research ethics, especially given prevailing views about payment for research participation. What seems more relevant is what the exploiter should have done *morally*. Dr Ann's below market rate for her services reflects a moral determination about what is just, given her obligations. This kind of comparison is useful when thinking through the Baltimore and AZT examples. Our intuitions about what a just researcher would do in that situation seem highly relevant to judgements about whether or not they have exploited their research subjects.

When the Belmont report discusses justice it describes it primarily in terms of distributive justice while not mentioning the importance of liberty as discussed by Rawls. One way of teasing out the appropriate normative baseline for MACE cases is in terms of an unfair set of liberties. If we consider the AZT trials and Baltimore lead abatement study wrong because they involve MACE then the appropriate normative baseline might be the appropriate liberties for these participants. The participants in the AZT trials would not have been exploited if their decision to take part was one that occurred when they could access appropriate care under similar conditions to those in other countries. The participants in the Baltimore lead abatement study would not have been exploited if they had agreed to participate when they were able to access reasonable housing.

A normative baseline of this kind does seem to be consistent with the wrongness of research arrangements of this kind. However, a normative baseline of this kind will not help those who want non-exploitation to be a principle of research ethics. If the normative baseline in MACE cases involves an appeal to justice then these cases are reasonably covered by the principle of justice. If research participants take part in public health research because their liberty to improve their situation in other ways is seriously limited then this is a case of injustice, even if we might also describe that transaction as MACE.

References

Annas, G. and Grodin, M. (1995) *The Nazi Doctors and the Nuremberg Code: Human Rights in Human Experimentation*. Oxford: Oxford University Press.

Annas G. and Grodin, M. (1998) Human rights and maternal child HIV transmission prevention trials in Africa. *American Journal of Public Health*, 88: 560–3.

Appelbaum, P. S., Roth, L. H., Lidz, C. W., Benson, P. and Winslade, W. (1987) False hopes and best data: consent to research and the therapeutic misconception. *Hastings Center Report*, 17(2): 20–4.

Arneson, R. (2001) Exploitation. *Mind*, 110: 888–91.

Bayer, R. (1998) Research to prevent maternal-fetal transmission of HIV: racist exploitation or exploitation of racism? *American Journal of Public Health*, 88: 567–70.

Beauchamp, T. (2007) The 'four principles' approach to healthcare ethics. In *The Principles of Healthcare Ethics*, 2nd edn, ed. R. Ashcroft, A. Dawson, H. Draper and J. McMillan. Chichester: John Wiley.

Beauchamp, T. and Childress, J. (1994) *The Principles of Biomedical Ethics*. Oxford: Oxford University Press.

Beecher, H. (1966) Ethics and clinical research. *New England Journal of Medicine*, 274: 1354–60.

Caplan, A. (1992) Twenty years after. The legacy of the Tuskegee Syphilis Study. *When Evil Intrudes, Hastings Center Report*, 22: 29–32.

Childress, J. F., Faden, R. R., Gaare, R. D., *et al.* (2002) Public health ethics: mapping the terrain. *Journal of Law and Medical Ethics*, 30: 17–18.

Council for International Organizations of Medical Sciences (CIOMS) in collaboration with the World Health Organization (WHO) (2002) *CIOMS International Ethical Guidelines for Biomedical Research Involving Human Subjects*. Geneva: CIOMS.

Daniels, N. (1985) *Just Health Care*. Cambridge: Cambridge University Press.

Dworkin, G. (1988) *The Theory and Practice of Autonomy*. Cambridge: Cambridge University Press.

Economic and Social Research Council (ESRC) (2006) *Research Ethics Framework*. Swindon: ESRC.

Emmanuel, E., Wendler, D. and Grady, C. (2000) What makes clinical research ethical? *Journal of American Medical Association*, **283** (20): 2701.

Faden, R. and Beauchamp, T. (1986) *A History and Theory of Informed Consent*. Oxford: Oxford University Press.

Feinberg, J. (1990) *Harmless Wrongdoing*. Oxford: Oxford University Press.

Gauld, R. and McMillan, J. (1999) Ethics committees and qualitative health research in New Zealand. *New Zealand Medical Journal*, **112**: 195–7.

Gostin, L. (1991) Ethical principles for the conduct of human subject research: population-based research and ethics. *Law, Medicine and Health Care*, **19**: 191–201.

Hope, T. and McMillan, J. (2004) Challenge studies of human volunteers: ethical issues. *Journal of Medical Ethics*, **30**: 110–16.

Institute of Medicine (1988) *The Future of Public Health*. Washington, DC: National Academy Press.

Karim, S. (1998) Placebo controls in HIV perinatal transmission trials: a South African's viewpoint. *American Journal of Public Health*, **88**: 564–6.

Lurie, P. and Wolfe, S. (1997) Unethical trials of interventions to reduce perinatal transmission of the human immunodeficiency virus in developing countries. *New England Journal of Medicine*, **337**: 1159–61.

McMillan, J. and Conlon, C. (2002) Developing world research and the Nuffield Council's Report. *Journal of Medical Ethics*, **30**: 204–6.

MacQueen, K. and Buehler, J. (2004) Ethics, practice and research in public health. *American Journal of Public Health*, **94**(6): 928.

Mastroianni, A. and Kahn, J. (2002) Risk and responsibility: ethics, *Grimes v Kennedy Krieger*, and public health research involving children. *American Journal of Public Health*, **92**: 1073–6.

Miller, F. and Brody, B. (2003) A critique of clinical equipoise: therapeutic misconception of the ethics of clinical trials. *Hastings Center Report*, **33**(3): 19–28.

Miller, P. and Weijer, C. (2009) The trust based obligations of physicians to patients in clinical research. In *The Limits of Consent: A Socio-legal Approach to Human Subject Research in Medicine*, ed. O. Corrigan, K. Liddell, J. McMillan, M. Richards and C. Weijer. Oxford: Oxford University Press.

National Commission for the Protection of Human Subjects of Biomedical and Behavioural Research (1979) *The Belmont Report: Ethical Principles and Guidelines for the Protection of Human Subjects of Research*. Bethesda, MD: Office of Protection from Research Risks, US Public Health Service.

Northington Gamble, V. (1997) Under the shadow of Tuskegee: African Americans and health care. *American Journal of Public Health*, **87**: 1773–8.

Pappworth, M. (1968) *Human Guinea Pigs: Experimentation on Man*. London: Beacon Press.

Punch, M. (1994) Politics and ethics in qualitative research. In *The Sage Handbook of Qualitative Research*, ed. N. K. Denzin and S. Yvonna. Lincoln. Newbury Park, CA: SAGE.

Rawls, J. (1972) *A Theory of Justice*. Oxford: Oxford University Press.

Research in Health and Behavioral Change (1989) *Changing the Public Health*. Chichester: John Wiley.

Royal College of Physicians (1996) *Guidelines on the Practice of Ethics Committees in Medical Research Involving Human Subjects*, 3rd edn. London: Royal College of Physicians.

Stoljar, N. (2007) Theories of autonomy. In *The Principles of Healthcare Ethics*, 2nd edn, ed.

R. Ashcroft, A. Dawson, H. Draper and J. McMillan. Chichester: John Wiley.

Van Willigenburg, T. (2007) Reflective equilibrium as a method in health care ethics. In *The Principles of Healthcare Ethics*, 2nd edn, ed. R. Ashcroft, A. Dawson, H. Draper and J. McMillan. Chichester: John Wiley.

Verweij, M. and Dawson, A. (2007) The meaning of 'public' in 'public health'. In *Ethics, Prevention and Public Health*, ed. A. Dawson and M. Verweij. Oxford: Oxford University Press.

Wade, D. (2005) Ethics, audit and research: all shades of grey. *British Medical Journal*, **330**: 473.

Wertheimer, A. (1996) *Exploitation*. Princeton, NJ: Princeton University Press.

Wertheimer, A. (2007) Exploitation in health care. In *The Principles of Healthcare Ethics*, 2nd edn, ed. R. Ashcroft, A. Dawson, H. Draper and J. McMillan. Chichester: John Wiley.

Wilkinson, M. and Moore, A. (1997) Inducement in research. *Bioethics*, **11**(5): 373–89.

World Medical Association (2008) *Declaration of Helsinki. Ethical Principles for Medical Research Involving Human Subjects*. 59th WMA General Assembly, Seoul, Korea, October 2008. Available at: http://www.wma.net/e/policy/b3.htm (accessed: 8/12/08).

Equity and population health
Toward a broader bioethics agenda

Norman Daniels

Introduction

In its early decades, bioethics concentrated on two important problem areas: (1) the dyadic, very special relationships that hold between doctors and patients and researchers and subjects; and (2) Promethean challenges, the powers and responsibilities that come with new knowledge and technologies in medicine and the life sciences, including those that bear on extending and terminating life. The dyadic relationships yield important goods, impose significant risks, are rife with inequalities in power and authority, and yet are bound by complex rights and obligations. They provide a rich field for ethics to explore. The Promethean challenges are the favourites of the media: how god-like can we become in our relations with people, with animals, and with our environment without losing our moral footing? They attract serious inquiries about how to use knowledge and technology responsibly for the individual and collective good. Unfortunately, they also form the frontline trenches for contemporary culture wars.

Bioethics' focus on the largely non-institutional examination of these dyadic relations and the emergence of exotic technologies means other important issues concerning population health and its equitable distribution were not addressed. (There are exceptions to this generalization.) The doctor–patient relationship and the researcher–subject relationship do have a bearing on population health, since medicine and medical research have impact on the health of individuals and populations. By not examining the broader institutional settings and policies that mediate population health, bioethics has sometimes been myopic, not seeing the context in which these relationships operate. Similarly, the focus on exotic technologies may blind bioethics to the broader determinants of health and thus to factors that have more bearing on a larger good both domestically and globally.

To motivate a broader bioethics agenda, I shall focus on equity in three problem areas: (1) health inequalities between different social groups and the policies needed to reduce them; (2) intergenerational equity in the context of rapid societal aging; and (3) issues of equity raised by international health inequalities and the international institutions and policies that have influence on them. Each area has both domestic and international implications.

There are good reasons for pursuing this broader agenda. The agenda aligns bioethics with the goal of more effectively promoting a fundamental good, improved population health, especially for those who enjoy less of it domestically and internationally. It focuses bioethics on the pursuit of justice. Justice obliges us to pursue equity and fairness in the promotion of health, but policy needs the guidance of ethics in determining what this means. These population issues provide the relevant institutional context in which we should think about the role of new technologies and the dyadic relationships I mentioned earlier. Finally, for bioethics to play this role, it must draw on, and train its practitioners in, a wider range of philosophical skills and social science disciplines.

What must we do to pursue equity in health?
Health egalitarians and health maximizers

I take 'health' to mean normal functioning, that is, the absence of pathology, mental or physical.[1] This biomedical account of health is clearly narrower than the widely quoted WHO (1946) definition: 'Health is a state of complete physical, mental and social well-being and not merely the absence of disease or infirmity.' The WHO conception erroneously expands health to include nearly all of well-being, so it may no longer function as a limit notion. People who actually measure population health, such as epidemiologists, concentrate on departures from normal functioning. As we shall see, understanding health as normal functioning is quite compatible with taking a broad view of the determinants of health revealed by the social determinants literature.

This characterization of health has implications for what counts as pursuing equity in health.[2] Every society has some healthy and some unhealthy people. One natural way to understand the goal of equity in health – the goal of health egalitarians – is to say that we should aim, ultimately, to make all people healthy, that is, help them to function normally over a normal lifespan.[3] Pursuing equality means 'levelling up' – bringing all those in less than full health to the status of the healthy.[4]

Surprisingly, the ultimate aim of health maximizers is identical to that of health egalitarians: We maximize population health if all people function normally over a normal

---

[1] This characterization is neutral between a value-free, stochastic account of normal functioning, such as Boorse's (1975, 1997), and a modestly normative, etiological (or evolutionary) account, such as Wakefield's (1992) account of mental disorders as harmful dysfunctions. Neither account views pathology simply as an 'unwanted condition' without providing a clear, objectively ascribable view of what makes it a dysfunction at some level within the organism.

[2] I side-step a debate about whether to measure all individual variation in health, later factoring in information about demographic sub-groups (Gakidou *et al.*, 2000), or to focus on health inequalities across important sub-groups, for example, by class or race or ethnicity (Braveman *et al.*, 2002).

[3] Rawls's social contract situation involves the simplifying assumption that all people are fully functional over a normal lifespan. We might take this to be an egalitarian default position (Rawls, 1971).

[4] My health egalitarian behaves like Parfit's (1995) 'prioritarian': one would not level down the better health of some to make them more equal with those in worse health (blind the sighted to equalize health states with the blind) if there were no reasonable off-setting gain to those who are in worse health. Doing so would frustrate the ultimate egalitarian goal of making all fully normal over a normal lifespan.

lifespan. Health is clearly different from income (and possibly well-being). There is no natural stopping point for income – the rich can always be richer – but health is a limit concept. Being completely healthy is being completely healthy. Despite convergence on ultimate aims, health egalitarians and health maximizers generally support different strategies or policies for achieving their common ultimate aim of producing a completely healthy population.[5] A maximizing strategy or policy will seek the highest achievable aggregate measure for resources invested, regardless of how the health is distributed. Someone concerned with equity in health will put important constraints on how the health is distributed.

Unsolved rationing problems

A family of unsolved distributive problems has been discussed by people in the social sciences and bioethics (Kamm, 1987, 1993; Brock, 1988; Daniels, 1993, 1994). In these problems, maximizing strategies are pitted against fairness or equity considerations. For example, when we select an intervention because it has the best cost-effectiveness ratio, we are maximizing health benefits at the margin regardless of how the benefits are distributed. Consider three ways this maximizing strategy conflicts with concerns about equity. First, it gives no priority to those who are worse off or in greater need. Most people want to give some priority to those who are worse off even if they do not want to give them complete priority. How much priority should we give? That is the priorities problem. Second, cost-effectiveness analysis (CEA) allows us to aggregate minor benefits to larger numbers so that they outweigh significant benefits to fewer people. Yet, even though most people accept some forms of aggregation, they reject unrestricted aggregation, refusing to allow, for example, life-saving treatments to a few to be outweighed by very minor benefits to very large numbers. The aggregation problem asks when should we aggregate? Third, CEA doggedly pursues 'best outcomes' while denying fair chances for some benefit to those with worse outcomes. Yet most people reject a strict maximizing strategy, preferring to give people fair chances at some benefit. How should we balance best outcomes against fair chances? This is the best outcomes/fair chances problem. We have considerable trouble agreeing on what the appropriate middle ground is in each of these problems.

Reducing health inequalities and unsolved distributive problems

The same distributive problems arise when we think about eliminating health inequalities. Five of the eight internationally negotiated Millennium Development Goals (MDG) are inequality reducing, aiming at poverty reduction or providing primary education to those who lack it. The three health targets, however, are stated in terms of reducing population aggregates, for example, mortality of children under age 5. Gwatkin (2002) models two extreme approaches to these aggregate goals. A maximizing approach aims at rapid achievement of the target goal by directing resources to those who are already better off but easier to reach with strategies for improvement. An egalitarian approach aims to help those who are worst off first, then the next worst off and so on. Programme incentives and the geo-politics

---

[5] I set aside ethical and conceptual problems that arise in the construction of summary measures of population health, which allow us to aggregate across various health conditions of different seriousness and length.

surrounding the MDG programme mean that the maximizing strategy is more likely to be implemented, since funders want rapid results, although it actually increases inequality in the population.

The unsolved distributive problems are raised in contexts where it is not morally problematic why those who are worse off are so – they are just sicker than the others for whatever reason. In the MDG problem, as in the concern about inter-group health inequalities more generally, the baseline distribution is itself morally problematic because there is some social responsibility for creating the basic health inequality. Racial disparities in the USA, ethnic disparities in the UK and gender inequalities in the prevalence of HIV/AIDS in sub-Saharan Africa may be clear examples. The injustice of the existing baseline may give extra weight to the concern that we minimize inequalities, giving impetus to efforts to draw attention to race disparities in health in the USA and to stronger efforts to reduce class disparities in the UK, Sweden and elsewhere in Europe. Indeed, the WHO Commission on the Social Determinants of Health encourages broad attention to health disparities and their origins in the inequitable distribution of various other goods.

How much should this consideration of the injustice of the baseline outweigh our concern that we are not achieving best outcomes in the aggregate? Some may object that if we single out some groups as 'more deserving' because they were wronged, then we are abandoning the principle that we ought to focus only on need in medical contexts. We should not, then, give priority to fixing the broken leg of the mugging victim over the skier. When the Chinese decided to give priority in access to antiretroviral treatments to victims of infected blood, they were criticized for stigmatizing as less deserving those people infected in other ways.

Moral disagreement about these conflicting concerns will be sharp. There will be disagreements about who is really responsible for the baseline and efforts to explain its injustice away (perhaps in the form of victim-blaming). The unsolved distributive problems are thus made even more difficult. Bioethics has barely risen to the challenge of solving them when they have morally neutral baselines. It must also address the added challenge posed by inequitable baselines.

Social determinants and health inequalities

Most Americans, and I suppose most British, who are asked, 'What does it take to assure people of equity in health?' will respond with what they take to be a truism, 'Give people equal access to appropriate medical care', for example through a universal coverage insurance scheme. At best, this apparent truism is but a small part of the answer; at worst, it is misleading in important ways.

Equal access to medical services does not by itself assure equity if we have made the wrong trade-offs in our health system between equity and the maximization of aggregate health benefits. Just as important, we cannot produce equity in health simply by distributing medical or even public health resources equitably. Health inequalities have more complex origins. We know from the longitudinal Whitehall studies of British civil servants of different employment ranks, for example, as well as from other studies, that health inequalities in a population may not decrease, and may increase, even with universal coverage (Marmot and Wilkinson, 1999). The Whitehall study involves a study population that suffers no poverty and has had basic education. Our health is thus affected not simply by the ease with which we can see a doctor or be treated in a hospital, and not simply by the reduction in risks that come from traditional public health measures – though these factors surely matter – but also by our social position and the underlying inequality of our society.[6]

If we accept as otherwise just the inequalities we allow in our society, but these inequalities contribute to health inequalities, then should we view these health inequalities as themselves just? Or are significant health inequalities across groups always grounds for altering the distribution of other goods? Our answer may depend on the kinds of other inequalities that we see producing health inequalities (Daniels *et al.*, 1999, 2000). Turn from class, for the moment, to race.

American data reveals a significant but complex independent effect of race – or racism – on health. African Americans have worse health than whites at every income and educational level. Institutional and overt racism must be included as further social determinants of health. For example, the increasing de facto residential segregation that we see in America contributes significantly to these inequalities. The complex pattern by race and ethnicity of key behavioural risk factors (diet, tobacco, alcohol, and substance use and abuse, violence) contributes to, but does not account for, race and ethnic inequalities in health. In addition, medical treatment patterns differ by race, a result, perhaps, of conscious and unconscious stereotyping. A society that has a legacy of caste structure and exclusion creates psycho-social stresses in many institutional settings (schools, the workplace, shopping malls) that are implicated in health inequalities. Similar issues affect many immigrant ethnic minorities in European countries.

Race inequalities seem to be the easy case. What about the socio-economic status (SES) induced inequalities we began with? We live in societies that tolerate and even encourage some significant degree of inequality – as incentives, as justifiable desert, as an expression of diversity. Should we count as unfair or unjust health inequalities that result from other social inequalities that we think acceptable or justifiable?

In earlier work (Daniels *et al.*, 1999), I argued that Rawls's principles of justice as fairness quite unexpectedly capture what the social epidemiological literature picks out as the key social determinants of health – ranging from effective political participation rights to education and early childhood training to significant restrictions on income and wealth inequalities to supports for the social basis of self-esteem. Conformance with them would flatten socio-economic gradients of health more than any we see around us. Social justice, that is, fair terms of social cooperation developed in abstraction from thinking about health, is good for our aggregate health and leads to a more equitable distribution of it.

This conclusion is portrayed in the following argument:

1. To maximize population health requires making all people healthy. Making all people healthy achieves complete equity in health. (This is a conceptual point.)
2. There is no social justice without equity in health. (This is a widely held normative belief.)
3. There can be no equity in health without social justice. (This is an empirical and causal claim that depends on what we know about the social determinants of health, combined with the hypothesis that distributing them in accord with Rawlsian principles of justice flattens health inequalities [Daniels *et al.*, 1999]).

---

[6] Because these additional social factors so crucially affect population health and its distribution, the distinction that labels health as a natural rather than as a social good, as in Rawls (1971) or Nagel (1977), is less clear.

4. Therefore, achieving the best level of population health requires (causally) that we pursue social justice more broadly.[7]

If social justice is important to population health and its fair distribution, then the policies aimed at equity in health must be intersectoral in scope. All socially controllable factors that affect the distribution of health become the concern of those pursuing equity in health. In a striking way, this perspective challenges one version of the view that we should treat health as a separate 'sphere' – focusing on health benefits without thinking about the contributions health makes across spheres.

We live in a non-ideal world that does not comply with Rawlsian principles of justice. We face important questions left unanswered by ideal theory. Many health improving interventions we may undertake have the property that they increase the levels of health of all parts of the population even as they may increase health inequalities (Mechanic, 2002). For example, black infant mortality rates (IMRs) were 64% higher than whites in 1954 but were 130% higher in 1998, even though white rates dropped by 20.8 per 1000 and black IMR dropped by 30.1 per thousand. Mechanic (2002) concludes from this and other cases that it is reasonable to accept increasing health inequalities that result from policies that improve population health as long as the health of all groups is being improved.

Suppose, however, that we have two interventions (whatever sector, whatever novel technology) that both raise the health of all groups. If intervention A does less for those who are worse off than B but much more for those much better off, then both satisfy Mechanic's criterion. We may have strong views about whether to pursue A or B, depending on further facts about the magnitude of the effects or other facts about the sizes of the groups and thus the total impact of the programs. If society is responsible for causing the initial inequality through unfair policies, it may have special obligations to give more weight to equity than maximization and to considering the speed at which it rectifies the effects of past injustice.

The complexity of inequality itself

Policy choices about reducing health disparities are especially complex because they are at the interface of claims about injustice and standard distributive problems about which reasonable people disagree. Unfortunately, another source of complexity derives from what Temkin (1993) has identified as the complexity of inequality itself.

Temkin describes situations in which two or more groups of individuals differ in their levels of well-being. He then asks the normative, not descriptive, question, which has the worse inequality? Specifically, someone who is worse off has a complaint about the unfairness of the inequality. The strength of that complaint depends on whether we compare those who are worst off (1) with those who are best off, (2) with all those better off than they

---

[7] Suppose we flatten SES gradients of health as much as the principles of justice would seem to require us to but there remain socio-economic inequalities that induce some health inequalities. Are these residual health inequalities just? Or must we eliminate all social or economic inequalities that contribute to health inequalities? Some might interpret the priority Rawls gives to opportunity as requiring this response. Then, Rawls's theory becomes more egalitarian than was supposed. Alternatively, we might come to understand the mechanisms through which health inequalities are produced by other inequalities and intervene to reduce them without having to reduce otherwise justifiable inequalities. On another reading, Rawls's theory may not specifically answer this question about residual health inequalities (see Daniels et al., 1999).

are or (3) with the average to determine the magnitude of their complaint. To determine when one inequality is worse than another, we must not only assess the strength of each complaint, but we must aggregate those complaints within each situation. There are three approaches to aggregation: a maximin egalitarian view, an additive view, or a weighted additive view about how to sum up complaints. The nine combinations of these bases for judging inequalities better or worse yield divergent judgments about cases, including ones with multiple groups and ones involving welfare transfers among groups. All nine approaches, for example, prefer to make the worst off individual or group better before adding comparable benefits to any of the other individuals or (equal-sized) groups, but they differ on judgments about other cases.

Temkin argues that none of these nine combinations can be dismissed outright as inconsistent or otherwise completely implausible. Consequently, Temkin's egalitarian must accept the fact that reasonable people will often disagree about when one situation is worse with regard to inequality than another. Since egalitarians will give more weight to reducing worse inequalities than ones that are not as bad, they will have reasonable disagreements about which inequalities to give priority to reducing. This explanation for the disagreement in judgments about when one inequality is worse than another may underlie some disagreements about how much priority to give worst off individuals or groups.

Broadening the bioethics agenda

Bioethics is not the right field to find the relevant policy levers to reduce health inequalities. That is a task of social epidemiologists and other social scientists. But bioethics should provide guidance, in light of the complexity we have discussed, to the policy decisions that involve different ways of trading off equity against maximization. There are two key dimensions to that body of work.

First, there is purely normative work trying to find consensus on principles that might guide us in the range of cases posed by our policy options, including those that arise in developing and disseminating new technologies. These bioethics agenda items bear on this normative work:

1. Advance the existing ethical work on the unsolved distributive problems.
2. Clarify when a health inequality is unjust.
3. Explain how that injustice affects the unsolved distributive problems.
4. Clarify what counts as a reasonable rate of progress toward reducing health inequalities.
5. Test the implications of (1)–(4) in the context of actual policy choices about reducing health disparities, including those that involve the dissemination of new technologies.

Second, bioethics must consider what to do when we cannot achieve consensus on principles that can resolve the disagreements we encounter in agenda items (1)–(5). All these problems must be solved in ways that are perceived to be fair and legitimate in real time. Where we lack consensus on distributive principles, we must rely on procedural justice to give us fair and legitimate resolution to moral disagreements. In effect, procedural justice must supplement principled approaches to problems wherever the principles we can agree on are too indeterminate or coarse-grained to resolve disputes.

Sabin and I developed an approach we call 'accountability for reasonableness' and have used it to examine medical resource allocation in managed care contexts in the USA (Daniels and Sabin, 2002). The approach appeals to key elements of deliberative democratic theory to characterize the features of fair process in a range of decision-making contexts and institutions. I have used it, for example, to address issues of equity in scaling up antiretroviral treatments in high prevalence countries in the context of the WHO 3 by 5 programme (Daniels, 2005). It is also being used to improve the legitimacy of decision-making about coverage of treatments within the catastrophic insurance scheme of the Mexican Seguro Popular. It is cited as a framework for ethical deliberation about the implications of cost-effectiveness analysis in a recent IOM report on regulatory contexts (Miller *et al.*, 2006). Others are using it to improve decision making in publicly managed systems in Canada, Norway, Sweden, New Zealand and the UK (where NICE's Citizens' Council derives some support from our approach). Still, there are many problems developing appropriate versions of this approach at the various institutional levels where policy regarding health inequalities is made and implemented.

My expanded agenda calls for bioethics to:

6. Develop the general account of fair process so that reasonable people who disagree can view policies as fair and legitimate.
7. Apply the account to the various institutional contexts at which they must be addressed.

Equity between age groups and birth cohorts in the context of societal aging

Societal aging, especially in developing countries, will emerge as a major public health problem of the twenty-first century. Societal aging intersects with and complicates two under-analysed problems of intergenerational equity. Though I have earlier written about the problems of equity between age groups and equity between birth cohorts, I underestimated the difficulty of integrating solutions to these problems in the face of persistent societal aging.

Societal aging is greeted as a crisis in many recent book titles (which refer to an 'age quake', 'age wave' or 'generational storm' to note a few (Peterson, 1999; Wallace, 2001; Kotlikoff and Burns, 2004)), even though it is a result of the success, not the failure, of widely pursued health and family planning policies aimed at reducing mortality and fertility rates. It is accentuated when some birth cohort is much larger than the one following it – as with the American post-war baby boom or the Chinese cohort that enjoyed dropping mortality rates that preceded the 'one child' policy. Societal aging is a global phenomenon that has broad impacts on social structure and not just health.

In the USA, Kotlikiff and Burns (2004) observe that 'walkers replace strollers'. By 2030, nearly 20% of the US population will be 65 or over, whereas only 4% were in 1900. By 2040, the number of Americans over 80 (26.2 million) will exceed the number of pre-school children (25 million) (Peterson, 1999). European countries, including the UK, have already reached 'zero population growth'. In Italy, the fertility rate (1.2) is well below the level at which a population can reproduce itself (2.1), and the working age population is already shrinking (as it also is in Japan) (CSIS Commission on Global Aging, 2002). America's fertility rate of 2.1 helps insulate it from the more extreme aging Italy faces. The UN predicts that Italy will have a median age of 54 by 2050, second only to Spain. But Italy is not alone. All the European G7 countries are below the replacement level in fertility rates. By 2050, half of Continental Europe will be 49 or older, and well before that, by 2030, one of every two adults in developed countries will have reached retirement age.

The UN projects that the ratio of working-age adults to elderly in the developed world will drop from 4.5 : 1 today to 2.2 : 1 in 2050.

While the proportion of the elderly in developed countries is due to double over the next 50 years, from 15% to 27%, it is due to triple in East Asia, from 6% to 20%. By 2050, there will be 332 million Chinese aged 65 years or over, equivalent to the world's elderly population in 1990 (Jackson and Howe, 1999). The two billion people over age 60 who will live in our aging world by 2050 will mostly be living in developing countries.

This rapid societal aging in developing countries takes place without the wealth and the sophisticated economic institutions that exist in developed countries. As one commentator noted, China will grow old before it grows rich, unlike the developed countries. And China is not alone. The rate of increase in the number of older people between 1990 and 2025 is projected to be eight times higher in developing countries, such as Colombia, Malaysia, Kenya, Thailand and Ghana than it is in the UK and Sweden (International Center for Longevity, 2006). By 2050, the transitional economies of Eastern Europe will have populations with 28% elderly, and Latin America will have over 17%, well over the current US rate (CSIS Commission on Global Aging, 2002).

Two effects of societal aging

Societal aging dramatically changes the profile of needs in a country, creating new and intensified forms of competition between age groups for scarce resources. It also reduces society's ability to sustain measures for meeting those needs, sharpening competition between birth cohorts. Together these effects bring questions about intergenerational equity to the fore that may have not been noticed under different demographic conditions.

We all know, for example, that the rapid growth of those over 75 – Bernice Neugarten's (1982) 'old-old', those elderly who face especially increased disability and dependency – will bring with it increased burdens for the management of chronic disease and long-term care. Despite the presence in some developed countries of publicly funded long-term care, most such care is provided by family members, so the burden of societal aging will increasingly fall on adult working children, usually women. Yet, nearly one-quarter of all the elderly in the USA in 1989 had no children, and another 20% had only one child. With more women in the workforce, the problem of providing family care is intensified, since women have traditionally been the primary care givers. Pressures will increase to provide costly public programmes – at the same time that the working age population is shrinking.

In developing countries, the problem is not the sustainability of the kinds of publicly supported social and medical services provided for the elderly in developed countries, but the sustainability of informal, social structures of support, such as the traditional patterns of care that involve aged parents living with adult children, as in Japan and China. China, for example, must face the specific consequence of the success of its very strict population policy: one child for urban couples, two for rural ones. Like the USA, China will have many elderly with no children and even more elderly who have only one child to support them. The Chinese refer to this as the '1–2–4' problem, one child must care for two parents and four grandparents. In 1996, the Chinese government made it a legal requirement that adult children support their elderly parents, obviously anticipating that traditional filial obligations would be strained to the breaking point by the new demographic realities. The law is not going to solve the problem. Nor would such a law work in other developing countries in which rapid aging, extensive urbanization and industrialization, and a lack of existing health care and income support systems of the elderly collide with traditional family values.

The increase in medical needs and the shift in the profile of those needs with societal aging is much broader than the problem of long-term care for frail elderly people. With societal aging there are increases in the prevalence of cardiovascular disease, chronic pulmonary disease, diabetes, arthritis and cancer, as well as Alzheimer's disease and other dementias. The increased cost of treating the greater prevalence of these illnesses imposes great strains on resources and intensified competition for them in developed countries. The problem will be even worse in developing country health care systems that have barely begun to gear up to meet the needs posed by chronic diseases. In poorly funded systems, beefing up medical services for the chronic illnesses of middle and older age means diverting resources from primary care and preventive care for the whole population.

Age groups and birth cohorts: two distributive problems

Age groups and birth cohorts are easy to confuse, for the term 'generation' is ambiguous between them. But they are different. Birth cohorts age, but age groups do not. At any given moment, an age group consists of a birth cohort; over time, it consists of a succession of birth cohorts.

The age group problem raises these questions: how do we treat age groups fairly within distributive schemes, such as health care systems? What is a just allocation of resources to each stage of life, given that needs vary as we age? When is a distributive scheme age-biased in an unfair way? Is age itself a morally permissible criterion for limiting access to new technologies?

Medicare in the USA recently approved three very expensive technologies: left ventricular assist devices (LVAD) as 'destination therapy' for patients ineligible for heart transplants but suffering from advanced congestive heart failure; lung volume reduction surgery (LVRS) for select patient groups with chronic obstructive pulmonary disease; and implantable defibrillators (Gillick, 2004). Only the last one fell within any usual cost-effectiveness threshold. No consideration of opportunity costs entered the deliberation. Since Medicare is a system only for the elderly, unlike universal coverage systems in other countries, equity issues in allocation over the lifespan were impossible to raise. We could, for example, produce more health for both the young and the old were proper screening and treatment for high blood pressure implemented instead. The billions spent on these technologies are arguably better spent on other forms of care for the elderly themselves.

How should we think about health care resource allocation across age groups? The key to thinking about this age group problem is the observation that we all age, though we do not change race or sex (Daniels, 1988). Treating people differently at different ages, provided we do so systematically over the lifespan, creates no inequalities across persons. Treating people differently by race or class or gender creates inequalities that are always in need of justification. Indeed, treating ourselves differently at different stages of life can make our lives go better over all – we invest in our youth, at some sacrifice of immediate revenues and pleasures, in order to be rewarded more later in life. We take from ourselves in our working years in order to make our later, retired years go better.

Prudent allocation over the stages of life should be our guide to fair treatment among age groups (even if prudence is not a general guide to justice). This 'prudential lifespan account' must be properly qualified by assuming we already enjoy just distributions across persons and that we will live with the results over our whole lifespan (Daniels, 1988). Specifically, we should allocate health care so that it promotes the age-relative fair share of opportunities (or capabilities).

Rationing by age on this view is permissible under some scarcity conditions because it would not be imprudent to so allocate. This argument does not rely on specific, contested intuitions about the fairness of age rationing (as do Williams' [1997] claim that the old have had their fair innings or Frances Kamm's [1993] claim that the young need more years more than the old). It relies only on the general prudential allocation model I used. Since reasonable people disagree about the acceptability of this model and about specific issues, such as age rationing, we will need fair procedures of the sort I noted before to resolve disputes about priority setting among age groups. Properly used, a transfer scheme based on prudential allocation or on some other view of fair outcomes that emerges from fair process would solve the age group problem.

A solution to the age group problem must also be compatible with solutions to the birth cohort problem. Imagine that over time different birth cohorts pass through a scheme that solves the age group problem to our satisfaction. These cohorts are each treated fairly, I proposed two decades ago, if they have comparable 'benefit ratios' as they age through the schemes. New technologies that were not available for the elderly when they were young but will be available over the lifespan of those now young pose a special problem of inter-cohort equity.

This approach to the birth cohort problem can adjust for temporary demographic shifts, such as those produced by the US baby boom cohort. It is less clear how it can be modified to accommodate persistent population decline. That is the new challenge we find in global aging.

The bioethics agenda I am proposing must:

8. Address the distributive issues raised by the age group problem, including the impact of new technologies on resource allocation over the lifespan; assess the permissibility of rationing by age; consider age-bias in health systems, such as the inadequacy of long-term care in the USA and elsewhere, and age bias in our methodologies, such as cost effectiveness analysis; and consider fair process where reasonable people disagree about these issues.

9. Address how persistent societal aging affects the complex problem of treating cohorts equitably while at the same time not undermining proper solutions to the age group problem.[8]

International equity and health

Earlier, I suggested that health inequalities are unjust if they arise from an unjust distribution (as specified by Rawls's principles of justice as fairness) of the socially controllable factors that affect population health and its distribution. Judged from this ideal perspective, there are indeed many health inequities – by race and ethnicity, by class and caste, and by gender – around the world. Health inequity is pervasive globally.

This account is unfortunately silent about important questions of international justice. When are inequalities between different societies unjust? What do better off societies owe as a matter of justice (not charity), by way of improving the health of the population in less

---

[8] Privatization strategies do not solve the problem – they just represent one conclusion about what such equity requires and they do so without allowing us to use a scheme that addresses the age group problem at the same time. In addition, privatization is not even a starter for lifespan health systems they way it is for income support.

healthy societies? Suppose countries A and B each do the best they can to distribute the socially controllable factors affecting health fairly, and there are no glaring sub-group inequities. Nevertheless, health outcomes are unequal between A and B because A has many more resources to devote to population health than B. Is the resulting international inequality in health a matter of justice? Suppose B fails to protect its population health as best it can, leading again to population health worse than that of A. Is the resulting health inequality a matter of international justice?

Recasting the problem as an issue of a human right to health and health care does not improve the situation for two reasons. First, the obligation to secure a right to health for a population falls primarily on each state for its own population. Although international human rights agreements and proclamations also posit international obligations to assist other states in securing human rights, the international obligations cannot become primary in the human right to health and health care. External forces cannot assure population health across national boundaries in the way they might intervene to prevent violation of some other rights, even when they can afford assistance.

Second, even when a right to health is secured in different states, health inequalities between them may exist. Since conditions do not always permit everything to be done to secure a right in one country that may be feasible in another, the right to health and health care is viewed as 'progressively realizable'.[9] Reasonable people may disagree about how best to satisfy this right, given the trade-offs priority setting in health involves. Consequently some inequalities may fall within the range of reasonable efforts at 'progressive realizability'. In addition, because of their unequal resources, different states may achieve unequal health outcomes while still securing a right to health and health care for their populations. Appealing to human rights does not tell us if these inequalities are unjust and remains silent on what obligations better off states have to address these inequalities.

Though nearly all people recognize some international humanitarian obligations of individuals and states to assist those facing disease and premature death, wherever they are, there is substantial philosophical disagreement, even among egalitarian liberals, about whether there are also international obligations of justice to reduce these inequalities and to better protect the rights to health of those whose societies fail to protect them as much as they might. Nagel, who affirms these humanitarian obligations, argues that socio-economic justice, which presumably includes the just distribution of health, applies only when people stand in the specific relation to each other that is characterized by a state. Specifically, concerns about equality are raised within states by the dual nature of individuals both as coerced subjects and as agents in whose name coercive laws are made (Nagel, 2005). Rawls (1999) also did not include international obligations to assure a right to health on the list of human rights that liberal and decent societies have international obligations of justice to protect.

This 'statist' view encounters a strong counter-intuition. Life expectancy in Swaziland is half that in Japan (40 versus 80+ [WHO, n.d.]). A child unfortunate enough to be born in Angola has 73 times as great a chance of dying before age five as a child born in Norway

---

[9] The UN Commission on Human Rights (2003) 'Urges States to take steps, individually and through international assistance and cooperation, especially economic and technical, to the maximum of their available resources, with a view to achieving progressively the full realization of the right of everyone to the enjoyment of the highest attainable standard of physical and mental health by all appropriate means, including particularly the adoption of legislative measures.'

(UNICEF, 2000). A mother giving birth in southern sub-Saharan Africa has a 100 times as great a chance of dying from her labour as one birthing in an industrialized country (WHO, 2007). Many of us think there is something not just unfortunate and deserving of humanitarian assistance, but something unfair about the gross inequality.

Those who claim the gross health inequalities are unjust have quite different, incompatible ways of justifying that view. For example, those who believe that any disadvantage that people suffer through no fault or choice of their own is unjust would assert that the disadvantage facing the Angolan child is therefore unjust. The underlying principle of justice is applied to individuals wherever they are in the cosmos and regardless of what specific relationships they stand in to others – contrary to the Rawls–Nagel account, which applies principles of justice to the basic structure of a shared society. The disadvantage of the Angolan child might also be thought unjust by those who, like Rawls or Nagel, think principles of justice are 'relational' and apply only to a basic social structure that people share, but who, unlike Rawls or Nagel, believe we already live in a world in which international agencies and rule-making bodies constitute a robust global basic structure that is appropriately seen as the subject of international justice developed perhaps through a social contract involving representatives of relevant groups globally (Beitz, 2000). Fair terms of cooperation involving that structure would, some argue, reject arrangements that failed to make children in low income countries as well off as they could be. Clearly, there may be more agreement about some specific judgments of injustice than there is on the justification for those judgments or on broader theoretical issues.

I shall examine briefly two ways of trying to break the stalemate between statist and cosmopolitan perspectives. One approach aims for a minimalist (albeit cosmopolitan) strategy that focuses on an international obligation of justice to avoid 'harming' people by causing 'deficits' in the satisfaction of their human rights (Pogge, 2002, 2005a). It is a minimalist view in the sense that people may agree on negative duties not to harm even if they disagree about positive duties to aid. This approach handles some international health issues better than others. A more promising (relational justice) approach, which I can only briefly illustrate, requires that we work out a more intermediary conception of justice appropriate to evolving international institutions and rule-making bodies, leaving it open just how central issues of equality would be in such a context (Cohen and Sabel, 2006).

Harms to health: a minimalist strategy

If wealthy countries engage in a practice or policy – or impose an institutional order – that foreseeably makes the health of those in poorer countries worse than it would otherwise be, specifically, making it harder than it would otherwise be to realize a human right to health or health care, then, Pogge (2005a) argues, it is harming that population by creating this 'deficit' in human rights. Since this harm is defined relative to an internationally recognized standard of justice, the protection of human rights, Pogge argues that imposing the harm is unjust. Moreover, if there is a foreseeable alternative institutional order that would reasonably avoid the deficit in human rights, there is an international obligation of justice to produce the rights-promoting alternative.

There remains some unclarity about how the baseline against which harm is measured is specified. When is there a 'deficit' in a human right to health? Whenever a country fails to meet the levels of health provided, say, by Japan, which has the highest life expectancy? Or is there some other, unspecified standard? Consider two examples.

The brain drain of health personnel

The brain drain of health personnel from low-income to OECD countries may exemplify Pogge's concerns. The situation is dire. Over 60% of doctors trained in Ghana in the 1980s emigrated overseas (WHO, 2003). In 2002, in Ghana 47% of doctors posts were unfilled and 57% of registered nursing positions were unfilled. Some 7000 expatriate South African nurses work in OECD countries, while there are 32,000 nursing vacancies in the public sector in South Africa (Alkire and Chen Alkire, 2004). Whereas there are 188 physicians per 100,000 population in the USA, there are only 1 or 2 per 100,000 in large parts of Africa. The brain drain does not cause the whole of the inequality in health workers, but it significantly contributes to it.

International efforts to reduce poverty, lower mortality rates and treat HIV/AIDS patients – the Millennium Development Goals (MDG) agreed upon in 2000 – are all threatened by the loss of health personnel in sub-Saharan Africa. An editorial in the Bulletin of WHO points out that the MDG goals of reducing mortality rates for infants, mothers and children under five cannot be achieved without a million additional skilled health workers in the region (Chen and Hanvoravonchai, 2005). The global effort to scale up antiretroviral treatments poses a grave threat to fragile health systems, for its influx of funds – hardly a bad thing in itself – may drain skilled personnel away from primary care systems that already are greatly understaffed.

What about causes? There is both a 'push' from poor working conditions and opportunities in low-income countries and a 'pull' from more attractive conditions elsewhere. Is this simply 'the market' at work, backed by a 'right to migrate'?

Pogge's argument about an international institutional order has more specific grip than the vague appeal to a market. When economic conditions worsened in various developing countries in the 1980s, international lenders, such as the World Bank and International Monetary Fund (IMF) insisted that countries severely cut back publicly funded health systems as well as take other steps to reduce deficit spending. In Cameroon, for example, in the 1990s, their measures included a suspension of health worker recruitment, mandatory retirement at 50 or 55 years, suspension of promotions and reduction of benefits. The health sector budget shrank from 4.8% in 1993 to 2.4% in 1999, even while the private health sector grew (Liese et al., 2004). As a result, public sector health workers migrated to the private sector and others joined the international brain drain. The international institutional order increased the push.

The 'pull' attracting health workers to OECD countries is also not just diffuse economic demand. Targeted recruiting by developed countries is so intensive that it has stripped whole nursing classes away from some universities in the south. In 2000, the Labour government in the UK set a target of adding 20,000 nurses to the NHS by 2004. It achieved the goal by 2002. The UK absorbed 13,000 foreign nurses and 4000 doctors in 2002 alone. Recruitment from EU countries was flat (many of these countries also face shortages due to aging populations), but immigration from developing countries continued despite an effort to frame a policy of ethical recruitment (Deeming, 2004). Arguably, even if there were a diffuse economic 'pull', in the absence of active recruiting, the harm would be much less.

The remedy for this harm is not a prohibition on migration, which is protected by various human rights. The UK has recently announced a tougher code to restrict recruitment from 150 developing countries. In addition it has initiated a US$100m contribution to the Malawi health system aimed at creating better conditions for retaining health personnel there. The UK has thus taken two steps that are intended to reduce both the push and the pull behind the brain drain. Other countries have not followed suit.

International property rights and access to drugs

The minimalist strategy becomes harder to apply in a clear way to other international health issues. The problem of international property rights and the incentives they create goes beyond the issue of access to existing drugs, such as the antiretroviral cocktails that were the focus of attention in recent years. Big Pharma has long been criticized for a research and development bias against drugs needed in developing country markets. Indeed, it has responded to existing incentives by concentrating on 'blockbuster' drugs for wealthier markets, including many 'me too' drugs that marginally improve effectiveness or reduce side effects slightly. Funding the research needed to develop a vaccine against malaria, for example, has fallen to private foundations.

Do intellectual property rights and the incentive structures they support create a foreseeable deficit in the right to health that can be reasonably avoided? Pogge (2005b) argues that they do. Nevertheless, many drugs developed by Big Pharma under existing property right protections have filtered into widespread use as generics on 'essential drug' formularies in developing countries. Health outcomes in those countries are much better than they would be in the absence of such drugs. Since many of these drugs would not have been produced in the absence of some form of property right protections, people are not worse off than they would be in a completely free market with no temporary monopolies on products.

Arguably, however, different property right protections and different incentive schemes would make people in these poor countries with poor markets better off than they currently are. Which schemes ought we to select? Pogge (2005b) proposes that we revise incentives for drug development by establishing a tax-based fund in developed countries that would reward drug companies in proportion to the impact of their products on the global burden of disease. For example, drugs that meet needs in poor countries with very high burdens of disease would pay more, even if the drugs are disseminated at a cost close to the marginal cost of production. The tax, he admits, would be hard to establish, but it would be offset in rich countries by lower drug prices. The programme could be limited to 'essential drugs' leaving existing incentives in place for other drug products. Even so, the tax and thus the incentives could vary considerably, presumably with consequences of different magnitude for the global burden of disease. How do we pick which alternative to use as a baseline against which a 'deficit' in the right to health is specified? Pogge does not tell us.

Leaving aside the problem of vagueness, Pogge's proposal cannot be justified by appealing to the 'no harm' principle alone. The proposed incentive fund would better help to realize human rights to health, as Pogge argues, but 'not optimally helping' is not the same as 'harming' and so the justification has shifted. There may well be good reasons for an account of international justice to consider the interests of those affected by current property right protections more carefully than those agreements now do – but that takes us into more contested terrain than the minimalist strategy.

International harming is complex in several ways. The harms are often not deliberately imposed, and sometimes benefits were arguably intended. The harms are often mixed with benefits. In any case, great care must be taken to describe the baseline against which harm is measured. Such a complex story about motivations, intentions and effects might seem to weaken the straightforward appeal of the minimalist strategy, but the complexity does not undermine the view that we have obligations of justice to avoid harming health.

In any case, international harming is only one of three causes of international health inequalities. International health inequalities are also the result of (1) domestic failures to promote population health adequately or fairly and (2) differences across countries in levels of human and natural resources and in the natural conditions that contribute to the prevalence of disease (such as malaria). Thus the minimalist strategy fails to address many inequalities that some believe raise questions of international justice.

The new terrain of global justice: where the action is

Although I noted the strong pull of the cosmopolitan intuition about the unfairness of international health inequalities, there is also a strong intuition that obligations of justice arise only when people stand in certain specified relations to each other ('relational justice'). If we abandon the idea that such relations can arise only within states, we may find attractive the view argued for by Cohen and Sabel (2006). They sketch three types of international relationships that might give rise to obligations of justice going beyond humanitarian concerns, international agencies charged with distributing a specific good, cooperative schemes and some kinds of interdependency. Each may give rise to obligations of justice, such as concerns about inclusion. These may range from an obligation to give more weight to the interests of those who are worse off if it can be done at little cost to others, to obligations of equal concern, perhaps yielding far more egalitarian obligations. I shall illustrate each of these relationships and the obligations they give rise to with examples focused on key issues of global health.

WHO plausibly illustrates the idea that institutions charged with distributing a particular, important good, such as public health expertise and technology, must show equal concern in the distribution of that good. The organization would be charged with being unfair if it ignored the health of some and attended more to the health of others. For example, this point about showing equal concern arises in other debates about the methodologies WHO employs. We saw that CEA ignores issues of equity in the distribution of health and health care (Daniels and Sabin, 2002). These criticisms of CEA thus challenge the unconstrained use of CEA by the WHO whether it is using the methodology to determine health policy within a specific country or across countries. WHO is constrained by its mission of improving world health to consider equity in distribution in all contexts in which it works – within and across countries.

Concerns about equity show up in programmatic discussions as well. WHO paid attention to equity in the distribution of antiretroviral treatments (ARTs) for HIV/AIDS. I noted earlier WHO's sponsorship of a Commission on the Social Determinants of Health, with its focus on equity. Both these examples illustrate behavior compatible with and required by the institutional charge to WHO. Either this is a misguided focus of energy for WHO, as seems to be implied by Nagel's strong statist view, or it is an implication of the obligation to show equal concern that arises within institutions charged with delivering an important good – whether they operate within states or across them.

Consider now the international bodies that establish rules governing intellectual property rights, including those that are key to creating temporary monopolies over new drugs. Such a scheme is 'consequential' in that it increases the level of cooperation in production of an important collective good, research and development of drugs, and it does so in a way that has normatively relevant consequences (Cohen and Sabel, 2006). Suppose we conclude that this mutually cooperative scheme generates considerations of equal concern, or at least that it must be governed by a principle of inclusion. Then we might view quite favourably Pogge's suggestion about structuring drug development incentives so that they better addressed the global burden of disease. Earlier, I said Pogge's proposal could not be defended on the minimalist grounds that it avoided doing harm because of the problem of specifying the relevant human rights baseline. Now, however, we have a new basis on which to defend the justice of Pogge-style incentives. Such an incentive scheme, supplementing existing property rights or modifying them appropriately, would greatly enhance the benefits to those who are largely excluded from benefit for a significant period of time, and it would do so at only modest cost to those profiting from the endeavour. Minimally, it illustrates what a more inclusive policy should include; one can build into it even stronger egalitarian considerations, if the cooperative scheme gives rise to concerns about equality and not simply inclusion. Exactly what form the policy would take, or the justification for it deriving from the form of cooperative scheme involved, remains a task for further work. With these issues worked out, we might then support Pogge's incentive schemes as a way of moving some countries closer to satisfaction of a right to health, connecting the effort to human rights goals as he does.

Consider again the example of the brain drain of health personnel from low- and middle-income countries to wealthier ones. Nagel (2005: 130) notes that nations generally have 'immunity from the need to justify to outsiders the limits on access to its territory', though this immunity is not absolute, since the human rights of asylum seekers act as a constraint. Still, the decisions different countries make about training of health personnel and about access to their territories have great mutual impact on them. There is an important interdependency affecting their well-being, specifically, the health of the populations contributing and receiving health personnel. The British decision in 2000 to recruit 30,000 new nurses from developing countries rather than try to train more greatly affected the fate of people being served by health systems in southern Africa. The under-funding of salaries for African nurses and doctors, in part a legacy of Structural Reform Programs imposed by the IMF and World Bank, but clearly continued by local governments, helps create the 'push' factor driving these workers abroad. Arguably, this relation of interdependence brings into play obligations of inclusion, perhaps those of equal concern, going beyond in any event humanitarian considerations. In addition to Pogge's 'no harm' or minimalist approach, we thus have available obligations of inclusion requiring us to consider the interests of all those in the interdependent relationship. These obligations can be translated into various policy options that address the brain drain: it may be necessary to restrict the terms of employment in receiving countries of health workers from vulnerable countries; it may be necessary to seek compensation for lost training costs of these workers; it may be important to contribute aid to contributing countries aimed at reducing the push factors; it may be necessary to prohibit active recruitment from vulnerable countries.

We might combine these relationships of interdependence with the relationships and obligations that arise from cooperative schemes. The International Organization for Migration, established in 1951 to help resettle displaced persons from the Second World War, now has 112 member states and 23 observer states. It 'manages' various aspects of migration, providing information and technical advice, and arguably goes beyond its initial humanitarian mission. Suppose it took on the task of developing a policy that helped to coordinate or manage the frightening health personnel brain drain. Minimally, it might seek internationally acceptable standards for managing the flow – standards on recruitment, on compensation, on terms of work. More ambitiously, it might seek actual treaties that balanced rights to migrate with costs to the contributing countries, countering at least some of the pull factors and even providing funds that might alleviate some of the push factors underlying the brain drain. In seeking these, it might work together with the International Labour Organization (ILO), with the World Trade Organization (WTO), with WHO and with the United Nations (UN). Such a cooperative endeavor would reflect the common interest in all countries of having adequate health personnel – and thus being able to assure citizens a right to health and health care – as well as the common interest in protecting human rights to dignified migration.

The fuller development of a plausible account of justice in these intermediary institutions is a task for the expanded bioethics agenda I have been charting:

10. Assess the implications of the obligation not to harm for reducing health inequalities internationally.
11. Develop an account of justice for the evolving international institutions and rule-making bodies that have an impact on international health inequalities.
12. Examine Promethean challenges from the perspective of their impact on international health inequalities and obligations of justice regarding them.

Preparing the field

The broader bioethics agenda I have described poses two distinct and significant challenges to the field. The first challenge is one of training. Many of the problems take us outside the more familiar domain of ethics and the clinical practice of medicine into the far less familiar terrain of political philosophy and a wide range of social sciences. The relevant philosophical literature is less familiar to many in the field and it would have to be mastered by both those who teach bioethics and those who engage in it. Some training programs in bioethics already include some of this material, but many would have to expand their focus.

The second challenge is political. An implication of my earlier argument is that social justice is good for population health and is essential to its fair distribution. But engaging in the pursuit of social justice and not simply justice in health care can be divisive in a novel way. Many people already agree that we have social obligations to give people equal access to an appropriate array of health care interventions. Perhaps this is because they see the threat of disease and disability as a part of the struggle of humans against nature. In that battle, we are united in our vulnerability. We hope that technology will rescue all of us. The Promethean battle of humans against nature – and our own human weaknesses – is in a certain sense unifying.

Many fewer people, however, understand the broad ways in which the distribution of other goods affect health inequalities, let alone agree about how to distribute those goods. Indeed, this is a context in which we cannot all easily unite against nature. Rather, there are divisions of interest and perspective among all of us, including across nations. Shifting a bioethics agenda to address the causes of health inequality can thus be politically divisive, both domestically and internationally.

Acknowledgements

This article is reprinted (with permission) from the *Hastings Center Report* (Daniels, 2006). It was originally adapted from a lecture delivered to the Nuffield Council of Bioethics (May 2005). I also draw on material from my book, *Just Health: Meeting Health Needs Fairly* (2008).

References

Alkire, S. and Chen Akire, L. (2004) Medical exceptionalism in international migration: should doctors and nurses be treated differently? *JLI Working Paper*, **7–3**: 1–10.

Beitz, C. (2000) Rawls' law of peoples. *Ethics*, **110**(4): 669–96.

Boorse, C. (1975) On the distinction between disease and illness. *Philosophy and Public Affairs*, **5**(1): 49–68.

Boorse, C. (1997) A rebuttal on health. In *What Is Disease?*, ed. J. M. Humber and R. F. Almeder. Totowa, NJ: Humana Press, pp. 1–134.

Braveman, P., Starfield, B. and Geiger, H. J. (2002) World Health Report 2000: how it removes equity from the agenda for public health monitoring and policy. *British Medical Journal*, **323**: 678–81.

Brock, D. (1988) Ethical issues in recipient selection for organ transplantation. In *Organ Substitution Technology: Ethical, Legal and Public Policy Issues*, ed. D. Matthieu. Boulder, CO: Westview Press, pp. 86–99.

CSIS Commission on Global Aging (2002) *Meeting the Challenge of Global Aging*. Washington, DC: Center for Strategic and International Studies. Available at: http://www.csis.org/gai (accessed: 27/8/05).

Chen, L. and Hanvoravonchai, P. (2005) HIV/AIDS and human resources. *Bulletin of the World Health Organization*, **83**: 143–4.

Cohen, J. and Sabel, C. (2006) Extra rempublicam nulla justitia. *Philosophy and Public Affairs*, **34**(2): 147–75.

Daniels, N. (1988) *Am I my Parents' Keeper? An Essay on Justice Between the Young and the Old*. New York: Oxford University Press.

Daniels, N. (1993) Rationing fairly: programmatic considerations. *Bioethics*, **1**: 255–71.

Daniels, N. (1994) Four unsolved rationing problems. *Hastings Center Report*, **24**(4): 27–9.

Daniels, N. (2005) Fair process in patient selection for antiretroviral treatment for HIV/AIDS in WHO's 3 by 5 program. *The Lancet*, **366**: 169–71.

Daniels, N. (2006) Equity and population health: toward a broader bioethics agenda. *Hastings Center Report*, **36**(4): 22–35.

Daniels, N. (2008) *Just Health: Meeting Health Needs Fairly*. Cambridge: Cambridge University Press.

Daniels, N., Kennedy, B. and Kawachi, I. (1999) Why justice is good for your health: Social determinants of health inequalities. *Daedalus*, **128**(4): 215–51.

Daniels, N., Kennedy, B. and Kawachi, I. (2000) *Is Inequality Bad for Our Health?* Boston, MA: Beacon Press.

Daniels, N. and Sabin, J. E. (2002) *Setting Limits Fairly: Can We Learn to Share Medical Resources?* New York: OUP.

Deeming, C. (2004) Policy targets and ethical tensions: UK nurse recruitment. *Social Policy and Administration*, **38**(7): 227–92.

Gakidou, E. E., Murray, C. J. L. and Frenk, J. (2000) Defining and measuring health inequality. *Bulletin of the World Health Organization*, **78**: 42–54.

Gillick, M. (2004) Medicare coverage for technological innovations – time for new criteria? *New England Journal of Medicine*, **350**(21): 2199–203.

Gwatkin, D. R. (2002) *Who Would Gain Most from Efforts to Reach the Millennium Development Goals for Health? An Inquiry into the Possibility of Progress that Fails to Reach the Poor. Health, Nutrition and Population Discussion paper*. Washington, DC: World Bank. Available at: http://poverty.worldbank.org/files/13920-gwatkin1202.pdf (accessed: 27/8/05).

International Centre for Longevity (2006) *Aging on the World Stage*. New York: ICL.

Jackson, R. and Howe, N. (1999) *Global Aging: The Challenge of The New Millennium.* Washington, DC: CSIS/Watson Wyatt Worldwide. Available at: http://www.csis.org/gai (accessed: 27/8/05).

Kamm, F. (1987) The choice between people, commonsense morality, and doctors. *Bioethics*, 1: 255–71.

Kamm, F. (1993) *Morality, Mortality, Volume I: Death and Whom to Save from It.* Oxford: Oxford University Press.

Kotlikoff, L. J. and Burns, S. (2004) *The Coming Generational Storm.* Cambridge, MA: MIT Press.

Liese, B., Blanchet, N. and Dussault, G. (2004) *The Human Resource Crisis in Health Services in Sub-Saharan Africa. Background Paper: World Development Report 2004.* Washington DC: The World Bank.

Marmot, M. and Wilkinson, R. G. (1999) *Social Determinants of Health.* Oxford: Oxford University Press.

Mechanic, D. (2002) Disadvantage, inequality, and social policy. *Health Affairs*, 21(2): 48–59.

Miller, W., Robinson, L. S. and Lawrence, R. S. (eds) (2006) *Valuing Health for Regulatory Cost-Effectiveness Analysis.* Washington, DC: National Academies Press.

Nagel, T. (1997) Justice and nature. *Oxford Journal of Legal Studies*, 17(2): 303–21.

Nagel, T. (2005) The problem of global justice. *Philosophy and Public Affairs*, 33(2): 113–47.

Neugarten, B. L. (1982) *Age or Need? Public Policies for Older People.* Beverley Hills, CA: SAGE.

Parfit, D. (1995) Equality or priority? Lindley Lecture at the University of Kansas.

Peterson, P. (1999) *Gray Dawn: How The Coming Age Wave Will Transform America – And The World.* New York: Three Rivers Press.

Pogge, T. (2002) *World Poverty and Human Rights: Cosmopolitan Responsibilities and Reforms.* Cambridge: Polity Press.

Pogge, T. (2005a) Severe poverty as a violation of negative duties. *Ethics and International Affairs*, 19(1): 55–83.

Pogge, T. (2005b) Human right and global health: a research program. *Metaphilosophy*, 36: 889–909.

Rawls, J. (1971) *A Theory of Justice.* Cambridge, MA: Harvard University Press.

Rawls, J. (1999) *The Law of Peoples.* Cambridge, MA: Harvard University Press.

Temkin, L. (1993) *Inequality.* New York: Oxford University Press.

UN Commission on Human Rights (2003) *Resolution 2003/28: The Right of Everyone to the Enjoyment of the Highest Attainable Standard of Physical and Mental Health.* Geneva: UNHR.

UNICEF (2000) *The State of the World's Children. Under-Five Mortality Rankings.* Copenhagen: UNICEF. Available at: http://www.unicef.org/sowc00/stat2.htm (accessed: 12/8/05).

Wakefield, J. C. (1992) The concept of mental disorder. On the boundary between biological facts and social values. *American Psychologist*, 47: 373–88.

Wallace, P. (2001) *Agequake: Riding the Demographic Rollercoaster Shaking Business, Finance and Our World.* London: Nicolas Brealey.

Williams, A. (1997) Intergenerational equity: an exploration of the fair innings argument. *Health Economics*, 6: 117–32.

World Health Organization (n.d.) *WHO Mortality Database: Tables.* Available at: http://www.who.int/healthinfo/morttables/en/index.html (accessed 23/8/07).

World Health Organization (1946) Preamble to Constitution of WHO, adopted by International Health Conference, NY 19–22 June 1946; entered into force 7 April 1948, never amended.

World Health Organization (2003) *International Migration, Health & Human Rights.* Geneva: WHO.

World Health Organization (2007) *Maternal Mortality in 2005: Estimates Developed by WHO, UNICEF, UNFPA, and the World Bank.* Geneva: WHO.

| Chapter | # Health inequities |

12

James Wilson

Introduction

The infant mortality rate (IMR) in Liberia is 50 times higher than it is in Sweden, while a child born in Japan has a life expectancy at birth of more than double that of one born in Zambia (Central Intelligence Agency, 2007).[1] And within countries, we see differences that are nearly as great. For example, if you were in the USA and travelled the short journey from the poorer parts of Washington to Montgomery County Maryland, you would find that 'for each mile travelled life expectancy rises about a year and a half. There is a twenty-year gap between poor blacks at one end of the journey and rich whites at the other' (Marmot, 2004: 2).

There are two types of questions that it is important to ask about inequalities in health such as these. The first are social scientific questions about the extent of inequalities in health and the factors which are causally responsible for these inequalities. Examples of social scientific questions to ask might be: how do infant mortality rates in the UK differ according to social class? What is the difference in life expectancy between Japanese who emigrate to the USA and those who remain in Japan? Why do civil servants in higher ranked jobs tend to live longer than civil servants in lower ranked jobs?

The second type are normative questions about the reasons we have to care about inequalities in health. Important normative questions to answer are: which inequalities in health should we care about (all inequalities or merely some of them)? When is an inequality in health unjust? How should we weigh our concern for equality in health against other factors such as maximizing the health achievement of community?

This chapter focuses on these normative questions. But I shall first briefly outline some of the main findings of the social sciences literature in order to put the normative questions in the right perspective. Much of the relevant literature has focused on the relationship between socio-economic status (SES) and health achievement, and I shall follow this lead in my summary.

The gradient in health

There is evidence of a socio-economic gradient in health in all countries for which statistics are available. In other words, as a person's SES increases, so her life expectancy

---

[1] The infant mortality rate in Liberia is 149.73 per 1,000; in Sweden it is 2.76. The life expectancy at birth in Japan is 82; in Zambia it is 38.4 (Central Intelligence Agency, 2007).

Public Health Ethics, ed. Angus Dawson. Published by Cambridge University Press. © Cambridge University Press 2011.

improves and so also do a range of other important health indicators.[2] The gradient is by no means confined to groups who suffer absolute deprivation. It also occurs within groups who are in absolute terms, fairly well off. For example the famous Whitehall studies showed a gradient in health among civil servants, all of whom were, in absolute terms, comfortably off (Marmot *et al.*, 1978). So it is not just that 'the poor', as a group have worse health, but also that, as we go up the social scale, each rung we ascend will increase life expectancy, and decrease the chance of developing many diseases, such as stroke or heart disease.[3]

The socio-economic gradient in health is less steep in some countries than in others (and also changes in severity in the same countries over time), which suggests that there must be social factors that can either flatten gradients or make them more vertiginous. And if the socio-economic gradient in health has social causes, then it seems plausible to think that it will be in our power to flatten it if we want to.

Does low socio-economic status cause ill health?

The correlation between low SES and ill health is robust. However, correlation is not causation. It does not follow logically from the fact that people with low SES tend to have worse health and lower life expectancies that having a low SES *causes* ill health. For all that we have so far seen, it might be ill health that causes low SES, or it might be that there is some further factor that causes *both* low SES *and* ill health, while neither low SES nor ill health cause one another.

Many people think that the direction of causation of health inequalities is important, because they think that it is morally worse if an inequality in SES causes an inequality in health, than if an inequality in health causes an inequality in SES. As Daniels *et al.* (2004: 63) put it, 'Many who are untroubled by some kinds of inequality are particularly troubled by health inequalities. They believe that a socio-economic inequality that otherwise seems just becomes unjust if it contributes to heath inequalities.' Because of this, much of the social sciences literature on health inequalities has been devoted to establishing that it is low SES which is responsible for poor health, rather than vice versa.

No one disputes that *some* of the correlation between SES and health is caused by the effects of ill health. For example, it is very plausible to think that, as a group, people

---

[2] The term SES is usually used to refer to 'the relative position of a family or individual on a hierarchical social structure, based on their access to or control over wealth, prestige and power' (Mueller and Parcel, 1981). However, when defined in this way SES is difficult to measure accurately and so studies tend to use something easier to measure as a proxy for SES. Popular candidates for proxy measures include level of education, current income, overall wealth, type of occupation or some combination of these measures (Shaver, 2007). Each of these measures has their advantages and disadvantages, and clearly the fact that different studies use different measures creates a degree of difficulty in comparing the results of different studies examining the relationship between SES and health (Braveman *et al.*, 2005). However the finding that there is a correlation between SES and health is sufficiently robust that it holds whichever way we measure SES, so I shall set this problem of measurement aside here.

[3] There are some (very few) conditions, such as breast cancer in European countries, which show a reverse socio-economic gradient. (A possible explanation for the reverse economic gradient in breast cancer is that having children later increases risk of breast cancer, and women with a higher SES tend to have children later. See Strand *et al.*, 2007.)

who are unable to work because of chronic illness will tend to have a lower income than people who are able to work. The interesting question is whether *all* (or even most) of the socio-economic gradient in health can be explained in this way. And in fact the evidence shows that the effects of this 'health selection' are fairly small in comparison to the overall size of the socio-economic gradient.[4]

Of course, there are other factors which might explain the correlation. One obvious factor could be that it is inequalities in access to health care which explain the social gradient in health. However, this does not seem to be a very significant cause of variation in health, given that we see a significant social gradient in health even in countries such as the UK, which have a nationalized health system. Another factor could be intelligence: it might be the case that more intelligent people will tend to do better in their jobs, and also will tend to take more health preserving behaviours than less intelligent people, so that intelligence will tend to influence both SES and health. Ultimately, though the question remains whether we can plausibly account for *all* the correlation of health and SES without allowing that low SES causes a significant proportion of the variation in health. And it seems that we cannot.

In addition, we have a number of possible models which seek to explain *how* low SES could cause ill health, by explaining how the social factors associated with lower SES could have a bad effect on health. Marmot (2004) hypothesizes that people of a lower SES tend to have less control over their working and living environments, and that this sense of lack of control leads to stress responses, which predictably cause conditions such as atherosclerosis and obesity. Wilkinson (1996) argues that it is income inequality that is the key factor which affects the size of the socio-economic gradient, and that other things being equal, the health of *all* members of society tends to be worse in an unequal society. This suggests that goods such as social capital and social cohesion play a role in governing health states – presumably ultimately via similar causal pathways to those hypothesized by Marmot.

There is very much more that could be said about the social sciences literature, in particular on the question of how low SES causes ill health. However, our focus is on the normative questions that arise about health inequalities, and as we shall see below, there is good reason to think that these questions of causation are only of tangential relevance to the fundamental normative question of which inequalities in health are unjust.

From social science to political philosophy

Until fairly recently, there was little interaction between social scientists working on the extent and causes of health inequalities and political philosophers seeking to answer normative questions about which inequalities are unjust. One reason for this was a failure (by both sides) to see how materials produced by the other could be relevant to the questions that they were asking. For instance, it is notable that Rawls, the most influential political philosopher of the second part of the twentieth century, scarcely addresses health at

---

[4] For example, Chandola *et al.* (2003) argue that in the Whitehall study, the data show that the effect of social position on health was over two and a half times greater than the effect of health on social position. Clearly the size of the causal effect of health on SES will vary from country to country and from situation to situation, depending on the level of support a society provides for those unable to work through illness. But nowhere is it plausible to attribute *all* the socio-economic gradient in health to health selection.

all, and where he does, questions of inequalities in health do not even enter onto his radar.[5] Meanwhile, Marmot (2004), who has done more than anyone to raise and to answer the social scientific questions, reports that it was only fairly recently that he realized that the normative implications of his work on inequality in health had already been separately explored at length by political philosophers.[6]

However, recent times have seen a change. Workers within empirical fields are becoming increasingly aware of the role that ethical thinking and particularly political philosophy can play, while political philosophers have become increasingly aware of the relevance of the social scientific literature. One of the major aims of this chapter is help to strengthen this dialogue.

The concept of a health inequity

Before going any further, we must make an important distinction between health *inequalities* and health *inequities*. I shall take health inequalities to be 'the generic term used to designate differences, variations, and disparities in the health achievements of individuals and groups' (Kawachi *et al.* 2002: 647), while I shall take health inequities to be those health inequalities that are, all things considered, unjust.

We need to make this distinction because it is plausible to think that there are at least some inequalities in health that are not unjust. And where an inequality is not unjust, it would be wrong to think that we have a duty to alleviate it or eliminate it.[7] To give an example, a recent study of 1000 major European and North American pop stars 1956–2005 revealed that they 'experience significantly higher mortality (more than 1.7 times) than demographically matched populations in the USA and UK' (Bellis *et al.*, 2007: 896), thus showing a significant health inequality between pop stars and the ordinary members of the public. But I think that few would feel that the researchers had thereby uncovered an inequity that the European and US governments should be in a hurry to address, given that pop stars' decreased life expectancy seems to be due in large part to their choices to adopt high-risk behaviours.

When dealing with concepts such as that of a health inequity, which imply a normative judgement about those things that fall under them, it is often useful to begin by clarifying the role that we think the concept should play before going on to specify which things should fall under the concept. For it is usually much easier to get a consensus on the role

---

[5] There is one passage which is particularly telling, where Rawls allows that health is equally as important a good as the primary goods which his theory of justice picks out to be distributed fairly. However he denies that we should treat health as one of the primary goods, on the grounds (1) that it is 'natural' rather than a social good (meaning that it is much less closely affected by changes in the basic structure of society than are the genuine primary goods such as rights, liberties and opportunities, income and wealth, and the social bases of self-respect), and (2) his theory of justice concerns only the justice of the basic structure of society (1971: 62). While this was a reasonable view of health to hold in 1971, the mass of literature produced on the social determinants of health over the past thirty years has clearly demonstrated that (1) is false. Rawls seems never to have revised his views to take account of the social determinants of health.

[6] As he (2004: 38) puts it, 'I read for the first time [in 1998], Amartya Sen's writings on Inequality . . . I felt like the man who had discovered he had been talking prose. I was intrigued to discover that some of the conclusions towards which my colleagues and I had been struggling towards on the basis of our evidence, were elegantly laid out there.'

[7] Of course, it would not necessarily be wrong to alleviate or eliminate it. My point is simply that we would not be *obliged* to do so.

that a normative concept should play than to get a consensus on what things should fall under that concept, and once we have this consensus it is easier to understand and to adjudicate the disputes that will then inevitably arise about which things should fall under the concept. So the rest of this section aims to clarify the role that the *concept* of a health inequity should play.

I shall briefly examine the two most influential definitions of a health inequity, the first by Whitehead Dahlgren (1992, 2006; Whitehead, 1990), and the second by Kawachi *et al.* (2002). I shall argue that neither is adequate, and will suggest a more precise definition.

In a widely cited article, Whitehead (1990: 5) defines health inequities as differences in health which are 'unnecessary and avoidable but, in addition are also considered unfair and unjust'.[8] Whitehead does not provide much by way of an explanation as to why the differences should have to be 'unnecessary and avoidable' as well as unjust, and it seems to me that these additional qualifications are unhelpful. For if we already thought that a given health inequality was unjust, we would usually be taken to be already making the claim that it amounted to a health inequity. So I do not think that being also told that the inequality was 'unnecessary and avoidable' would add anything. Conversely, if we did not know whether a difference in health was inequitable, discovering that the difference was unnecessary and avoidable would not provide a reason in and of itself to think that the difference in question was inequitable. For instance, when competent adults undertake dangerous sports such as mountaineering, they knowingly increase their risk of death and injury. This increased risk creates a health inequality between mountaineers and non-mountaineers which is unnecessary and avoidable, but not unjust (and hence not inequitable) (Kawachi *et al.* 2002: 648). So at the very least, adding the claims that the differences have to be 'unnecessary and avoidable' *adds* nothing to the definition of health inequity.

However, things are worse than this. The assumption that health inequities by definition are 'unnecessary and avoidable' has led Whitehead and Dahlgren and those who have followed them to make some very implausible claims about what kinds of things could and could not count as health inequities. Whitehead and Dahlgren's (2006: 2) underlying thought seems to be that it is only where 'social processes . . . produce health differences rather than these being determined biologically', that it makes sense to say that there is a health inequity, and that hence only inequalities which are caused by *social* as opposed to *natural* factors are even candidate health inequities. Their argument for this claim seems to be as follows:

> Human beings vary in health as they do in every other attribute. We will never be able to achieve a situation where everyone in the population has the same type and degree of illness and dies after exactly the same life span. This is not an achievable goal, nor even a desirable one. Thus, that portion of the health differential attributable to natural biological variation can be considered inevitable rather than inequitable.
>
> (Whitehead, 1990: 6–7)

The thought seems to be that inequalities which are due to human activity are avoidable *because* they are caused by human action, whereas inequalities caused by nature are not

---

[8] It is unclear why there is a reference to differences which are *both* unfair *and* unjust, given that she does not make any distinction between these two terms, which are in any case close to synonymous in ordinary usage. I shall assume that we should delete unfair, and simply leave ourselves with the idea of *unjust* differences.

caused by human action and so we are powerless to do anything about them. There are two mistakes contained in this: first, it does not follow that just because something has a social cause that we will be able to successfully stop it by social intervention. (It is by no means clear that we will be able to stop climate change, for instance.) Second, it does not follow from the fact that something is caused by 'nature' either that we are powerless to stop it, or that we should refrain from trying to stop it. (Presumably all of medicine could legitimately count as trying to stave off what would otherwise be the inevitable operation of nature, as John Stuart Mill [1874] points out.)

Moreover the conclusion does not follow from the premises. For, even if it would be unjust and undesirable to attempt to equalize health achievement across a society, it would not follow that people who are born with worse health have *no* claim to some form of rectification on grounds of justice. For example, we may not be in a position to give someone who is blind sight, and clearly it would be undesirable to blind the rest of the population to restore equality. But there are other things we can do, such as ensuring that buildings are arranged for easy navigation by blind people, or ensuring that all official documents are available in braille, which many people take to be required by justice. Hence the fact that we cannot alleviate blindness does not mean that we have to say that it is merely down to 'nature', and that the disadvantage to the blind person should be considered inevitable rather than inequitable.

Further, much of the mainstream philosophical writing on justice over the last 30 years has taken it as axiomatic that undeserved disadvantages due to bad luck (such as being born blind, or without the use of one's legs, or having a very low life expectancy) *do* raise issues of justice, and that undeserved disadvantages of this kind give the affected individuals claim for rectification under egalitarian justice. This position has now come to be known as 'luck egalitarianism'. See for example, Dworkin (1981a, 1981b), Arneson (1989) and Cohen (1989). For critiques of this position, see Anderson (1999) and Scheffler (2003).

This means that Whitehead and Dahlgren must either allow that health inequities account for only some of the inequalities in health achievement which a just society should be concerned about, or they must be committed to the claim that luck egalitarianism's central claim is false, and that in fact it is only inequalities with a social cause which are of concern for egalitarian justice. Both of these options seem inappropriate for an account of the *concept* of a health inequity. Absent any account of why we should treat unjust inequalities with social causes differently from unjust inequalities with natural causes, it looks arbitrary to suggest that we should address them separately. And it would seem to be a mistake to build a controversial claim about the nature of egalitarian justice into our concept of a health inequity. While such controversial positions might be true, they need to be argued for as the *best* accounts of health inequity, rather than simply presupposed as following from the very concept of a health inequity.

Where does this leave us? I take it that the only part of Whitehead and Dahlgren's original definition of a health inequity still standing is the idea of an *unjust* inequality. This idea forms the kernel of the second major definition of health inequity in the literature, namely that 'Health inequity refers to those inequalities in health that are deemed to be unfair or stemming from some form of injustice' (Kawachi *et al.*, 2002: 647). This is, I shall suggest, much better, but still in need of a little more refinement.

Kawachi *et al.*'s definition suggests that health inequalities which *stem from* injustice should count as health inequities. However, it is unclear why we should accept this. For not every inequality which stems from an injustice is itself unjust. Some inequalities which stem from injustices will be trivial and morally insignificant, while other inequalities might even benefit those who have been unjustly treated. (For instance, a society which allowed men, but not women, to smoke would treat women unjustly. However, the health inequalities in women's favour to which this would no doubt lead would not rightly be considered to be health inequities.)

So it seems too strong to suggest, as Kawachi *et al.* seem to, that *all* inequalities which stem from injustice are themselves inequitable. Rather, it is only when an inequality which stems from injustice adversely affects something that we already think we have reason to care about from the perspective of justice, that we think it is unjust. Hence inequalities in health that stem from injustice will count as health inequities only if we already have a reason to think that inequalities in health are something that we ought to care about from the perspective of justice. And we ought to care about inequalities in health from the perspective of justice only if such inequalities are either unjust in themselves or contribute to states of affairs which are unjust in themselves. So if we build into our definition of a health inequity the claim that inequalities in health which stem from injustice are inequitable, we risk begging the question.

It follows, I take it, that a concern with health equity is purely and simply a concern for justice in the distribution of health achievement. So a health inequality is a health inequity if and only if it is an inequality which a just society would seek to counteract. The key question then is *which* health inequalities are unjust?

Two dimensions of egalitarian justice

I shall assume that the correct account of justice is in some broad sense egalitarian, and that a just society should seek to treat all its citizens as equals.[9] There is a dispute in egalitarian justice as to the appropriate scope of obligations of justice: cosmopolitans such as Pogge (2008) argue that obligations of justice are global, while others such as Rawls (1999) and Nagel (2005) argue that obligations of socio-economic justice fundamentally apply only within societies. We shall not enter into this dispute here, but I should point out that the outcome of this debate will have a major impact on which types of health inequalities could count as inequities. For if there are no strict obligations of global socio-economic justice, then health inequalities between nations will not count as health inequities.

There are two axes along which theories of justice vary. First, there is the 'what' dimension: *what* good or goods need to be distributed fairly to each in order to ensure

---

[9] Egalitarianism in this broad sense has come to be central to the way we think about justice. Whereas in former times the idea that some form of *inegalitarianism* – that for example, took men to be worth more than women, white more than black citizens, or rich more than poor was expressed and even defended, the thought that a just society ought to treat all its citizens as equals enjoys overwhelming support today. In Sen's (2004: 22) words, 'a theory of justice in the contemporary world would not have any serious plausibility if it did not value equality in some space – a space that would be seen as important in that theory'. This is not to say that in the world as we encounter it women are *in fact* treated as equals to men; and the poor are *in fact* treated as equals to the rich, but rather that where such things occur they are widely recognized to be unjust. Defending this intuition of fundamental human equality is beyond the scope of this chapter. (I go some way towards defending it in Wilson [2007a, 2007b]). For the best current overview and defence of the idea of fundamental human equality, see Waldron (2000).

that a society is just? Second, there is the 'how' dimension: *how* should we distribute those goods which are the appropriate concern of egalitarian justice? (Hurley, 2007).

Cohen (1989: 906) famously labelled the 'what' question the question of the currency of egalitarian justice: '[w]hat aspects of a person's condition should count in a *fundamental* way for egalitarians, and not merely as a cause of or proxy for what we regard as fundamental?' For instance, a crude egalitarian might take financial wealth to be the only currency of egalitarian justice, while more sophisticated egalitarians argue that the relevant currency is opportunity for welfare, or access to advantage.[10] The key normative question for us is whether *health* matters in a fundamental way for egalitarian justice. If it does not, then talk of *health* inequities risks being needlessly imprecise and potentially misleading, given that the relevant inequity will not lie in the maldistribution of health, but rather in the maldistribution of another, more fundamental good. I take up the question of health and egalitarian justice in the following section.

The key question posed by the 'how' question is how we should seek to distribute those goods which *are* of fundamental concern for egalitarian justice. There are three main approaches within the broadly egalitarian framework. *Strict egalitarians* take it that our goal (insofar as we are concerned with egalitarian justice) should be to *equalize* the amount of those goods that are of fundamental importance to justice which each person receives. Importantly, strict egalitarians believe that it can be legitimate to 'level down' – namely to remove goods which are of fundamental importance from the perspective of justice from those who are better off, just to make the distribution more equal, even if no individual person's life is made better by this. *Prioritarians* take it that it is not an equal distribution of goods per se which matters, but rather how each individual person is faring relative to how they might be faring. According to the prioritarian, we should give priority (either absolute or weighted) to improving the condition of those who are worst off in the distribution of those goods which are of fundamental importance from the perspective of justice. This avoids the counterintuitive result of levelling down. Lastly, *sufficientarians* take it that what matters from the perspective of justice is that each person have *enough* of the goods that are of fundamental importance for justice, and that once this threshold has been reached, a person has no more claims on justice. As we shall see below, how to apply these answers to the 'how' question to the domain of health is a complex question.

Is health of fundamental importance for egalitarian justice?

It is implausible to think that health is the *only* currency of egalitarian justice. For there seem to be goods which are important to a just society which are neither reducible to fair distribution of health achievement, nor valued only for their contribution to fair distribution of health achievement. For example, it would seem strange to describe a society which was rife with racism and discrimination, and prevented women from voting or from holding political office, but yet where fortuitously everyone had the same level of health

---

[10] Focusing only on financial wealth is a crude view, first because financial wealth is not important in itself, but rather only important for the goods it gives access to. Second, different people will have different levels of efficiency in converting money into things that do matter for their own sake. (For instance, if we gave the same amount of money to all persons, this money would go much less far for someone who requires expensive equipment to counteract a disability, than it would for someone who lacked this disability.) Cohen (1989) defends access to advantage, while Arneson (1989) defends opportunity for welfare, as the appropriate currency of egalitarian justice.

achievement as one which was just in an egalitarian sense. Nor is it much more plausible to claim that health is the most important good that a just society should be aiming at. For this would seem to turn our commitment to health into a 'bottomless pit', as there will always be further interventions we could make that would marginally improve health, which would have to be bought at the cost of our commitment to goods other than health[11] (Dworkin, 2000: 309).

It follows that egalitarian justice must care about more than merely health. There are two major options. Either there is a single currency of egalitarian justice, and this currency is not health (and so health is important from the perspective of justice only for the impact that it has on this currency), or there are multiple (and mutually irreducible) currencies of egalitarian justice, and health is but one of them.[12] In this section, I shall examine three well worked out versions of these options. First, Dworkin's monistic approach, which takes there to be a single currency of egalitarian justice, which is not health. Second, the pluralistic capabilities approach of Nussbaum and Sen, according to which the capability to live a healthy life of a normal length is one of the currencies of justice. And lastly, I will look at Daniels' approach, which aims to argue that while health is not itself a currency of egalitarian justice, it is so closely related to something that is a currency of egalitarian justice (namely opportunity), that we ought to treat health as special from the perspective of justice.

Before getting to this, we must briefly address two issues. First, health is a good which is much more difficult to redistribute than others we are usually concerned about from the perspective of justice. Second, there is a question about *which* health inequalities we should be focusing on: only those which arise between different socio-economic groups, or also those which arise between individuals considered separately?

Distributing health

Most of the goods we might be concerned about from the perspective of justice are divisible and redistributable, and so it is easily possible to remove some of them from those who have too much, and bestow more on those who have too little. For instance, if we want to combat an unjust income inequality, we can quite easily redistribute money from the rich to the poor, by taxing the rich and then giving the resulting money to the poor. Or if we find that there is an unjust distribution of liberty (as, for example, in a society which allowed men, but not women to own property), we could change the law so that both men and women would equally have the liberty to own property.

However, if we were to uncover an unjust distribution of health, it would be rather more difficult to address it by redistribution, as health is not (in general) directly transferable

---

[11] The World Health Organization (WHO) definition of health, namely that health 'is a state of complete physical, mental and social well-being and not merely the absence of disease or infirmity' makes it less implausible to think that health so defined could be the most important good for a just society to focus on. However this is due to the fact the definition of health is simply too all-encompassing to be useful as a definition of *health*. (For the debate on the WHO definition of health, see further Callahan [1973] and Bok [2004]).

[12] There is also a third possibility, which I shall set aside: it might be the case that there are multiple currencies of egalitarian justice, and that health is not one of them. From the perspective of our interest in health inequalities, this would be normatively little different from the first option: in both cases health would be only indirectly relevant to justice.

from one person to another.[13] So we can only rectify unjust distributions of health indirectly. One such way would be to ensure a just distribution of the social determinants of health. While ensuring a just distribution of the social determinants of health would clearly help to produce a just distribution of health, it would not fully rectify any current injustice, given that many of the ill health conditions which are caused by an unjust distribution of the social determinants of health will not be reversible. For example if someone has atherosclerosis as a result of working for a long time in a stressful environment in which they experienced little control over what they were doing, then allowing them decent working conditions would not undo their atherosclerosis.[14] Another way of counteracting the effects of unfairly poor health would be by compensating those people with unfairly poor health with a different and more readily redistributable good (such as money, free health care or free mobility equipment). However, it is far from clear that ill health can be fully compensated by being provided with other goods (see 'Deciding between these approaches', below).

The upshot seems to be that even if we do think that health is an appropriate currency of egalitarian justice, it will not be easy, and may in fact be impossible, to bring it about that there is an equitable distribution of health.

Individual and group inequalities in health

Until fairly recently, researchers who have been interested in health inequities have assumed that the relevant inequities that we should be worrying about are inequities between groups rather than individuals, so that they have thought it was a cause for concern if certain groups (such as African Americans) do worse than other groups (such as white Americans). However, Murray *et al.* (1999, 2000) argue that we should also be interested in inequalities in health between individuals. Unless we do so, they argue, we fail to attend to the inequalities *within* these groups, and thus 'mask part of the inequality present in the population' (Murray *et al.*, 1999: 537).

It seems to me that it is only if we are committed to the view that health is a fundamental currency of justice and we think that inequalities with natural as opposed to social causes can be unjust that we ought to be concerned about individual health inequality. (If these conditions held, it would follow that each individual was owed a fair share of health. It would then simply be false to say to an individual that we had treated him justly with respect to health because the social class or race of which he was a member was sufficiently healthy.)

However, if we do not think that health is a currency of justice, we will find it much more useful to know for social policy purposes the kinds of questions that social scientific researchers have tended to concentrate on, namely how inequalities in health correlate with other variables, such as social class that *are* of fundamental concern for justice. Knowing about individual inequalities in health will not tell us very much about what we would need

---

[13] Unless, that is, we redistribute healthy organs from one person to another person with less healthy organs. However this would be such a gross violation of the self-ownership of the people from whom the organs were taken that it can be safely set aside as a solution to how to distribute health justly (Segall, 2007: 358).

[14] In addition, as we saw earlier, arguably there are some unjust distributions of health which do not have a social cause, so these would remain untouched by addressing the social determinants of ill health.

to do to make society more just, given that justice will depend on the distribution of goods other than health (Hausman *et al.*, 2002; Hausman, 2007). In addition, measurements of individual health inequalities do not allow us to filter out what is caused by social factors from what is caused by natural factors, and so they will be a useful measure only if there is no normative difference between these two types of health inequalities (Asada and Hedemann, 2002).

Monistic approaches

Any view of justice that takes there to be a single currency of justice will be forced to conclude that this single fundamental currency is not health. So all monistic approaches to justice present a standing challenge to the normative significance of health inequalities. We shall take Dworkin's (1981a, 1981b) account as an example of a monistic approach to egalitarian justice. Dworkin picks out resources as the currency of egalitarian justice. He uses the concept of resources in a broad way to include not just 'external' resources such as land and money, but also talents, which are theorized as 'internal' resources. Disability and ill health are understood as negative internal resources.[15]

Dworkin's view has two main implications for the study of health inequities. First, our duty would be to ensure a *fair share of resources* for each person. Health is only one such resource, and can reasonably be traded against other goods. So the fair distribution of resources would not require us to take health to be a special case, and to seek to equalize it separately from other goods.

Second, in Dworkin's view (in common with other luck egalitarians) the distinction between the natural and social is not of normative significance, and so should not be presupposed in a theory of justice. What matters according to Dworkin is whether someone can fairly be held responsible for the shortfall in their combined bundle of internal and external resources. If a person suffers a shortfall for which they cannot be held responsible, then this requires rectification, regardless of whether the cause of the shortfall is natural or social. So, for example, on Dworkin's view, the natural inequality in life expectancies between women and men would raise a prima facie case for rectification.[16]

In addition, Dworkin (along with other luck egalitarians) does not think that justice requires us to equalize advantages or disadvantages which result from choices that competent adults make. Hence on Dworkin's account disadvantages in terms of health or other resources caused to individuals by their competent choices to drink heavily or to not take

---

[15] Dworkin (1981b: 312) denies that ill health and disability give someone a *direct* claim to equalization of resources, on the ground that this would amount to a 'slavery of the talented', and he argues that justice requires only that each person be given sufficient resources to enable them to purchase insurance against ill health and disability. However, it is questionable whether Dworkin's argument for this claim is consistent with his broader position, as Cohen-Christofiadis (2004) argues. For a good overview of the debate on egalitarianism and disability, see Wolff (2008).

[16] There are two reasons why Dworkin would be unlikely to suggest that we take steps to remedy this gender based health inequality. First, his theory requires us to equalize resources, not health. The natural inequality in life expectancies *favours* women, and so if anything will help to counteract the gender imbalance of resources which is likely to result in a male dominated society. Second, it is difficult to see how we could systematically favour one sex over another in the distribution of health care related resources, without violating the core idea of egalitarian justice, namely that each should be entitled to treatment as an equal (Sen, 2004: 24).

exercise do not call for rectification. This would mean that we would need to work out to what extent (if any) individuals can fairly be held responsible for the types of health disadvantage which are correlated with, for example low SES.[17]

Capabilities approaches

Capabilities theorists, of whom Sen (1999, 2004) and Nussbaum (2000) are the pre-eminent exponents, differ in two fundamental ways from Dworkin. First, they believe that resources are the wrong distributive space to be working in. They argue that what is of value is people being able to function in various characteristically human ways, such as using their practical reason, or playing, or living a healthy life of an ordinary length, rather than the amount of resources at their disposal. Capabilities theorists argue it would be a mistake for a society to attempt to *provide* everyone with the given functioning, as someone may legitimately choose not to exercise it. (For example, someone may wish to fast for religious reasons, and at such a time it would be wrong for a society to force them to have the functioning of being well nourished.) So capabilities theorists argue that we should focus on providing each person with the *capability* to function in the valued way, not ensure that they do actually function in this way.

Second, they argue that we should be pluralists when it comes to justice: there are a plurality of capabilities which are jointly necessary for a flourishing human life, and we cannot fully compensate a shortfall in one capability with a superfluity of another. Given this broad pluralistic framework, the argument for why health is a functioning that matters fundamentally for egalitarian justice is simple. In Sen's (2004: 23) words:

> . . . health is among the most important conditions of human life and critically significant constituent of human capabilities which we have reason to value. Any conception of social justice that accepts the need for a fair distribution as well as efficient formation of human capabilities cannot ignore the role of health in human life and the opportunities that persons respectively have to achieve good health – free from escapable illness, avoidable afflictions and premature morality.

Approaches inspired by Rawls

Rawls (1971, 2005) argues that there are two principles of justice which determine the justice of the basic structure of society. First, and foremost, the liberty principle, which states that each individual has an equal right to protection by a fully adequate scheme of basic liberties. Second, a two-part principle governing which social and economic inequalities are acceptable, namely that such inequalities must first be open to all under conditions of fair equality of opportunity (the opportunity principle), and second the resulting advantages must be to the advantage of the least advantaged members of society (the difference principle).

As we have already mentioned, Rawls does not theorize a place for health in his theory of justice. There are at least three ways that we might account for health within the broad context of Rawls' theory of justice. First, we could do what Peter (2001) does, and argue that

---

[17] Solving the problem of how to determine which actions people can reasonably be held responsible for is a difficult problem for the luck egalitarian. For an interesting (though controversial) approach to solving it, see Roemer (1993). For further discussion of personal responsibility and health inequities, see Wikler (2004).

Rawls' theory of justice is already adequate as it stands, and that we should understand health inequities to be those inequalities in health which are the result of unjust social arrangements.[18] Second, we could conceive of health as a primary good, to be distributed (insofar as this is possible) according to the difference principle.[19]

Third, we could do what Daniels (1985, 2008; Daniels *et al.*, 2004) does, and account for health by reference to the opportunity principle. Daniels argues that we should greatly extend the opportunity principle so that it is not simply a matter of getting a fair opportunity to compete for jobs and offices (as in Rawls' vision), but rather becomes a matter of guaranteeing to each individual a fair share of the normal range of opportunities for someone with their talents. Health (argues Daniels) is a necessary condition for someone being able to access the normal opportunity range for their talents, and so a commitment to fair equality of opportunity commits us to treating health (and health care) as 'special'. Treating health and health care as special amounts to focusing on these as goods to be equalized on their own quite apart from our more general commitments to egalitarian distribution.

Deciding between these approaches

Daniels' approach claims an impressive pedigree; Rawls's theory of justice is by general consensus the best worked out and most comprehensive theory of justice that we currently have, and so to provide an account of justice and health which dovetailed neatly with Rawls would be very desirable.

However, there are two problems which Daniels' account struggles to overcome. First, it is far from clear that the importance of health and health care are correctly explained in terms of their impact on opportunity (Segall, 2007). Second, Daniels' account appears to be internally inconsistent. Daniels' argument for the specialness of health depends on the claim that health is a condition for the possibility of a normal opportunity range, whereas other goods (such as wealth) implicitly are not. He then draws the conclusion from this that whereas other goods can be distributed according to the difference principle, or even according to the free market, health and health care must be governed by the more stringent opportunity principle. However, the literature on the social determinants of health which we reviewed above shows that health is pervasively determined by the distribution of other goods, such as workplace culture, levels of income equality, the amount of social capital in a society. Hence it follows that someone's share of the normal opportunity range is significantly determined by the distribution of these other goods. And given that health

---

[18] Peter describes this as an 'indirect' account of health inequity. It threatens to share the same problem we saw with Kawachi *et al.*'s (2002)'s definition of a health inequity, namely that it becomes unclear why we should treat the health inequalities which result from unjust social arrangements as *health* inequities. Peter (2001: 164) acknowledges this and adds that 'an indirect approach will need some justification for why health is considered a relevant indicator and such a justification will draw upon the good of health', but does nothing further to explain how we should relate this conception of the good of health to a Rawlsian approach to justice. It is unclear how she can ultimately avoid a commitment to either a position analogous to Dworkin's (which says that health matters only for the influence it has on other factors which are directly relevant to justice), or a position analogous to the capabilities approach (which makes health one of the currencies of justice).

[19] This seems to be Veatch's (1999) position.

does not have the asymmetrical causal role that his argument requires, 'we cannot argue from it for the view that health makes special demands of justice because it has an asymmetrically fundamental causal role in as a condition of opportunity for other goods' (Hurley, 2007: 328).

This, as I see it leaves Daniels with a dilemma. Either he can expand his account of what he takes to be special, so that all the social determinants of health now count as special too because of their impact on opportunity (but, this would have results which are unattractive for egalitarianism in general[20]) or, he could drop his claim that health is special – but this would be to give up the essence of his position on health and justice.[21]

It is more difficult to determine whether a monistic account such as Dworkin's or a pluralistic account such as Sen or Nussbaum's provides the best way of accounting for the place of health in a theory of justice. Ideally, we would want a theory of egalitarian justice that was both fully sensitive to all those feature(s) that make us equals, and all those goods that need to be distributed fairly if a society is to be a just one (call this the accuracy requirement), and enabled us to make useful comparative judgements about which of two situations departs more fully from what justice requires (call this the indexing require-ment). The main problem is that the accuracy and the indexing requirements conflict. The indexing requirement will tend to push us towards a monistic currency of justice. This is because, 'if two goods, or two forms of advantage and disadvantage, cannot be compared, then they cannot be placed on a common scale, and so it will become impossible, in many cases, to say whether one person is worse off or better off than another' (Wolff and de-Shalit, 2007: 23). And clearly this problem will only get worse as we increase the plurality of incommensurable goods which we allow as currencies of justice.

However, the accuracy requirement will tend to push us towards acknowledging a plurality of goods, none of which is fully reducible to the others. Wolff and de-Shalit point out that if some form of monism about justice were true (for the sake of convenience, assume that the sole currency of justice was resources in Dworkin's sense), it would follow that *any* disadvantage relevant to justice could be fully rectified by providing a suitable amount of this one currency. However, this seems not to be the case, particularly if the disadvantage to be suffered is an increased risk of early death, or chronic ill health. And so we seem forced by a concern for accuracy to admit that there are multiple goods which are of relevance to justice (Wolff and de-Shalit, 2007: 21–35).

This, I take it leaves us with a very difficult problem to solve in normative political philosophy. I would (tentatively) suggest that we should favour accuracy over indexing here, as there seems little point in starting our accounts of justice from a theory of value we already know to be inadequate. Although the indexing problem for a plurality of different goods looks to be very difficult to solve, it is plausible to hope that we may be able to make

---

[20] As Segall (2007: 360) explains, the claim that health is special 'mandates that entitlement to health care should not be curtailed due to inferior or superior wealth. . . . But while this feature ("working both ways") appears attractive when it comes to medical care, it appears considerably less attractive with regard to the other social determinants of health. Egalitarians typically do want to allocate more (social bases of) self-respect to those who have less of other goods (for example income, looks) and conversely, allocate more income to those who have smaller bundles (compared to others) of other social (and natural) assets. But treating the social determinants of health as special prohibits this.'

[21] I examine Daniels' position in greater depth in Wilson (2009).

some progress on it in the future.[22] And if we *do* allow that there is a plurality of goods which should count as currencies of egalitarian justice, then it seems overwhelmingly plausible that health should be one, given both its importance for human life in its own right, and its status as a precondition for many other important functionings.

The how of health equity

Egalitarian justice in the broad sense has its basis in the idea that we should treat persons as equals. Even leaving aside disputes about *which* goods should count as currencies of justice, there are different interpretations of how egalitarians in this broad sense should aim to distribute those goods that are agreed to be currencies of justice. There are three main positions developed in the literature: strict egalitarianism, which argues that distributive equality is an end in itself; prioritarianism, which argues that we should give priority in the distribution of goods to those who are worst off; and sufficientarianism, which argues that justice requires only that we ensure that each person has a sufficient quantity of the thing being distributed.[23]

Strict egalitarianism

Strict egalitarians believe that the best distribution of those goods that are currencies of justice is an equal one, and that there is a value to equal distributions in and of itself, even where no individual is made better off by such distributions. If we cared only about equality in health, then we would prefer a society in which there was very little inequality in health, but where life expectancies were lower, to one in which everyone lived longer, but there was much greater inequality in health. For the purposes of simplicity, let us say that we have a choice of two societies: in society A, everyone (rich or poor) dies at the age of 60, while in society B, all the poor die at 65, while all the rich die at 90.[24] Strict egalitarians argue that, insofar as we are egalitarians, we should favour society A to society B, as it has a more equal distribution of health.

However, while it is certainly true that society A has a more equal distribution of health, it is far from clear that we should choose it over society B, given that moving from society B to society A would be levelling down. No one is better off in society A than they are in society B, as both the poor and the rich have a higher life expectancy in society B. And in fact society A makes both rich and poor *worse off* than they would otherwise be. Many take this to be a strong intuitive complaint against strict egalitarianism.

Strict egalitarians (such as Temkin, 1993) make two moves to attempt to ward off the levelling down objection. First, they argue that equality is only *one* of the values which we should deploy when deciding how goods should be distributed all things considered. So while society A may be better from the perspective of equality, there may nonetheless be

---

[22] Wolff and de-Shalit (2007: 89–107) propose a practical strategy for solving indexing problems in real world solutions, which looks like a promising avenue for further research.

[23] In this section I shall assume that health is a currency of justice in the relevant sense. I do not take it that this has been established by the argument in the previous section. I make this assumption simply because, unless health is a basic currency of justice, there will be little further to be said about how we should go about distributing health justly.

[24] For the purposes of simplicity I am making the rather unrealistic assumption that there are no individual health variations *within* the groups.

compelling reasons to favour society B, all things considered. Second, they argue that the levelling down objection presupposes a person-affecting requirement, namely that one situation cannot be better than another unless there is a person for whom it is better; however this requirement is false.

The strict egalitarian's first response may well appear to be dodging the issue: what we are attempting to work out is the overall principle or principles by which to distribute those goods which are the currencies of justice. To be told that strict egalitarianism is but one principle that needs to be weighed against as yet to be specified others, is not perhaps as helpful as one would have liked.

The problem with the strict egalitarian's second reply is that, as Hurley (2007) points out, it is not true that all objections to levelling down presuppose the person-affecting requirement. So even if the person-affecting requirement were false, it would not follow that levelling down in health is acceptable. If a good which is a currency of justice is not only good for the person who has it, but is also impersonally good, then there would be reasons to object to levelling down in respect of that good that are separate from the person affecting requirement. Hurley (2007: 332–3) argues that health is just such a good:

> Health is a distinctive type of flourishing, with a specific natural character and basis . . . It is not just good for people to be healthy rather than unhealthy; it is also good in itself for there to be healthy people rather than unhealthy people.

If this is true, then there is an intuitively obvious objection to levelling down in health which does not rely on the person affecting principle, namely that 'leveling down wastefully throws away the higher reaches of good' (2007: 332). And so the objection to levelling down seems to stand, at least when we are distributing health.

Prioritarianism

Thinking about the problem of levelling down has led many to the view that the core commitments of egalitarian justice in health should not be strict egalitarianism, but rather to what has come to be known as *prioritarianism*, namely that we should give priority to improving the condition of those who are worst off (Parfit, 1997). Rawls' difference principle is an explicitly prioritarian principle of justice, namely that social and economic inequalities are to be to the greatest benefit of the least advantaged members of society.

Prioritarianism is very appealing as an account of what we owe to one another when it comes to health. However, while it may be true in most obvious cases that we should give priority to alleviating the condition of the worst off, giving an *absolute* priority to improving the condition of the worst off can have counterintuitive implications. For it may well be the case that it is much less cost effective to attempt to improve the condition of those who are the very worst off, than to attempt to improve the conditions of some other groups who are slightly better off. (This is often the case in health care, where those who are worst off frequently require very expensive treatments which only succeed [if at all] in improving their condition marginally.) And so a focus on giving priority to the worst off will sometimes conflict with considerations of cost-effectiveness and efficiency.[25]

---

[25] The underlying worry here is similar to the levelling down objection. But where the levelling down objection concerns cases where *no one* gains and there is a significant loss to some, this objection concerns cases where there is a slight benefit to some, but a much more significant loss to others.

Prioritarians can address this challenge from efficiency in one of two ways: either they can deny that considerations of efficiency have any role to play here, and claim that even if *much more* good could be done to those who are less badly off, we should still focus our efforts on those who are worst off. Or they can shift to a position which has come to be known as *weighted prioritarianism*, which claims that priority to the worst off is to be given a high (but not absolute) weighting, so that in certain circumstances priority to the worst off can legitimately be overridden by the demands of efficiency.

Sufficientarianism

Sufficientarians (Frankfurt, 1987; Crisp, 2003a, 2003b) argue that priority is only to be given to those who are worse off than a certain threshold, and that if everyone is above this threshold, benefits to those who are comparatively better off count equally to those who are comparatively worse off. The policy implications of a sufficientarian approach to health would clearly depend on what we took the relevant threshold to be for health achievement. If the threshold was set high (for instance to 90 years of healthy life), then a sufficientarian approach would not be distinguishable in practice from a prioritarian approach. However, if the threshold was set low (for instance, to 50 years of moderately healthy life), then socio-economic conditions which caused someone to die at 55 or 60 would not deprive someone of a share of healthy life to which they were entitled by justice.

Crisp (2003a, 2003b) argues that we should set the level of sufficiency through the exercise of compassion from the perspective of an impartial observer. However, this seems not to be a very complete answer, given that what we reasonably feel compassion for is closely related to what we feel is to be expected. And indeed, it is hard to see how there could be a nonarbitrary way of deciding how long a life was 'long enough'. As Hooker (2008: 190) puts it, 'As long as a pleasant, intellectually active, socially interactive life is possible, I cannot see why anyone's "needs" expire at 70 years, or at 100 years, or at 150 years.' So it may be that when we are thinking about the length of life, there is no relevant sufficiency threshold. It is more plausible to think that there could be an objective standard for when a life of a given length is sufficiently healthy. But even here we would face the very difficult task of deciding what that level should be, a problem the prioritarian (who only needs to determine who is worse off) does not face.[26]

I take it that these difficulties give us some reason to favour prioritarianism over sufficientarianism when we are distributing health, even if only on pragmatic grounds.

Conclusion

Social scientists working on health inequalities have often thought that it is simple to identify health inequities. For example, Dahlgren and Whitehead (2006: 3) forthrightly state that:

> In today's Europe, working out what social differences in health are fair and unfair is unnecessary. Essentially, all systematic differences in health between different socioeconomic groups within a country can be considered unfair and, therefore, classed as health inequities. There is no biological

---

[26] As Hooker (2008) reminds us, 'All prioritarianism has to do is determine who is worse off, and this seems much easier than determining whether *y's* getting *x* is something that *y* needs or merely something that would benefit *y* . . . Crisp needs to defend a line; prioritarianism has no line to defend.'

reason for their existence, and it is clear that even systematic differences in lifestyles between socioeconomic groups are to a large extent shaped by structural factors.

This chapter has argued that things are rather less clear cut than this, and that it is a much more complex matter to determine which inequalities in health should count as inequities. Which inequalities in health should count as inequities is, we argued, on analysis a matter of which inequalities in health are unjust.

We saw that there are two different dimensions to theories of egalitarian justice. First, there is the question of which goods we should take to be the currencies of justice. Here we argued that, despite the indexing problems it causes, there is reason to favour a pluralistic account of the currencies of justice over a monistic account, and that if we adopt a pluralistic theory of justice it is overwhelmingly plausible to think that health should be one of the currencies. Second, there is the question of how we ought to distribute those goods that are currencies of justice. Here we suggested that when we are distributing health, an approach that gives priority to those who are worst off may be preferable both to a strict egalitarian one, and a sufficientarian one.

Assuming this is correct, it follows that justice requires us above all to concentrate on improving the condition of the worst off, and that what makes one person worse off than another will be, among other things, their health state. Flattening socio-economic gradients in health will be one important way of improving the condition of those who are worst off, especially as so doing will also require us to distribute goods other than health more equitably.

References

Anderson, E. (1999) What is the point of equality? *Ethics*, **109**: 287–337.

Arneson, R. (1989) Equality and equal opportunity for welfare. *Philosophical Studies*, **56**: 77–93.

Asada, Y. and Hedemann, T. (2002) A problem with the individual approach in the WHO health inequality measurement. *International Journal for Equity in Health*, **1**(2). Available at: http://www.equityhealthj.com/content/1/1/2 (accessed: 14/02/11).

Bellis, M., Hennell, T., Lushey, C., Hughes, K., Tocque, K. and Ashton, J. (2007) Elvis to Eminem: quantifying the price of fame through early mortality of European and North American rock and pop stars. *Journal of Epidemiology and Community Health*, **61**: 896–901.

Bok, S. (2004) Rethinking the WHO definition of health. *Harvard Centre for Population and Development Studies: Working Paper Series*, **14**: 7.

Braveman, P., Cubbin, C., Egerter, S., Chideya, S., Marchi, K., Metzlr, M. and Posner, S. (2005) Socioeconomic status in health research: one size does not fit all. *Journal of the American Medical Association*, **294**: 2879–88.

Callahan, D. (1973) The WHO definition of 'health'. *Hastings Center Studies*, **1**(3): 77–87.

Central Intelligence Agency (2007) *The World Factbook 2007*. Available at: https://www.cia.gov/library/publications/the-world-factbook/ (accessed: 18/07/08).

Chandola, T., Bartley, M., Sackera, A., Jenkinson, C. and Marmot, M. (2003) Health selection in the Whitehall II study, UK. *Social Science & Medicine*, **56**(10): 2059–72.

Cohen, G. (1989) On the currency of egalitarian justice. *Ethics*, **99**(4): 906–44.

Cohen-Christofiadis, M. (2004) Talent, slavery and envy in Dworkin's equality of resources. *Utilitas*, **16**(3): 267–87.

Crisp, R. (2003a) Equality, priority, and compassion. *Ethics*, **113**: 745–63.

Crisp, R. (2003b) Egalitarianism and compassion. *Ethics*, **113**: 119–126.

Dahlgren, G. and Whitehead, M. (1992) *Policies and Strategies to Promote Equity in Health*. Copenhagen: WHO Regional Office for

Europe. (Document number: EUR/ICP/RPD 414 (2). Available at: http://whqlibdoc.who.int/euro/-1993/EUR_ICP_ RPD414(2).pdf (accessed: 18/07/08).

Dahlgren, G. and Whitehead, M. (2006) *Levelling Up (Part 1): A Discussion Paper on Concepts and Principles for Tackling Social Inequities in Health.* Copenhagen: WHO Regional Office for Europe. Available at: http://www.who.int/social_determinants/resources/leveling_up_part1.pdf (accessed: 18/07/08).

Daniels, N. (1985) *Just Health Care.* Cambridge: Cambridge University Press.

Daniels, N. (2008) *Just Health.* Cambridge: Cambridge University Press.

Daniels, N., Kennedy, B. and Kawachi, I. (2004) Health and inequality, or why justice is good for our health. In *Public Health, Ethics and Equity,* ed. S. Anand, F. Peter and A. Sen. Oxford: Oxford University Press, pp. 63–92.

Dworkin, R. (1981a) What is equality? Part 1: equality of welfare. *Philosophy and Public Affairs,* **10**: 185–246. (Reprinted in Dworkin 2000.)

Dworkin, R. (1981b) What is equality? Part 2: equality of resources. *Philosophy and Public Affairs,* **10**: 283–345. (Reprinted in Dworkin 2000.)

Dworkin, R. (2000) *Sovereign Virtue: The Theory and Practice of Equality.* Cambridge, MA: Harvard University Press.

Frankfurt, H. (1987) Equality as a moral ideal. *Ethics,* **98**: 21–42.

Hausman, D. M. (2007) What's wrong with health inequalities? *Journal of Political Philosophy,* **15**, 1: 46–66.

Hausman, D. M., Asada Y. and Hedemann T. (2002) Health inequalities and why they matter. *Health Care Analysis,* **10**, 2: 177–91.

Hooker, B. (2008) Fairness, needs, desert. In *The Legacy of H. L. A. Hart,* ed. M. Kramer and C. Grant. Oxford: Oxford University Press.

Hurley, S. (2007) The 'what' and the 'how' of distributive justice and health. In *Egalitarianism: New Essays on the Nature and Value of Equality,* ed. N. Holtung and K. Lippert-Rasmussen. Oxford: Oxford University Press, pp. 308–34.

Kawachi, I., Subramanian, S. and Ammeida-Filho, N. (2002) A glossary for health inequalities. *Journal of Epidemiology and Community Health,* **56**: 647–52.

Marmot, M. (2004) *Status Syndrome: How Your Social Standing Directly Affects Your Health and Life Expectancy.* London: Bloomsbury.

Marmot, M., Rose, G., Shipley M. and Hamilton, P. (1978) Employment grade and coronary heart disease in British civil servants. *Journal of Epidemiology and Community Health,* **32**: 244–9.

Mill, J. (1874) *On Nature.* (Originally published in Mill's collection *Nature, The Utility of Religion and Theism.* Now most conveniently available at: http://www.lancs.ac.uk/users/philosophy/texts/mill_on.htm [accessed: 18/07/08].)

Mueller, C. and Parcel, T. (1981) Measures of socioeconomic status: alternatives and recommendations. *Child Development,* **52**: 13–30.

Murray, C., Gakidou, E. and Frenk, J. (1999) Health inequalities and social group differences: what should we measure? *Bulletin of the World Health Organization,* **77**(7): 537–43.

Murray, C., Gakidou, E. and Frenk, J. (2000) Response to P. Braveman *et al. Bulletin of the World Health Organization,* **78**(2): 234–5.

Nagel, T. (2005) The problem of global justice. *Philosophy and Public Affairs,* **33**(2): 113–47.

Peter, F. (2001) Health equity and social justice. *Journal of Applied Philosophy,* **18**(2): 159–70.

Nussbaum, M. (2000) *Women and Human Development: The Capabilities Approach.* New York: Cambridge University Press.

Parfit, D. (1997) Equality and priority. *Ratio,* **10**: 202–21.

Pogge, T. (2008) *World Poverty and Human Rights,* 2nd edn. Cambridge: Polity Press.

Rawls, J. (1971) *A Theory of Justice.* Cambridge, MA: Harvard University Press.

Rawls, J. (1999) *The Law of Peoples.* Cambridge, MA: Harvard University Press.

Rawls, J. (2005) *Political Liberalism,* expanded edn. New York: Columbia University Press.

Roemer, J. (1993) A pragmatic theory of responsibility for the egalitarian planner. *Philosophy and Public Affairs*, **22**(2): 146–66.

Scheffler, S. (2003) What is egalitarianism? *Philosophy and Public Affairs*, **31**(1): 5–39.

Segall, S. (2007) Is health care (still) special? *The Journal of Political Philosophy*, **15**(3): 342–61.

Sen, A. (1999) *Development as Freedom*. Oxford: Oxford University Press.

Sen, A. (2004) Why health equity? In *Public Health, Ethics and Equity*, ed. S. Anand, F. Peter and A. Sen. Oxford: Oxford University Press, pp. 21–34.

Shavers, V. (2007) Measurement of socioeconomic status in health disparities research. *Journal of the National Medical Association*, **99**(9): 1013–23.

Strand, B., Kunst, A., Huisman, M., *et al.* (2007) The reversed social gradient: higher breast cancer mortality in the higher educated compared to lower educated. A comparison of 11 European populations during the 1990s. *European Journal of Cancer*, **43**(7): 1200–7.

Temkin, L. (1993) *Inequality*. Oxford: Oxford University Press.

Veatch, R. M. (1999) Justice, the basic social contract and health care. In *Contemporary Issues in Bioethics*, 5th edn, ed. T. Beauchamp and L. Walters. Belmont, CA: Wadsworth, pp. 368–74.

Waldron, J. (2000) Basic equality. Delivered as the Sir Malcolm Knox Lecture at the University of St Andrews, May 2000. Available at: http://weblaw.usc.edu/ academics/assets/docs/waldron.pdf (accessed: 18/07/08).

Whitehead, M. (1990) *The Concepts and Principles of Equity and Health*. Document number: EUR/ICP/RPD 414. Copenhagen: WHO Regional Office for Europe. Available at: http://whqlibdoc.who.int/ euro/-1993/EUR_ICP_RPD_414.pdf (accessed: 18/07/08).

Wikler, D. (2004) Social and personal responsibility for health. In *Public Health, Ethics and Equity*, ed. S. Anand, F. Peter and A. Sen. Oxford: Oxford University Press, pp. 109–34.

Wilkinson, R. (1996) *Unhealthy Societies: The Afflictions of Inequality*. London: Routledge.

Wilson, J. (2007a) Nietzsche and equality. In *Nietzsche and Ethics*, ed. G. von Tevenar. Oxford: Peter Lang, pp. 221–40.

Wilson, J. (2007b) Transhumanism and moral equality. *Bioethics*, **21**(8): 419–25.

Wilson, J. (2009) Not so special after all? Daniels and the social determinants of health. *Journal of Medical Ethics*, **35**: 3–6.

Wolff, J. (2008) Disability among equals. In *Philosophy and Disability*, ed. K. Brownlee and A. Cureton. Oxford: Oxford University Press.

Wolff, J. and de-Shalit, A. (2007) *Disadvantage*. Oxford: Oxford University Press.

Index